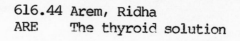

The Thyroid Solution

T H E
THYROID
S O L U T I O N

A Mind-Body Program for Beating Depression
and Regaining Your Emotional and Physical Health

RIDHA AREM, M.D.

BALLANTINE BOOKS

NEW YORK

The case histories included in this book are based on the author's experience with his patients, although patients' names and personal information have been changed to protect their privacy. The opinions and recommendations in this book are those solely of the author. Baylor College of Medicine and affiliated teaching hospitals share no responsibility whatsoever for the writing or publication of any portion of this book. The information contained in the book is provided for educational purposes only. You need to seek the advice of your health care professional before you use any recommendation found in this book.

A Ballantine Book
Published by The Ballantine Publishing Group

Copyright © 1999 by Ridha Arem, M.D.

www.randomhouse.com/BB/

A CIP record for this book is found at the Library of Congress

Text design by Ann Gold

Manufactured in the United States of America

First Edition: June 1999

10   9   8   7   6   5   4   3

To the very special people who enriched my heart with love:
my very dear parents, my beloved wife, and my two wonderful sons.
It is my hope that this book will inspire my sons
to dedicate themselves to helping and loving others.

CONTENTS

PART III
Women's Thyroid Problems:
Your Symptoms Are Not All in Your Head

PART IV
Diagnosing and Treating Common Thyroid Disorders:
The Journey to Wellness

Acknowledgments

So many people have made the writing of this book possible. First of all, my deepest gratitude goes to the patients who have taught me what books and articles could not and to those who were kind enough to share their experiences with me for this book. These patients have made an invaluable contribution toward helping others. The hard work and dedication of researchers and psychiatrists from around the world who have studied thyroid disease were critical in enabling me to understand and interpret the intricate interactions between the mind and thyroid. A special thank-you goes to my mentor, Professor Raymond Michel, who in the early 1950s was one of the researchers who discovered T3, the most active form of thyroid hormone. Professor Michel ingited my passion for learning the role thyroid hormone plays in our bodies.

There is no doubt that without the unshakable support and understanding of my wife, Noura, I would not have been able to carry out the project of writing this book. I would like to thank my administrative assistants, Julie Murphy and Maile Louie; the staff of the Endocrine Laboratory at the Methodist Hospital; and the medical and nursing staff at Baylor College of Medicine, Internal Medicine Consultants. Their support over the years has been tremendous.

I am indebted to everyone who, in the initial stages of the writing, read portions of the manuscript and helped with their suggestions, critiques, and editing. Maralyn Robinson, Laura Russell, Sabrena Belz, and Katherine van der Pol, to name a few. I want to particularly thank Dr. Lauren Marangell, Director of Mood Disorders Research at Baylor College of Medicine and Dr. Paul Ladenson, Chief of Endocrinology at Johns Hopkins University School of Medicine, for thoroughly reviewing the manuscript and providing me with the most insightful advice and suggestions. I also thank Gillian Ford, author of *Listening to Your Hormones*, for her guidance. It was certainly a joy working with Mark Mayell, who did an outstanding job of refining and organizing the manuscript. Sandi Gelles-Coles did a remarkable job helping me with the preparation of the proposal. My gratitude to my agent, Angela Rinaldi, cannot be expressed in words. Her help and guidance at every stage of this endeavor were priceless. I deeply appreciate the thoroughness and talents of my editor at Ballantine, Leslie Meredith. Her suggestions were always on target. I also wish to thank the entire team at Ballantine—in particular, Catherine Elliott and Adrian Wood. Their support and help enabled me to remain in good spirits throughout the tedious process of delivering this book.

Finally, I would like to thank all the typists for keeping pace with the progress of the work and the active members of the American Foundation of Thyroid Patients and other patient support organizations in the United States and abroad for their help and their commitment to patient education.

Introduction

In the space of a week a few years ago, I saw two patients, Stacy and Murielle, whose experiences ultimately inspired me to write this book. As the chief of Endocrinology and Metabolism at a major teaching hospital associated with Baylor College of Medicine in Houston, I've treated many patients with thyroid conditions. As an associate professor of medicine and the director of an endocrine laboratory, I've also done much original research into the effects that the thyroid gland, located in the front of the neck, has on the body. Yet Stacy and Murielle gave me a new perspective on the many mysteries of the thyroid and its functions..

Stacy came to me for a second opinion on her ailment, a condition called Graves' disease, which results in an overactive thyroid. She asked me to recommend a book for "civilians" dealing with the psychological and emotional aspects of thyroid disease. Stacy had already studied all the books suggested by the Thyroid Foundation of America, the principal patient resource organization for thyroid conditions. She had also browsed through the health and medicine sections of a number of large bookstores. Stacy had been suffering from her thyroid condition for four years, and the consequent mental and emotional symptoms had contributed to the collapse of her marriage and the loss of her job. She was determined to learn how her thyroid condition had affected her mind and how she was likely to feel in the future. Although I mentioned a number of scientific studies, I realized that I knew of no popular books directed at a general audience that addressed this important issue.

Shortly after Stacy's visit, I saw Murielle, a young psychologist who was suffering from depression. "My energy level is so low," she told me. "It seems like all I can do is just to try to stay focused because I'm tired. I want to work less, and I've come to dread doing really hard, complex cases with a lot of personality problems."

Although her background gave her some experience in dealing with questions of mind and mood, Murielle was unsure about the cause and cure of her own depression. Because she was aware that depression and tiredness could also be symptoms of a thyroid imbalance, she began to wonder whether her symptoms were thyroid related. Unlike Stacy, Murielle turned out not to have a dysfunctioning thyroid gland. Instead, she was suffering from a brain chemistry disorder related to an imbalance of thyroid hormone levels in the brain. Although Murielle had tried several antidepressants, she wasn't able to regain fully her happiness, energy, and sense of overall well-being until she began taking a thyroid hormone medication in addition to an antidepressant. Thus, even though Murielle did not have a thyroid condition per se, for her, thyroid hormone treatment along with an antidepressant was the solution for full recovery.

In the course of my treatment of her, Murielle asked me a number of good questions, among them where she could go to learn more about how the thyroid and the hormones it releases into the bloodstream affect the brain and nervous system, thus directly or indirectly altering mood, emotions, and behavior. Again, there was no book I could recommend that addressed, in layperson's terms, the intricate relationships among thyroid ailments, emotions, and thought patterns. My increasing awareness of the desperate need of patients like Stacy and Murielle to learn more about their condition compelled me to begin writing this book.

The intent of *The Thyroid Solution* is twofold. First, it aims to introduce readers to the many ways that the thyroid can affect brain chemistry. In recent years, scientists have made remarkable headway in showing how brain chemicals, such as the well-known neurotransmitter serotonin, can influence everything from mood to appetite. Yet even many physicians do not understand how essential thyroid hormones are to normal brain chemistry. It is time for thyroid hormones to be recognized as key brain chemicals, whose actions and effects are similar in many ways to those of serotonin and other neurotransmitters. These effects include relieving emotional states such as depression, as Murielle discovered, as well as aiding other communications between mind and body, including regulating metabolism, sexuality, fertility, appetite, weight, and mental clarity.

Second, this book aims to provide thyroid patients, as well as their partners, families, and friends, with useful, practical information that may help them understand and cope with the difficulties and emotional suffering induced by thyroid diseases. *The Thyroid Solution* details a mind-body program that will help you, the patient, halt the escalation of symptoms and become well again. It also teaches you how to work with your doctor to obtain an accurate diagnosis and to achieve and maintain an optimal thyroid balance, with treatment.

One in ten Americans—more than 20 million people—suffers from thyroid dysfunction. Thyroid hormone imbalance, along with its fraternal twin, clinical depression, may be the common cold of emotional illness. Yet most victims don't realize that thyroid ailments have *any* mental or emotional components. They just know that they don't feel like themselves—and haven't felt right for a long time. This book is directed to these individuals, and I am confident that it can help them regain their emotional health..

Addressing Conditions and Concerns

Like any organ in the body, the thyroid gland can be affected by a wide range of disorders—from the common and rampant condition called Hashimoto's thyroiditis, the leading cause of hypothyroidism (underactive thyroid), to rare and unusual conditions such as Riedel's thyroiditis (a condition in which fibrous tissue replaces healthy thyroid tissue). The main function of the thyroid gland is to produce thyroid hormone, a crucial chemical that affects metabolism and other bodily functions. Thyroid hormone is also part of the brain chemistry mix that regulates moods, emotions, cognition, appetite, and behavior.

A complete home-reference book on thyroid disease would describe in detail all thyroid conditions, both unusual and common. But that would leave little room to detail the hidden and often misunderstood effects of the most common thyroid hormone imbalances, which affect millions of people. For that reason, the main focus of this book is on conditions that result in the types of thyroid hormone imbalance most people are concerned about. Nevertheless, I have included useful information on various thyroid conditions, including goiters, lumps, thyroid cancer, thyroid eye disease, and many others. If you suffer from one of these conditions, this information will help guide you as you seek a diagnosis or receive treatment.

The Thyroid Solution also differs from many other thyroid books in its depiction of thyroid patients and their real-life challenges and concerns as patients have revealed them to me in my more than fifteen years of working with them and helping them to heal. This is the first book to explain the hidden suffering that many patients have difficulty expressing and the first to provide new ways of helping address and heal this suffering. It is my hope that their stories will help you identify symptoms of your own that you may have dismissed as unrelated to a thyroid condition. Further, their stories of regaining physical, mental, and emotional wellness may inspire you to find the answers and treatment you need.

How You Can Use This Book

Part I of *The Thyroid Solution* describes the emerging knowledge about the thyroid-mind connection and how thyroid imbalance is likely to affect not only your physical health but also your mood, emotions, and behavior. It highlights the types of thyroid conditions that could result in a thyroid imbalance and outlines their potential effects on your emotional and physical health. Here you'll find out how to recognize hypothyroidism (underactive thyroid) and hyperthyroidism (overactive thyroid) and work with your physician to obtain the proper diagnosis. Part I also shows you how neuroscientists have come to view the thyroid gland as an "annex to the brain," since the brain uses thyroid chemicals for a wide range of brain functions. You will also learn how dealing with stress, maintaining a healthy and stable mood, and coping with life depend to a great extent on whether the thyroid functions properly and on whether the right amount of thyroid hormone is properly delivered and dispersed in the brain. Stress and thyroid imbalance go hand in hand: thyroid imbalance affects your perception of stress, and stress can trigger an imbalance. This relationship between the thyroid, the immune system, and brain chemistry is intricate, and stress management is important in preventing flare-ups of thyroid imbalance. You will learn how the effects of thyroid imbalances are both physical and mental, although many physicians tend to focus only on the physical effects. You will also learn the many deplorable reasons why thyroid imbalances often remain undiagnosed and misdiagnosed. One reason is that patients suffering from a thyroid imbalance often have symptoms of mood disorders and anxiety and therefore may be misdiagnosed as depressed or anxious. A brain thyroid hormone imbalance can be caused by either a malfunctioning gland or a disruption in the way the hormone is dispersed in the brain. Either way, different types of depression and anxiety disorders can result. Thyroid hormone balance in the brain is crucial for maintaining stable mood, emotions, and behavior. Thyroid hormone can be used as a bona fide antidepressant. When natural or synthetic forms of the hormone are administered in the right dose along with certain antidepressants, almost miraculous mood-boosting effects may result. This can be especially true for people who are suffering from depression and have not fully responded to the conventional antidepressants, such as Prozac and other selective serotonin reuptake inhibitors.

Part II presents in-depth information on how thyroid imbalances may affect your weight, your sex life, and relationships.

Because thyroid imbalances can intrude in your personal life and affect both your sex life and relationships with devastating effects, it is important for you to learn how to discuss these intimate effects with your doctors. Such effects do not necessarily end after the imbalance has been treated, so you will also learn how to cope with these problems and how to ask your partner for the support you need.

Part III is devoted to women's health issues, especially infertility and miscarriage, postpartum depression, and premenstrual syndrome and menopause. A thyroid imbalance will cause or intensify premenstrual syndrome during the reproductive years and will affect the way a woman feels at menopause. Forty million women will enter menopause in the next two decades, and a significant number of them will become afflicted with a thyroid imbalance. Nearly 10 to 12 percent of postmenopausal women will experience hypothyroidism. Because the symptoms of menopause and those of thyroid imbalances share many similarities, it is important for women to know when to suspect a thyroid condition and when to consider estrogen therapy.

Even minute thyroid imbalances can result in infertility, and the depression engendered by this infertility is often worsened by a thyroid imbalance. Women may also lose the desire for sex. I'll explain the interplay between the effects of infertility and thyroid imbalance on the mind and how you can break the costly, vicious cycles generated by thyroid disease.

Part IV is the most directly practical section of *The Thyroid Solution*. It provides tools for you to determine how healthy your thyroid is and what to do if you do suffer from a thyroid imbalance. It also describes the most popular lab tests for measuring how much thyroid hormone you have in your system as well as the pros and cons of simpler self-diagnosis techniques. Here we also examine a major controversy in the field: Can you have a thyroid imbalance even though your blood tests seem normal? You'll find an extensive summary of other medical conditions that may increase your risk of suffering from a thyroid imbalance in the future. These are the same conditions that you will need to watch for if you have already been diagnosed with a thyroid disorder and treated for it. And you will learn some of the most common problems that can arise during the course of treating both hypothyroidism and hyperthyroidism, from side effects associated with the use of conventional thyroid drugs to the many problems that may occur if you're being treated with radioactive iodine.

You will learn how to work with your doctor to obtain the most appropriate treatment for your condition. You will also learn how to prevent the memory lapses and other cognitive problems, as well as depression, that may persist after thyroid imbalances have been treated. These lingering effects of thyroid imbalances often haunt millions of people even after their blood tests have returned to normal with treatment, and you may need to be persistent in seeking a cure for them. Many of my patients have benefited from following the "Circle of Wellness" model I provide for recovering from the long-term effects of a thyroid imbalance.

Whether you suffer from hypothyroidism, thyroid-related depression, fibromyalgia, or lingering effects, if you have been searching for a way to alleviate your symptoms and regain overall health, an innovative treatment protocol that I have developed by combining two major thyroid hormones may well revolutionize the way you treat your thyroid. *The Thyroid Solution* is the first book for laypeople to discuss this treatment and to show its benefits.

Finally, I present a comprehensive plan for maintaining your thyroid's overall health. The many lifestyle choices you make every day can prevent or alleviate thyroid imbalances. We look at the optimal diet for thyroid health—a diet that, not coincidentally, also supports the health of other glands and organs. You'll also learn the most thyroid-friendly nutrients and the benefits of antioxidant and essential fatty acid foods and supplements. We pay special attention to the thyroid-specific mineral iodine and medications that can affect your thyroid. Further discussions focus on the benefits of exercise or regular physical activity, and why alcohol and nicotine are especially damaging to the thyroid.

The concluding chapter offers eight ways to educate doctors and laypeople about the crucial links between thyroid, mind, and mood to benefit our country's overall public health. Patients need to begin asking for routine testing of their thyroids, and the inception of public screenings, like those that are becoming commonplace for cholesterol levels, would immensely benefit individuals and our population as a whole.

A Mind-Body Approach to the Thyroid

Ultimately, this book lets readers know what I try to emphasize to my patients: thyroid disease isn't a purely physiological disease—it is a biopsychiatric one, a mind-body ailment. Many thyroid imbalances can be controlled just as other mental disorders are now, by correcting brain chemistry (in this case, either too much or too little thyroid hormone) and restoring patients' wellness and peace of mind. Further, thyroid hormone can help depressed and anxious patients stabilize their brain chemistry when conventional antidepressants have failed.

If I had my way, everyone who had not been feeling at his or her best for some time would be routinely screened for thyroid imbalance. Those patients diagnosed with a thyroid imbalance who, after a reasonable period of treatment with thyroid hormones, didn't feel like their old selves again would be put on the mind-body program detailed in this book.

The key to correcting thyroid imbalances has changed from simply diagnosing and chronicling physical symptoms to concentrating on the emotional aspects of the disease. Thyroid dysfunction can inflict brutal blows to the brain and create changes that have long-term—sometimes permanent—ill effects on your health and peace of mind. When I treat the long-term emotional and mental effects of thyroid disorder, I use both medication and personal therapy—the best of laboratory-based and listening-based patient care. My intention with *The Thyroid Solution* is to bring groundbreaking information and hope to all those thyroid patients who still suffer from mental anguish that has not been sufficiently explained or understood by physicians.

PART I

THE EMERGING MIND-THYROID CONNECTION:

How a Tiny Endocrine Gland Intimately Affects
Your Mood, Emotions, and Behavior

1

THYROID IMBALANCE:

A Hidden Epidemic

Could you have an overactive or underactive thyroid and not even know it? Millions of Americans—and a high percentage of women in menopause and perimenopause (the decade or so before menopause during which hormonal, emotional, and physical changes begin)—do. Thyroid imbalances are not always easy to recognize. Only recently have physicians even begun to accept that minimal thyroid imbalances have an important effect on mental and physical health.

Do you have any of the following symptoms?

- Always fatigued or exhausted
- Irritable and impatient
- Feeling too hot or too cold
- Depressed, anxious, or panicky
- Bothered by changes in your skin or hair
- At the mercy of your moods
- Inexplicably gaining or losing weight
- Losing your enthusiasm for life
- Sleeping poorly or insomniac

Are you feeling burned out from having acted on an excess of energy for several months? Are you listless, forgetful, and feeling disconnected from your friends and family? Are people telling you that you've changed? Are you taking Prozac® or a similar drug for mild depression but still feeling that your mind and mood are subpar? Or have you been treated for a major depression in the past five years?

If you suffer from more than one of these symptoms or answered yes to one or more of these questions, you could be one of the many people with an undiagnosed thyroid condition. Although some of these symptoms may seem contradictory, all of them can be indications of a thyroid imbalance.

You could also be one of the many people who has been treated for a thyroid imbalance but still suffers from its often-overlooked, lingering effects—effects that may continue to haunt you even after treatments have presumably restored your thyroid levels to normal. If you've ever been treated for a thyroid imbalance, answer these questions:

- Do you feel better but still not quite your old self?
- Do you have unusual flare-ups of anger?
- Are you less socially outgoing than you used to be?
- Are you less tolerant of the foibles of family and friends?
- Do you suffer from occasional bouts of mild depression?
- Do you have frequent lapses in memory?
- Are you often unable to concentrate on what you're doing?
- Do you feel older than your chronological age?

If you've had a thyroid problem in the past but still answer yes to one or more of these questions, it is quite likely that your symptoms are thyroid-related. You don't have to suffer any longer. *The Thyroid Solution* will show you how you can work with your physician to heal these lingering symptoms.

The Thyroid and the Mind

At any given time in the United States, more than 20 million people suffer from a thyroid disorder, more than 10 million women have low-grade thyroid imbalance, and nearly 8 million people with thyroid imbalance remain undiagnosed. Some 500,000 new cases of thyroid imbalance occur each year.[1] All of these people are vulnerable to mental and emotional effects for a long time even after being diagnosed. Incorrect or inadequate treatment leads to unnecessary suffering for millions of these people. But these are numbers. Behind the numbers are the symptoms and ravaging mental effects experienced by real human beings.

The 1990s have seen a major increase in the recognition and detection of previously unsuspected thyroid diseases among presumably healthy people. This stems in part from improved medical technology, which has led to the development of sensitive methods of screening and diagnosing thyroid disease. It also stems from the increased public awareness that thyroid disease may remain undiagnosed for a long time and that even mild thyroid dysfunction may affect your health.[2] Recently, some medical associations such as the American Association of Clinical Endocrinologists have initiated public screenings for thyroid disease, much as cholesterol testing has become available in shopping malls and other public places. At any given time, more than half the patients in our population with low-grade hypothyroidism remain undiagnosed. In a recent thyroid-screening program involving nearly two thousand people that I directed in the Houston area,[3] 8 percent of those tested had an underactive thyroid. Many people screened had never heard of the thyroid gland but rushed to be tested when they recognized that they were suffering many of the symptoms listed in the announcement of the screening. The public's awareness of thyroid disease was boosted by press reports about former president George Bush and his wife Barbara, Russian president Boris Yeltsin, and Olympic track champion Gail Devers when they were diagnosed with thyroid disease. Thanks to these factors, people with nonspecific, undiagnosed complaints are becoming increasingly likely to ask their physicians whether their symptoms might be related to an undiagnosed thyroid disorder.

As an endocrinologist who has focused his research, teaching, and patient care on thyroid conditions, I realized early on in my practice that taking care of thyroid patients was not as easy as I had expected. Treating and correcting a thyroid condition with medication may not always make the patient feel entirely better. I discovered that to care fully for my patients, to help them heal completely, I had to treat their feelings as well as their bodies. If they didn't feel better even though their lab tests said they were cured, I learned to listen to them, believe them, and work with them to help them become wholly cured. In taking care of thyroid patients, the physician's role is not merely to address physical discomfort, test the thyroid, and make sure blood test results are normal (indicating that the right amounts of the various thyroid hormones are circulating in the body). Addressing the effects of thyroid disorders on the mind, helping patients cope with their condition, and counseling them sympathetically are equally important.

Many physicians treat dysfunctioning thyroids, but few of them listen to the person attached to the gland. They concentrate on the blood levels. For these physicians, once the lab results say that a patient appears stabilized, the case is closed. Yet many patients go on to suffer for years from a variety of symptoms left over from the thyroid imbalance. A recent survey conducted in our outpatient endocrine clinic revealed that nearly a third of patients with underactive thyroid glands continue to have symptoms after their thyroid hormone blood levels are normal. Physicians should be treating the still-suffering patients with new protocols for as long as it takes for the mental effects to subside. The reality today, however, is that millions of patients suffer needlessly while their doctors continue to treat thyroid dysfunction as a simple physical disorder rather than what it is: a complex blow to the body and brain.

In general, primary care physicians have not been adequately trained to detect and manage thyroid disease and may lack the expertise needed to diagnose and treat a wide range of thyroid disorders.[4] They also receive little teaching on the effects of thyroid disease on mental health or on understanding the interplay between the mind and the thyroid.

The majority of practitioners of internal medicine and family medicine complete their residency without having had a rotation (or semester) in endocrinology. Many physicians leave their training programs with inadequate knowledge of thyroid disorders and inadequate experience in diagnosing and treating these disorders. Physicians who do receive training in endocrinology realize that thyroid conditions are more widespread than most people think and are also some of the more complex problems in medicine.

Recently I talked with several residents who were about to complete their training in internal medicine. They had also just finished a two-month rotation in endocrinology (including attendance at outpatient clinics). One outstanding resident, who was about to start a primary care practice, pointed out the inadequate training for primary care physicians in diagnosing and treating thyroid conditions. He confessed:

> I didn't see many thyroid patients during my three years of training prior to attending your outpatient clinics. The patients I recall were those who came into the hospital with acute thyroid conditions or patients with medical conditions known to be related to thyroid disease. In these cases, the diagnosis was easy to make based on obvious signs and symptoms. But even in the outpatient setting, we residents seldom look for subtle indications of thyroid disease.

Because both the physical and mental symptoms of thyroid disease masquerade as signs of many other illnesses, getting the proper diagnosis can sometimes take a long time. Often symptoms are misdiagnosed and mistreated. Until patients find the right doctor, they are left alone to deal with devastating effects, which may include depression or even upsetting changes in personal behavior. Inexperienced and poorly trained physicians sometimes make their patients feel crazy or hypochondriacal when they report their symptoms. The doctors may give them antidepressants and a pep talk instead of blood tests, proper medication, and counseling on how to cope with their problems. Female hypothyroid patients may be given estrogen replacement therapy instead of thyroid hormone. Yet what male and female patients really need is a program of medication *and* counseling. Thyroid imbalance can quickly escalate into a destructive brain chemistry disorder— as powerful and pervasive as major depression, an anxiety disorder, or manic-depression.

Once the brain has been denied thyroid hormone or oversupplied with it because of thyroid disease, it takes a long time to recover. If the symptoms are ignored, they can intensify. A vicious cycle occurs wherein the patient gets depressed, the thyroid disease worsens, physical and emotional effects multiply, and mental health suffers further. This cycle is not widely understood or recognized, and many physicians do not know how important it is to halt the cycle—or indeed *how* to halt it.

To understand how we got to this sad state of affairs, it is instructive to take a look at how perceptions of the thyroid and knowledge of its functions have evolved over the past century.

Changing Views of the Thyroid

The Swiss artist Arnold Böcklin (1827–1901) painted a portrait of a woman who appeared quite depressed. Her unsmiling face was sad and lifeless, and her eyes had a detached look. The most striking thing about her appearance, however, was that the front of her neck was swollen. The swelling was so evident that Böcklin drew attention to it with his use of color and lighting. As a layman, he recognized that she had a physical illness and that she was depressed, but it is doubtful that he made a connection between her physical and mental states because even physicians and psychiatrists did not begin to understand the true reason for this connection until the late nineteenth century. In fact, the chicken-or-the-egg riddle was at work: health care professionals did not know whether mood disorders and emotional problems were the *result* of thyroid disease or the *cause* of thyroid disease.

Even before the thyroid gland was shown to play a role in regulating metabolism, it was recognized as "the gland of the emotions." In fact, the relationship between the thyroid gland and the mind was thought for years to have merely an anatomical basis: the thyroid is physically close to the brain. The thyroid was believed to protect the brain from overheating, which could result from increased blood flow to the brain when a person was upset. Dr. Robert Graves was the first to provide the classic description of what is now known as Graves' disease. In his description of this "newly observed affection of the thyroid gland in females,"[5] he highlighted symptoms of the nervous system and used the term *globus hystericus* because of the many psychiatric manifestations exhibited by his patients. Dr. Caleb Parry, who had recognized the condition before Graves but expired before his observations were published, wrote: "In more than one of these [patients], the affliction of the head has amounted almost to madness."[6]

For decades, in fact, Graves' disease was considered to be a mental illness rather than a true thyroid disorder. The early label "crystallized fright" illustrates that this condition was seen as some kind of mental illness that follows a psychological trauma. Among the first physicians to focus on the physical symptoms of the condition was Baron Carl Adolph von Basedow. In 1840, he described four patients with protruding eyes, goiter, and rapid heartbeat. He was also the first to describe pretibial myxedema, a brownish swelling over the legs that occurs in a small number of patients with Graves' disease. Whereas the term *Graves' disease* has prevailed in the English-speaking world, *von Basedow's disease* is the term used in Germany and some other European and African countries.

Nearly half a century after Graves' observations, the British physician Dr. William Gull[7] described for the first time the physical and mental consequences of an underactive thyroid. His writings suggested that some of the effects of hypothyroidism were significant mental changes leading to a severe slowing of the mind. Since then it has become clear that the main function of the thyroid gland is to produce thyroid hormone, which regulates the functioning of our body and at the same time is a bona fide brain chemical that regulates mood, emotions, and many other brain functions. Doctors now have come to understand that the basis of the thyroid-mind connection, which was, for a long time, a mystery, is at least in part related to too little or too much thyroid hormone circulating in the body. A patient with a thyroid imbalance may experience physical effects such as skin problems, irregular heartbeat, congestive heart failure, high blood pressure, muscle dysfunction, and gastrointestinal disturbances. Thyroid hormones regulate the metabolic rate, a concept so well popularized that most people associate thyroid imbalance with metabolism and weight problems. And yet, for many people, the emotional and mood-related consequences of a thyroid imbalance are more drastic than the physical ones.

Paradoxically, whereas nineteenth-century physicians first described and demonstrated the significance of such mental symptoms, many modern-day physicians who treat thyroid patients tend to view thyroid disease only as a glandular disorder with *physical* symptoms.

Why Thyroid Imbalances Are Frequently Unsuspected

Patients with dysfunctional thyroid glands often go to their primary care physicians and describe an array of symptoms, both physical and emotional. Physicians are expected to find the root of the suffering and alleviate the symptoms with treatment. Primary care physicians, however, may have neither the time nor the expertise to deal with conditions involving a combination of physical and emotional symptoms. When patients describe symptoms such as fatigue and anger, many doctors fall back on the catchall diagnoses of stress, anxiety, or depression.

Even when doctors correctly diagnose their thyroid patients, they often fail to give the patients adequate information about their condition and symptoms. Patients may continue to suffer mental anguish because many physicians minimize the seriousness of the physical and mental consequences of thyroid imbalance. Patients may be infantilized or made to feel foolish for asking "too many questions" about "minor considerations" such as forgetfulness or mood swings. As a result, many patients find themselves isolated and misunderstood.

Some physicians may perceive important symptoms of hypothyroidism as trivial, primarily because a large percentage of the population complains of varying degrees of tiredness,[8] lack of interest in life, and weight problems. Not only do symptoms of hypothyroidism and hyperthyroidism begin in an insidious fashion, but they can also involve different bodily organs. When physical symptoms of thyroid disease are prominent, the physician may focus on the specific organ or organs involved instead of searching for a general body imbalance and an underlying condition. The primary care physician may order tests only if he or she feels that the symptoms strongly indicate a thyroid disorder.

Let's take a look at the main reasons why doctors misdiagnose thyroid imbalances.

Stress, depression, anxiety, tiredness, and other emotional or mental states can mask a thyroid imbalance. The doctor on whom you rely to detect and treat your thyroid condition is usually the same doctor responsible for detecting and even treating most mood disorders. Depression is the most common condition seen in general medical practice.[9] Researchers estimate that, at any given time, 10 percent of the population suffers from depression; over a lifetime, the prevalence may be as high as 17 percent.[10] Most patients with mental health problems seek help from primary care physicians rather than psychiatrists.[11] Quite often these physicians have received no training or inadequate training in assessing, detecting, and managing subtle mental disorders. Doctors in health maintenance organizations accurately diagnose fewer than 50 percent of those patients with unequivocal depression.[12] Even among those who are correctly diagnosed with depression, only a small portion receives adequate treatment for a sufficient time.[13]

During physicians' training, their exposure to psychiatric problems takes place primarily in emergency rooms and less frequently in hospital wards. But they receive virtually no formal training in outpatient psychiatry.

Quite often, patients with thyroid disease will describe symptoms that may indicate depression but without recognizing that they are depressed. Some doctors may dismiss these symptoms as unimportant. Under some managed care systems, doctors cannot spend additional time talking to patients who may be depressed because they do not have time or do not get reimbursed for that time. Getting into the emotional aspects of somebody's life can be a drain on physicians' energy, so many will actually avoid trying to understand the roots of a patient's anxiety or depression. Internists and family practitioners may feel uncomfortable dealing with mental anguish and may stick to the familiar territory of performing a physical examination, obtaining laboratory test results, and prescribing medications.

Some doctors may tell their patients "You're doing too much" if they complain about tiredness, depression, and weight gain. One patient of mine, Margaret, a twenty-seven-year-old financial broker, told me of her experience with a previous physician. At the time, Margaret had become continually exhausted and moody and had gained twenty pounds. At first, she felt embarrassed to go see her doctor, thinking, "Who goes to the doctor because they're tired?" After three months of suffering, however, she did go to see her physician. He examined her and advised, "Exercise more and don't eat so much." According to Margaret, "I told him I was exercising more than anyone I know. He probably didn't believe me. The second time that I told him about my tiredness, he was flippant and said, 'I don't think you're sick.' "

Margaret was frustrated, angry, and depressed for months. Thankfully, her stepmother suggested that Margaret get a thyroid test. Margaret was finally diagnosed with an underactive thyroid.

When obvious precipitating reasons for depression are present—such as a difficult divorce, a stressful job, or other personal problems—a doctor is unlikely to consider a thyroid dysfunction as a possible cause or a contributing factor to the depression. The patient, family members, and the doctor become convinced that the overwhelming stress and life situations are responsible for the symptoms. Yet, as we'll see in Chapter 2, stress itself can trigger a thyroid imbalance and contribute to depression. Stress generated by the effects of thyroid hormone imbalance can lead to an escalating cycle of stress/illness/stress. Stressful life events may then be blamed for what are really thyroid-related symptoms, allowing these symptoms to linger and intensify. I recommend that everyone who has experienced a major stressful event, such as a difficult divorce or the death of a loved one, and has ongoing anxiety symptoms have his or her thyroid tested.

Doctors are even more likely to miss a thyroid problem and misdiagnose you if you have previously suffered from depression, panic attacks, or any other mood disorder. Symptoms of a thyroid imbalance are then likely to be attributed to the mood disorder, and the physician searches no further. One patient told me, "I learned quickly after I had been in the psychiatric hospital the first time what not to tell doctors, because once they hear that you had a mental condition, they disregard everything else you say."

Depression and anxiety disorders are the most common psychiatric conditions in the general population as well as the most common mental effects of thyroid disease. Therefore, patients with thyroid imbalance may see a psychiatrist rather than a medical practitioner. Because depression and anxiety disorders can cause the same physical symptoms as thyroid imbalance (such as a rapid heartbeat, increased sweating, and lack of sleep), psychiatrists are likely to come up with a psychiatric diagnosis when they see a thyroid patient. Often psychiatrists do not perform physical examinations that could lead them to detect physical causes for mental symptoms.[14] One study showed that when psychiatrists use conventional psychiatric criteria to assess hyperthyroid patients, they diagnose nearly half of the patients as depressed or suffering from an anxiety disorder.[15] Unfortunately, some psychiatrists do not always assess their patients for an underlying thyroid condition that might explain their fatigue, lack of interest in life, and inability to function as before.

The apparently close link between depression and thyroid imbalance has wide-ranging consequences. For a person like Rachel, a young wife and real estate agent I treated recently, uncovering that link was crucial for overall health and happiness. Before her true, thyroid-related condition was identified and treated, Rachel showed many of the signs of clinical depression. "I was always tired," she related.

> I couldn't exercise anymore, and that was very frustrating. I would come home and fall asleep. If I wasn't sleeping, I was doing nothing more than watching TV. I didn't cook. I didn't clean. I didn't even let the dog out. I also put on twenty pounds in one month and lost a lot of hair, which was terrible for my looks and my self-esteem. I became cold and was constantly turning up the thermostat. Jimmy, my husband, couldn't believe I was so cold. I just had no willpower. I had to take a broker's license test, which cost my firm $2,000, but I couldn't even get motivated to study for it. I just wanted to go home and put on my nightgown and sit there on the couch. I lost interest in having any social life with my husband. I didn't want to see anyone. We quit going out. Our sexual relationship went to zero, too.

Given Rachel's symptoms, it is not surprising that for a long time she was diagnosed as depressed. Yet many of these same symptoms are associated with an underactive thyroid, and when Rachel was treated for her thyroid imbalance, she began to improve. "I gradually woke up and began to feel good," she said. "I didn't feel groggy or rushed anymore. I started eating right. I was more active and doing moderate exercise, and I lost thirty pounds. My husband and I went dancing, and I reunited with my friends again. They all asked, 'Where were you?' " For Rachel to fully answer that question, she would need to understand more about the interplay of thyroid, mind, and mood. Clearly, an underactive thyroid frequently causes depression, and an overactive thyroid tends to result in an anxiety disorder. Nevertheless, anxiety is also common in hypothyroid patients, and some patients with an overactive thyroid suffer from depression. Although when hyperthyroid patients suffer from depression, the bouts of depression tend to be short-lived, some of these patients may have persistent, lingering depression that fulfills the psychiatric criteria for depression.

Patients aren't totally aware of the full range of their symptoms or don't communicate them to their doctors. Patients themselves sometimes unintentionally hinder a proper diagnosis by failing to volunteer all of their complaints to their doctors. The statement "I'm tired and exhausted" usually reflects only surface symptoms. The symptom of fatigue may hide a multitude of feelings and emotional problems that patients may be reluctant to reveal. Most people have difficulty analyzing and clearly expressing how they feel or how their mind has been affected. Often we are not taught to recognize how our hearts feel, and many of us are taught to ignore or discount our emotions. We frequently lump all discomfort and mental suffering into "I'm tired, I'm exhausted, and I can't function the way I used to." Also, we tend to dismiss any mental or physical dysfunction as temporary.

Many people experiencing fatigue, lack of interest in life, and an inability to function as they once did suffer for years. They adjust to these feelings and are able to work and take care of responsibilities at home. But inside they are hurting. They have to struggle to appear normal to those around them. They live in a state of denial or self-dismissal and may not seek help or treatment for their symptoms.

Some of this self-dismissal stems from the stigma our culture puts on any and all mental conditions. The prevailing view that mental suffering is less serious than physical suffering may cause some persons with a thyroid imbalance to hide their anxiety, depression, or pain and not seek medical help. Others may fear ridicule from friends and relatives if they do seek treatment.

One patient who was suffering from lingering depression due to hypothyroidism told me, "I knew I was depressed and something was inadequate within me. I didn't want my family to know. I didn't want my company to know. I didn't have health insurance coverage for depression treatment, so I couldn't afford proper help." Many patients who seek psychiatric care may encounter significant difficulties in obtaining life and disability insurance. Many people with depression choose not to be diagnosed and treated because they know they will be discriminated against when they change jobs.

A second-year law student whom I evaluated for a possible thyroid disorder had suffered from a severe anxiety disorder for two years. He had correctly diagnosed his anxiety disorder a year earlier but had not reached out for help. "I could not go see a psychiatrist because later on, when I sit for my bar exams, just having a record saying I saw a psychiatrist will affect my entire career." This patient turned out to have an overactive thyroid due to Graves' disease.

I cannot emphasize enough how important it is for you to seek help as soon as possible after the onset of your symptoms rather than accepting them and doing nothing about them.

The wide range of physical symptoms can mask a thyroid imbalance. Another reason why doctors may miss a diagnosis of thyroid disease is that thyroid patients' mental suffering may be buried amid the multiple physical effects of thyroid disease. When physical symptoms of thyroid disease are quite prominent, doctors may treat patients for those specific symptoms and fail to diagnose the thyroid condition that is causing the symptoms. For instance, rapid heartbeat is a common symptom of an overactive thyroid that often leads physicians to consider heart disease. But if the heart evaluation is normal, doctors often dismiss the patient as anxious.

Judy, a forty-one-year-old divorced woman whose mother had died three years previously, was experiencing many symptoms of anxiety and depression. Even more disturbing to her were frequent palpitations and weakness in her arms and legs. Hyperthyroidism may be associated with muscle weakness, which should not be confused with the intermittent general weakness accompanying acute anxiety. In Judy's words:

> I had been experiencing rapid heartbeats for about three years. I was nervous and impatient. I had shaky hands. My doctor told me it might be nerves. He put me on the anxiety-reducing drug Xanax. One time I got up at night to go to the bathroom, and when I started walking, I felt like I was going to fall over. I felt like I was losing control. I was nauseous. I called a friend and asked him to come and get me. When I went in the first time, the doctor in the emergency room said I was under tension.
>
> I kept having the same symptoms. I went to the hospital several times, and the doctors gave me a beta-blocker to slow my heart down, but it wasn't enough. I kept waking up at night with palpitations.

The doctors ended up scheduling a twenty-four-hour heartbeat-monitoring test.

It took a long time for Judy to be diagnosed with Graves' disease. The physicians who saw her on numerous occasions were focusing on her heart.

After her overactive thyroid was treated, all her symptoms, including the rapid heartbeat, resolved.

Thyroid hormone imbalance affects the functioning of most bodily organs. How severely it affects organs, however, differs from one person to the next. Imagine two people having the same level of hypothyroidism. They may have some symptoms in common, such as dry skin, constipation, and weight gain. One of them, however, may have severe headaches, which then become the main concern for both the patient and the physician. Joint and muscle pain is another symptom that often triggers unnecessary testing and leads to the wrong diagnosis. Doctors frequently consider neurological or rheumatological conditions in such patients rather than a thyroid disorder. Because many of the emotional and physical symptoms of an underactive thyroid are also symptoms of fibromyalgia and chronic fatigue syndrome (conditions that typically cause severe fatigue), hypothyroid patients may also end up being misdiagnosed with one of these two conditions.

Patients who undergo repetitive testing for rheumatological or neurological conditions and are referred to different specialists often become frustrated because the testing fails to produce a firm diagnosis. In the meantime, the patients' symptoms of depression and their feelings of being out of control may increase. Undiagnosed thyroid patients typically go from physician to physician, searching for the reason for their symptoms.

Gynecological and hormonal symptoms can mask a thyroid imbalance. Women with a thyroid imbalance frequently seek help from their gynecologists because their symptoms, both physical and mental, have evolved concurrently with the onset of heavy or irregular menstrual periods (hypothyroidism) or loss of menstrual periods (hyperthyroidism). Doctors frequently attribute menstrual problems to gynecological or hormonal changes, however, and often tell women they are becoming menopausal or are perimenopausal.

Janet had been suffering from hypothyroidism for more than a year, but her gynecologist focused on Janet's heavy bleeding. Janet ended up having a hysterectomy after four years of trying various reproductive hormonal preparations. According to Janet:

> The gynecologist gave me hormone samples to try for three months. I was still having heavy periods, and nothing felt better, so I went back. I got another type for three months. Four times I went and tried different hormones. Then I had a hysterectomy. I kept gaining weight. My hair was falling out. I felt out of control. I said, something is not right here. Finally, after almost two years, a doctor diagnosed me with hypothyroidism.

Angela, a thirty-five-year-old sales manager in a department store, told of how she suffered from numerous symptoms for which she could find no explanation for a long time:

After I had my second child, I stayed home for the first year of his life, and then I went back to work. There were times that I had a feeling of ill-being, sinking. If I didn't lie down and go to sleep, I felt like I was going to fall down and sleep where I was. I developed more symptoms, such as the migraines. My internist put me on Valium, which I stopped because it made me feel drowsy, but I then began to take Xanax twice a day and another drug for anxiety.

Angela was also suffering from impaired short-term memory, moodiness, anger, and frustration, partly due to thyroid hormone imbalance and partly as a result of anxiety from not knowing what was happening to her. When her menstrual periods became heavier and started lasting seven to eight days, she became concerned that all her symptoms were gynecological.

She says, "My mother told me, 'Your symptoms sound like you have early menopause. Go and see your gynecologist!' I complained to my gynecologist about my periods getting longer. She suggested using hormones to correct the problems, but my symptoms grew worse."

Angela's experience shows how the mental suffering due to hypothyroidism may be incorrectly attributed to reproductive hormonal problems. When estrogen or progesterone treatments do not help alleviate symptoms but actually make them worse, it is very important to get tested for a thyroid imbalance.

Women's health care still lags behind men's, and thyroid symptoms are often dismissed as unimportant "female complaints." In recent years, the question has arisen as to whether internists and family practitioners are adequately trained to provide care for women and to understand their health needs fully. Women's health considerations differ from men's because of differences both in reproduction and in hormonal, psychosocial, and socioeconomic factors.

A study published in the *Journal of Women's Health* in 1993 suggests that the detection of thyroid abnormalities among fifteen- to sixty-four-year-old women often depends on the competence of family and general practitioners and gynecologists. The study showed that women in general receive the majority of their health care from family and general practitioners (54.9 percent), while internists accounted for only 21.5 percent and gynecologists for 23.6 percent of visits.[16] However, women's general physical examinations were largely performed by gynecologists (57.3 percent).

An American College of Physicians task force has defined the minimum competencies for physicians who take care of women and has recommended enhancing the competencies pertaining to women in the field of internal medicine. Competency in the field of thyroid disease is not yet emphasized, despite the fact that thyroid disorders predominantly affect women. Women are more likely than men to be misdiagnosed, perhaps because many doctors often attribute women's complaints to anxiety. Because of time constraints, doctors may dismiss women who express "too many symptoms" when they detail their history. Some uninformed and socially backward doctors misperceive the emotional effects of a thyroid imbalance as "typical female complaints." Or they believe the symptoms are hypochondriacal. Such prejudices can result in failure to diagnose a thyroid imbalance.

Leslie Laurence and Beth Weinhouse, in *Outrageous Practices: The Alarming Truth about How Medicine Mistreats Women*, recount the story of a woman with an overactive thyroid caused by Graves' disease. It was twenty years before a physician finally made the correct diagnosis.[17] According to the patient, "They didn't look thoroughly enough because I'm a woman."

Although prejudices against women in health care are not unique to thyroid disorders, dismissing the symptoms of thyroid imbalance in women is probably more severe than any other common condition that doctors deal with. The complex interplay between premenstrual hormonal changes, menopause, the postpartum period, reproduction, and thyroid imbalance has not been significantly addressed in women's health care. We need to raise our awareness of the deficiencies in providing optimal care for women afflicted with thyroid disease.

Physicians are not well trained to do thyroid exams. Many primary care physicians often ignore the thyroid gland in routine examinations. The gland is not examined by touch, because the physicians either have not been taught the art of palpating the thyroid or are focusing on the patient's other complaints.

One physician in training told me, "The only time I had specific instruction on examining a thyroid gland was in medical school. I can't recall any point in my internship or residency when an attending physician, other than one endocrinologist, reviewed that exam with me." Often when doctors take a health history during a physical, they don't ask about the patient's thyroid. As the trainee said, "There is a lot of emphasis on rectal exams and what should be recorded on the patient's chart, but a thyroid exam is not a mandatory part of a physical exam. It is amazing that a simple thing like examining a thyroid, which is very important in the everyday practice of medicine, is not reinforced. Yet other sophisticated procedures, which may never be performed by general practitioners in their practice, are strongly emphasized."

She went on to say, "I have had many attending physicians, even senior physicians, admit that they don't feel comfortable doing a thyroid exam. They admit that this is because they were never taught well, or they haven't done it routinely in their practice, and so they are out of the habit of being able to interpret their findings. This ignorance is passed on from one generation to the next."

The simple touch examination, or palpation, of the thyroid gland is quite important in finding clues to the presence of thyroid disease. Approximately 5 percent of the population have a nontoxic goiter (an enlargement of the thyroid gland not associated with thyroid dysfunction), and another 5 percent have palpable thyroid nodules (distinct lumps), some of which may harbor thyroid cancer. Palpation allows physicians to evaluate the size and the consistency of the gland. For example, if a person has symptoms of an underactive thyroid, a goiter may provide a clue that the patient is suffering from Hashimoto's thyroiditis, causing hypothyroidism. With this condition, the thyroid gland is quite often enlarged and slightly tender. Again, in a patient having a rapid heartbeat, nervousness, anxiety, agitation, and a recent weight loss, the thyroid exam may reveal a goiter that would be consistent with an overactive thyroid due to Graves' disease.

Physicians may dismiss patients' self-diagnosis. Even when patients determine on their own that their symptoms might be due to a thyroid condition, some doctors may resist the idea. Molly, who had gained a lot of weight and was exhausted from her hypothyroidism, told me:

> Before I was originally diagnosed as being hypothyroid, I had read about it in a magazine. I kept telling my family physician that I had a lot of these symptoms. He never checked my thyroid. He told me, "You just want thyroid hormone because you think it will make you lose weight." That wasn't what I was looking for at all. I was just looking for an answer to why all these things were happening to my body. He finally agreed to do tests, and sure enough, I was hypothyroid.

The search for a correct diagnosis can be lengthy. To determine whether someone has an underactive thyroid, the person must be tested with TSH (thyroid-stimulating hormone), the pituitary hormone that regulates the functioning of the thyroid gland. The TSH test is much more reliable for detecting an underactive thyroid than the measurement of thyroid hormone levels in the blood. Jane, a twenty-eight-year-old nurse enrolled in an HMO, told her primary care physician about her classic symptoms of a thyroid imbalance: decreased sexual desire, hair falling out, troubles with vision, dry skin, and lack of concentration. On her insistence, he ordered a T4 test (which measures the levels of T4, one of the two thyroid hormones produced by the thyroid gland), whose results came back within the normal laboratory range, whereupon he declared that Jane could not have thyroid disease. However, he had not checked her TSH.

She says, "Being told that nothing was wrong with me made me think I might be crazy. I have a history of people trying to deny me my feelings, trying to tell me that what is going on in my body is not real." When her

TSH level was later measured by an endocrinologist, she was diagnosed as hypothyroid.

As you can imagine, having your doctor dismiss your symptoms as unimportant, transient, or irrelevant would generate a great deal of anxiety. Not only would you question your own experience and judgment, but you would still be suffering from the very real problems that caused you to go to your doctor in the first place! Thyroid patients may feel that they are perceived as hypochondriacs or even come to think they actually are imagining things. Yet at some level, they do know that their body is not acting the way it should. Therefore, when they ultimately obtain a proper diagnosis that confirms that there is something medically wrong with them, they are almost universally relieved that their symptoms were not just "in their mind" and that they were not "going crazy."

Important Points to Remember

- Thyroid imbalances have such a wide range of effects on body and mind that thyroid conditions can hide or masquerade as many physical and emotional disorders.
- At any given time, more than half the people suffering from a thyroid imbalance are either undiagnosed or misdiagnosed.
- Do not necessarily rely on your primary care physician to detect and treat your thyroid disorder. Many primary care physicians have been inadequately trained in this field or lack the expertise to deal with complex cases. Be persistent in asking for the right testing and follow-ups.
- If you are experiencing emotional problems, talk about them openly with your doctor. Discuss *all* of your symptoms. Much of the suffering generated by thyroid imbalances can be easily corrected.
- Remember, although thyroid imbalances can cause depression, anxiety, and mood swings, you may *not* need a psychiatrist.

2

STRESS AND THYROID IMBALANCE:

Which Comes First?

At the end of a lecture I gave recently to a third-year medical class, a student named John came to me and said that his twenty-three-year-old wife, Christy, had been experiencing "odd symptoms" for the previous year and that her primary care physician could find nothing wrong with her. "I'm wondering whether she has a thyroid condition, because she has many of the symptoms you described," he said. In my first encounter with Christy, she told what was happening to her. Her scenario was typical of what many thyroid patients go through.

Christy traced her symptoms to a period the year before when she and John had married and she had started law school. About that time, she began to gain weight and be extremely fatigued. At times, she felt her heart was beating fast; she was moody and would cry for no reason. Christy was having a hard time functioning and frequently felt "strange" in her body, which is often typical of panic attacks. She attributed her symptoms to the stress of being newly married and feeling torn between her husband and her studies. Her mother frequently blamed her for having brought her symptoms down on herself, saying that Christy shouldn't have started law school and gotten married at the same time.

Her primary care physician was initially concerned that Christy's palpitations might indicate a heart problem, but her electrocardiogram turned out normal. Once he learned more about Christy's schedule, the doctor, like her mother, suggested that her symptoms were due to stress. When Christy finally consulted me, I determined through blood tests that she had an underactive thyroid.

Christy told me:

Before this time, I was a relaxed person. But suddenly anything would set me off. Even little annoyances or problems seemed like the end of the world and had to be resolved right then. Even though I'm not a devoted cook, if John didn't finish the meal I served, I would fly off the handle. I overreacted to everything, and John wouldn't know from minute to minute what might set me off. This went on for an entire year.

Clearly the stress Christy was feeling was actually creating more stress. Her thyroid imbalance made her unable to deal with the minor stresses that had never affected her previously.

Christy had suffered unnecessarily for a year. Once her thyroid levels became well balanced with treatment, Christy became more able to deal equitably with the stress she faced.

"I don't get upset over silly things anymore. I'm feeling great, doing well in school now and at home without feeling stressed-out. John is happy, too. Recently he said, 'You're back; you're nice again.' "

Christy's story illustrates how dramatically thyroid hormone imbalance can affect a person's ability to deal with stressful events, even the small ones that would normally just be minor parts of daily life. Indeed, the relationship between stress and illness is more apparent in thyroid disorders than in any other medical condition. Thyroid imbalance is an ideal example of the interrelations between mind and body because it reveals how difficult it is to separate out whether the mind or the body is the origin of illness.

How your mind handles stress dictates whether you will recover quickly or fall into an emotionally and physically depleting stress-illness-stress cycle. Laid-back persons who handle difficult situations relatively easily are not likely to be swept up in such cycles. Those who find stressful situations difficult to bear might easily end up with a thyroid hormone imbalance once stress, and reactions to it, occur. *But these people should not be blamed for their illness.* They did not, as Christy's mother had told her, bring this illness on themselves. Different people handle stress differently, and you cannot avoid stress. It is an inevitable part of life.

Think of stress as a long bar with many notches in it. At one end of the bar are small notches that represent minor stresses, like an argument with a colleague, a child spilling soda on the sofa, or too much paperwork. In the middle of this bar are bigger notches representing life events such as the loss of a job, feelings of financial insecurity, or marital troubles. At the opposite end of the bar are large gashes—traumatic events, such as being a victim of violence or abuse or serving in combat. How your mind and body respond to a stressful event, however, may have more to do with how you *perceived* the event than with the precise nature of the event.

You feel, integrate, and react to stressful events through responses in your brain chemistry. The body responds to happy or upsetting events in an area of the brain called the limbic system, the same area that controls mood and emotions. This is also the part of the brain where thyroid hormone is delivered in great amounts. Within the limbic system, thyroid hormone is a major chemical player.

Thyroid imbalance, whether from a deficiency or an excess of thyroid hormone, generates a myriad of emotional, mood, and cognitive effects that both weaken the ability to cope with stress and compound an inability to cope with stress. Disturbed emotions inevitably generate new stress, which can be expressed as anger, irritability, depression, and maladjusted behavior. Upsetting situations that grow out of this regenerated stress are perceived in an amplified way, leading to a feeling of being constantly stressed-out.

Even a laid-back person can easily fall into the stress trap if his or her thyroid gland becomes dysfunctional, simply because thyroid hormone is one of the chemicals that regulates how we perceive and emotionally respond to stress. Symptoms of thyroid imbalance are often assumed to be symptoms of stress or the consequence of major stressful events. The similarity between stress reactions and symptoms of thyroid hormone imbalances causes a problem that is common among thyroid patients: their imbalance may go unrecognized for a long time before it is considered as the source of their suffering. Both patients and physicians blame the symptoms of thyroid imbalance on stress rather than on a chemical imbalance that is affecting the patient's body and mind.

How Stress Can Trigger a Thyroid Imbalance

It is crucial to understand that a mental state or stress can trigger and worsen thyroid disease and that you can learn ways to help yourself get well. My thyroid patients often ask, What caused or triggered this condition? Even though stress is not the only possible catalyst, it is in many patients an obvious one. Yet physicians often fail to emphasize stress as a triggering factor.

Physicians Deepak Chopra, Andrew Weil, and Bernie Siegel have emphasized the importance of attitude and mind-related techniques (such as meditation and guided relaxation) to help avoid or overcome illness and have increased our understanding of the relationship between stress and illness. *Anatomy of an Illness*, Norman Cousins's account of his mind and spirit's triumph over illness, was among the first memoirs to bring to public awareness the incontrovertible connection between good spirits and good health. Since its publication in the late 1970s, much research has supported this connection.

Research has further enhanced our understanding of how stress affects the mind and body. Under stress, the brain emits chemical messages that trigger major responses of the endocrine system. One such response is the overproduction of the stress hormone cortisol by the adrenal glands. Repeated overproduction of this hormone and other chemicals results in many of the deleterious effects associated with stress.[1] If you handle stress well, the response of the endocrine system is minimal and short-lived. But if you are stressed for a long time; experience major upheavals, setbacks, or traumas; or have difficulties coping with stress, your endocrine system becomes chronically challenged and causes health problems.

Various organs of the endocrine system are designed to respond to stress. These responses, however, occur at the expense of the immune system.[2] In studies conducted on the effect of arguing and hostility, psychologist Janice Kiecolt-Glaser showed that the more hostile people are during marital arguments, the more suppressed are their immune systems.[3] High levels of stress—and more important, an impaired ability to cope with stress—cause the immune system to weaken and make the body more vulnerable to infections. Stress causes viral and bacterial infections to stay with you longer. One experimental study showed that people experiencing a great deal of stress who are injected with a virus are more likely to become ill from the virus than are people with little or no stress.[4] The weakening of the immune system resulting from stress is primarily determined by brain chemistry, which uses the endocrine system and its chemicals as messengers. The person is now more vulnerable to infection and disease. The immune system will attack the invading virus, but if the virus has a molecular structure that mimics the makeup of the thyroid gland, when the immune system produces antibodies to attack the virus, it will mistake the thyroid gland for the virus. The key player in this scenario is the immune system.

With that in mind, it is easy to understand that if you deal with stress well, and if your coping mechanisms are strong, the cascade of brain chemicals and hormones emitted in response to stress is tempered. The adverse effects on your immune system will then be minor. The difference between a person who successfully interprets and deals with stress and the rest of us is that the more relaxed among us are less likely to experience disturbances of the immune system and other ailments resulting from too much cortisol. Those whose bodies have trouble managing stress and, in response, become depressed tend to develop problems.

The biochemical cascade that links the brain to the immune system is at the root of how mental stress triggers thyroid imbalance. The two most common underlying causes of thyroid dysfunction are disorders of the immune system:

1. Hashimoto's thyroiditis, the most prevalent disorder resulting in thyroid hormone deficiency
2. Graves' disease, the most common condition causing an excess of thyroid hormone production

Both of these thyroid ailments are recognized as autoimmune conditions because they reflect a pattern in which the body attacks itself. In each case, the immune system produces antibodies and other chemical substances that attack the thyroid gland and alter its functions. Many people never experience symptoms of an abnormal thyroid, however, despite having glands with immune reactions characteristic of Hashimoto's or Graves' disease.

Although these two conditions cause opposite reactions in the gland, people affected by one or the other have in common the same genetic abnormality. This explains why, in many cases, more than one member of the same family may be affected. Genetic predisposition to thyroid and other autoimmune disease is an important factor—but not the only one—in determining who is vulnerable to a thyroid imbalance.[5] If one of two identical twins has Graves' disease, for instance, the odds that the other twin will have the condition as well are perhaps only fifty-fifty. Genetic factors may also provide a clue as to why Graves' disease occurs seven to ten times more frequently in women than in men. As with other autoimmune diseases, some of the genes that predispose people to this condition may be located in the X chromosome.

In addition to the genetic predisposition, the fluctuation of hormones such as estrogen and progesterone plays a role in triggering these disorders. This is illustrated by the fact that, before puberty, both sexes are equally apt to develop an autoimmune disease, whereas after puberty, women become much more vulnerable to such conditions. Researchers believe that this is because women have higher levels and greater fluctuations of sex hormones compared to men. Some evidence indicates that estrogens aggravate autoimmune thyroiditis while testosterone suppresses the immune attack.

Hashimoto's thyroiditis causes gradual destruction of the thyroid gland and leads to an underactive or even moribund gland. The condition's fraternal twin, Graves' disease, results from an immune system that produces antibodies that stimulate the gland and make it overproduce thyroid hormone. Stress is one of the precipitating events that may disrupt the functioning of the immune system and thereby trigger the production of these thyroid-harming antibodies.

Among the infectious agents that have been linked to autoimmune thyroid disease are Coxsackie B virus, *Yersinia enterocolitica*, and *Escherichia coli*. Recently infections with *Helicobacter pylori* (the bacterium that results in gastritis and ulcer) have been found in a high percentage of people with autoimmune thyroid disease.[6]

People suffering from autoimmune thyroid diseases are more predisposed to other autoimmune conditions, such as pernicious anemia, insulin-dependent diabetes, lupus, rheumatoid arthritis, Addison's disease, and vitiligo (a blanching and loss of pigmentation in certain areas of the skin). Stress and psychological reactions to stress also affect these autoimmune conditions. However, the ability of mental stress to trigger an autoimmune attack and affect its severity is more clearly established with Graves' disease than with any other autoimmune condition.

A wide variety of stressful situations may serve as the trigger. For example, when I saw my patient Ron for the first time, he had already been treated for hyperthyroidism due to Graves' disease. His symptoms lingered, however, and his hormone levels were still not in balance, so I asked him to describe the circumstances that led to his disorder. In his words:

> I was in the military and living near the base with my wife. I was working two jobs trying to put her through school. One job was teaching, which kept me busy from six in the morning until three in the afternoon. I slept from four until seven, then I'd get up and go to the commissary, where I would stock shelves until about one A.M. We had borrowed money from my wife's family to put a down payment on a house and were being pressed to pay back the loan. The pressure was unbearable. My boss in the teaching job was verbally abusive and openly belittled me. It was a totally stressful situation.

Ron traced his early symptoms to this time in his life. "I couldn't tolerate the heat. I was sweaty all the time, and my heart pounded constantly. I had muscle contractions and chest pains. At night, I would be sleeping and then jump up out of bed. I went to the doctor at the base. He kept saying it was stress-related and I might want to see a psychologist."

As is often the case, Ron became short-tempered and found it hard to control himself around his children. He quit his second job, which made it more difficult to repay the loan. That situation, in turn, put even more pressure on him. His symptoms lingered. Each time he went back to the doctor, he was told his condition was stress-related. Unable to cope any longer, he left the army.

The Escalation Cycle

In many patients like Ron, detailed histories obtained when they are finally diagnosed reveal that major stress events, sometimes quite remote, probably triggered their conditions. Doctors may blame this event for the patient's symptoms. This misdiagnosis or lack of diagnosis may lead to lingering symptoms and finally escalation and perpetuation of the stress. Often physicians are faced with a Gordian knot: they can only guess whether symptoms are primarily due to a thyroid imbalance. If the treatment does not get to the root of the problem or find a way to break the cycle, however, the symptoms will go on endlessly.

Much of the cycle of symptoms takes root in the period before the patient is diagnosed. A mild dysfunction triggered by a stressful event becomes a more severe dysfunction with more stress. The additional stress results in illness, leading to more stress. The onset of one disease giving rise to another that subsequently affects the first is the pattern doctors face in diagnosing and treating thyroid imbalance. Yet this escalating cycle could easily be halted in its early stages if both physicians and patients became more aware of it. Interrupting this cycle by diagnosing the thyroid imbalance early and addressing the stress issues related to it prevents unnecessary physical and mental suffering, personal problems, and undue stress, enabling the patient to feel better faster.

Kimberly's struggle with a thyroid condition illustrates the perils for the patient entangled in the cycle. An attractive thirty-four-year-old woman, Kimberly was referred to me for Graves' disease by her gynecologist. Kimberly was certain that her symptoms had begun some two years earlier, approximately four months after she started a new job. Prior to that, she was happy and relaxed. She said:

> I thought the job would take me further in my career in management, but the pressure was too much. After trying to keep up, I began to realize it wasn't the right job for me. My self-esteem began to suffer.
>
> I was stressed-out and became anxious and depressed. I seemed to be sick all the time and exhausted, which I related to being ill for most of the winter. I became belligerent, noncooperative at work, and angry and overactive at home. My husband thought I was having a breakdown. He insisted I see a psychiatrist.

Kimberly slowly became entangled in a chain of events that affects many thyroid patients, sometimes for years, both before and after diagnosis. The psychiatrist treated her with antidepressants, which can cause patients with an overactive thyroid to feel worse. Kimberly noticed a puffiness around her eyes, and she lost weight. But because these symptoms were insignificant in relation to the problems that seemed to be pulling her world apart, she ignored them. The antidepressants did not help, so the psychiatrist put Kimberly on an antianxiety medicine. Meanwhile, her self-confidence was eroding daily at work, and the humiliation leaked into all areas of her life. Eventually she was fired.

At this point, Kimberly "went a little crazy," to use her expression. She interviewed for many jobs but came across as insecure and unfocused. No one would hire her. To fill the void, she tackled hundreds of extra tasks at home and performed them badly. Her husband had to take over the management of the children's activities. Arguing with her husband became part of Kimberly's daily life. The loss of her job and the reduced income became a source of marital tension. At some point, she began to suffer rapid heartbeats and consulted a cardiologist. He diagnosed her symptoms as stress-related. Her psychiatrist noticed that Kimberly had developed tremors and suggested she see a neurologist. Tests came back negative. Even so, Kimberly says, "I cried. I didn't care that there was nothing wrong. I just wanted someone to help me."

Kimberly's disease was spiraling. From the time the stress of the new job triggered her Graves' disease, to the mood disorder that followed, to the physicians' confusion about the root of her problem, Kimberly had run around the circle of thyroid disorder many times, with each symptom leading inevitably to the next. Depression followed stress, a disturbed immune system caused a worsening of the overactive thyroid, stress and the effects of hyperthyroidism led to exhaustion, and uncontrollable behaviors caused low self-esteem, which produced further stress. The cycle became self-reinforcing.

An astute gynecologist was the first physician to consider testing Kimberly's thyroid. By treating Kimberly's thyroid condition and addressing the stress issues, we were eventually able to interrupt this stress cycle. It wasn't quick and easy, however. The mental anguish had altered Kimberly emotionally, affecting her brain chemistry. Organically, she had gone through a change. It took weeks to normalize her thyroid hormone levels. Kimberly gradually regained her equilibrium through much support from home, good therapy, and an antidepressant medication. Sadly, her troubles could have been stopped at many points if both she and her doctors had not been confounded by the confusing mind-body symptoms of thyroid disease.

Until quite recently, researchers were unable to determine conclusively that stress is a major trigger of Graves' disease. This is ironic because, in the first cases of Graves' disease ever diagnosed, it was noticed that major stress had precipitated the cycle. The Irish physician Caleb Parry, the first to recognize the condition, described "Elizabeth S., aged 21," who "was thrown out of a wheelchair in coming fast down a hill . . . and was very much frightened. From this time she has been subject to palpitations of the heart and various nervous affections. About a fortnight after, she began to observe a swelling of the thyroid gland."[7]

It is often difficult for researchers and physicians to determine whether stress has been precipitated by thyroid imbalance or vice versa. There is just no way to pinpoint when the thyroid condition began in an individual unless blood levels of thyroid hormones were measured before the onset of stress.

Despite these difficulties, researchers have recently been able to establish a clear-cut link between stressful events and the onset of Graves' disease. One study, for instance, concluded that factors such as change in work conditions, change in time spent on work, and hospitalization of a family member for a serious illness (factors that could not have been caused by the thyroid condition) were all associated with the occurrence of Graves' disease.[8] Another recent study conducted at the University of Tokyo on 228 patients with newly diagnosed Graves' disease concluded that stress increased the occurrence of Graves' disease by 7.7-fold in women.[9] The study also showed that smoking (perhaps an indication of stress) increased the risk for Graves' disease, too. Divorce, marital difficulties, death of loved ones, and financial troubles are also possible triggers of Graves' disease.

The difficulties facing researchers are even greater with Hashimoto's thyroiditis, which causes an underactive thyroid. Hashimoto's disease is much more common than Graves' disease, affecting more than 10 percent of women. Many people suffering from Hashimoto's thyroiditis have an enlarged thyroid or a goiter but no other symptoms. They often have high blood levels of antithyroid antibody, which is produced by the immune system. Doctors use this antibody as a marker for the disease (see Chapter 14). Many patients with Hashimoto's thyroiditis have a minimally underactive gland, causing tiredness, dry skin, and a feeling of being colder than usual. Because the symptoms of Hashimoto's thyroiditis are more insidious than those of Graves' disease, few researchers have seriously attempted to establish that stress could trigger this condition or the resulting imbalance.

Nevertheless, endocrinologists routinely see patients with hypothyroidism whose symptoms began "coincidentally" with either stress (or what the patients described as stress) or depression. As with Graves' disease, physicians must wonder whether the stress or depression triggered Hashimoto's thyroiditis and the resulting underactive thyroid, or vice versa. Does the sharp increase in Hashimoto's thyroiditis at menopause occur only because of hormonal changes, or does it occur because stress and depression are more common around this phase of the reproductive cycle? Does the high frequency of thyroid imbalances after delivery of a baby result only from an immune system temporarily vulnerable because of hormonal swings, or does the stress of having to care for a new baby and the concomitant depression trigger the imbalance?

The effects of depression on the immune system are similar to those caused by stress. Therefore, the sequence of chemistry interactions that leads to the triggering of an autoimmune thyroid disorder is also likely to occur during depression. Physicians are only beginning to pay attention to this scenario. A recent, provocative study showed that women suffering from postpartum depression are more likely to have Hashimoto's thyroiditis than women who do not experience postpartum depression—even when the hormone levels of the depressed women are normal.[10]

Another extremely important component of the relationship between Hashimoto's thyroiditis and mental stress is illustrated by a study that revealed that people hospitalized for depression have a higher frequency of Hashimoto's thyroiditis than the general population, even when their thyroid hormone levels are normal.[11] Until recently physicians blamed hypothyroidism for causing depression and assumed that treating the underactive thyroid would reverse the depression. But sometimes the opposite is true: in many people, when physicians treat the thyroid imbalance, the depression—which might have been the source rather than the consequence of the thyroid imbalance—persists unless treated and addressed in its own right. Physicians should begin to suspect that depression, a form of major stress, might be the triggering event in many patients with Hashimoto's thyroiditis. Those patients exhibit the same escalation phenomenon described in patients with Graves' disease. For people suffering from either condition, steps to halt the cycle are the same: correct the thyroid hormone imbalance and address issues of stress and depression.

The accompanying diagram illustrates the complex set of interactions between brain chemistry and the thyroid that can contribute to the stress-illness escalation cycle.

THE BIOCHEMICAL BASIS OF THE ESCALATION CYCLE

Stress →→→→→→→ Brain chemistry ←←←←←←←←
←←←←←←←
↓   ↑
↓   ↑
Genetic predisposition, →→→→→→→→→ Immune system → ↑
viral and   ↓   ←   ↑
bacterial infections   ↓   ↑
↓   ↑
↓   ↑

Substances attacking   ↑
the thyroid   ↑
(antibodies and others)   ↑
↓   ↑
↓   ↑
Hashimoto's and Graves'   ↑
↓   ↑
↓   ↑
Thyroid imbalance →→→→→→→↑

The Brain and Thyroid Function

The amount of thyroid hormone produced by the thyroid gland compensates for the amount used by cells. The amount of thyroid hormone manufactured by the thyroid gland is primarily governed by the pituitary gland, which is situated at the base of the brain and produces thyroid-stimulating hormone, or TSH. The amount of TSH delivered to the thyroid gland tells the thyroid how much thyroid hormone to manufacture.

The pituitary gland senses any increase or decrease in thyroid hormone levels in the blood and reacts to the change by adjusting the production of TSH. Therefore the pituitary sees that the levels of thyroid hormones in the circulating blood remains normal and constant—and sees that the right amount of thyroid hormone is delivered to organs and to the brain. For instance, if the thyroid gland becomes damaged and produces less thyroid hormone than normal, the pituitary senses the decrease in thyroid hormone levels and releases more TSH. This stimulates the thyroid gland to produce more hormone and correct the deficiency. If, on the other hand, the level of thyroid hormone is excessive, the pituitary senses the change and decreases its TSH secretion, telling the thyroid gland to limit its production. For this reason, TSH has become the most widely used and most reliable test to diagnose a thyroid imbalance, even when it is minimal. TSH is also used to monitor treatment with thyroid hormone.

But the brain, when necessary, can have a say on how much thyroid hormone should be produced. Some areas of the brain, including those involved in regulating mood and behavior, can control the function of the pituitary. The intermediary between these regions of the brain and the pituitary is the hypothalamus, which communicates with the pituitary by emitting a chemical called thyrotropin-releasing hormone, or TRH. These areas of the brain send messages to the thyroid gland by making the pituitary increase or decrease the production of TSH. For example, the body's perception of cold is transmitted to the brain through brain chemicals that then communicate with the pituitary, telling it to increase the TSH level as a reaction to low temperature so that the thyroid produces more thyroid hormone and the body will generate more heat. If you starve yourself or fast for a prolonged time, or face extreme physical stress such as surgery or a major illness, your brain instructs the pituitary to produce less TSH so that your thyroid manufactures less thyroid hormone. This defense mechanism slows your metabolism and the rate of organ destruction. The brain is, in effect, protecting the body against starvation by lowering its metabolic rate. This also explains how the thyroid slows its function if you are suffering from an eating disorder, such as anorexia nervosa. The brain perceives an eating disorder as a potential threat to the body's energy reserves and will make the thyroid lower metabolism and preserve as much energy as possible for survival. After a major stressful event, such as a war situation, the brain may send signals to the thyroid gland to increase its production of thyroid hormone for a long time, which, in theory, will allow the person to be hypervigilant. (See the accompanying diagram showing how the brain regulates the thyroid system.)

BRAIN REGULATION OF THE THYROID SYSTEM

Brain	Brain chemicals
	↓
Hypothalamus	TRH
	↓ (+)
Pituitary gland	TSH
	↓ (+)
Thyroid gland	Thyroid hormones (T4 and T3)

The Thyroid and Postwar Syndromes

Many people who have been engaged in combat subsequently experience a multitude of mental and physical symptoms, such as shortness of breath, fatigue, headaches, chest pain, rapid heartbeat, diarrhea, troubled emotions, and sleep disturbances. These symptoms have been noted among veterans since the American Civil War and have been seen after most major wars, including the Vietnam War and the Persian Gulf War.[12]

"Postwar psychoneurosis" or, more familiarly, post–traumatic stress syndrome, is a complex condition that mixes depression, anxiety, and a host of other symptoms. Although many studies have been devoted to finding the cause for this syndrome, few researchers have carefully studied the possible link between thyroid function, wartime stress, and subsequent thyroid disease. Evidence supports the notion, however, that this syndrome reflects, to a great extent, the levels of both thyroid hormones and cortisol that were produced in response to the stress of combat.

When you experience a major stress that you interpret as a significant threat, the brain relays a chain of signals to the endocrine system that may go on indefinitely. One of the typical reactions is the stimulation of the thyroid gland to produce higher amounts of thyroid hormone. This prolonged stimulation explains why you remain superalert, frightened, and anxious for a long time after a major event such as combat or physical or sexual abuse. The effects of the increase in thyroid hormone levels in relationship to the levels of cortisol explain to a great extent the symptoms experienced by people suffering from post–traumatic stress syndrome, such as those who fought in combat or lived through a war.[13]

Combat veterans who experienced major stress have persistently high thyroid hormone levels at times and can feel extremely anxious as a result. They are unusually watchful or wary, angry, and irritable; they may have sleep or concentration problems. In essence, high levels of thyroid hormone, which are part of the self-preservation response that occurs during a major life-threatening situation, produce this extreme alertness.

People who experience combat or live in war-torn areas are not only at risk for experiencing post–traumatic stress syndrome. They also seem to become at risk for experiencing Graves' disease because of the effects of the stress on the immune system. For instance, doctors noted a significant increase in the incidence of Graves' disease during the Franco-Prussian Wars of 1870. During and following World War I, doctors observed a higher frequency of Graves' disease. For instance, at Camp Upton in New York, doctors noted that many people who were labeled as having a war neurosis had clear-cut symptoms of Graves' disease. The same doctors found that an overactive thyroid was responsible for some of the cases of "war neuroses" that they were treating.[14] During World War II, an increase in the frequency of overactive thyroid was also noted among refugees from Nazi prison camps and among the people of occupied Denmark.[15]

Former president George Bush may be an example of someone involved in a wartime situation who ends up suffering from a stress–thyroid imbalance–stress cycle. Did, in fact, the stress of the Gulf War trigger or unmask the president's Graves' disease?

The speculation about stress triggering President Bush's overactive thyroid was prompted by the fact that his symptoms became evident approximately two months after the Gulf War cease-fire (February 24, 1991). While jogging at Camp David on Saturday, May 4, Bush experienced shortness of breath and an irregular heartbeat. This led doctors at Bethesda Naval Hospital to test his thyroid, which was found to be mildly overactive. Prior to the diagnosis, President Bush had experienced a few symptoms, which began two to three weeks before his admission to the hospital. Toward the end of March, he had decided to lose weight and exercise more. However, Bush's loss of seven to eight pounds over a two-week period was disproportionate to his dieting and exercise. His secretary had also noted a trembling of Bush's right hand, which caused some difficulty writing. Bush's entourage at the time—including his wife, his trusted aide Patty Presock, General Brent

Scowcroft, and others on the White House and residence staff—had not noticed any emotional distress prior to diagnosis of the president's Graves' disease.

There has also been speculation that President Bush's overactive thyroid had preceded the war. Some news reporters described the president as animated by an incredible level of energy immediately after Iraq's August 2, 1990, invasion of Kuwait.[16] His heightened interest in sports activities at the time, his fast pace, and overactivity led some to speculate that Bush might have been suffering from an overactive thyroid as far back as August 1990— almost six months prior to the war. This would put the onset of Graves' disease during the months of preparation leading up to the war, one of the most intense periods in Bush's presidency.

It must be noted that a number of alternative mechanisms have been identified that may well have played a more important role in triggering Bush's ailment. Two years before President Bush was diagnosed with Graves' disease, first lady Barbara Bush had been diagnosed with the same condition. Cases in which partners are diagnosed with Graves' disease are known as "conjugal Graves' disease."[17] Conjugal Graves' disease may be due to environmental factors, such as toxins in the home or workplace, or even too much iodine and other chemicals in the water. The search for such factors in the White House was fruitless. Viral infections are also considered environmental in nature and can be implicated if there is a genetic predisposition, which both George and Barbara Bush could have.

(Coincidentally, the Bushes' dog, Millie, was suffering from lupus. When the news broke that the Bushes and their pet all had autoimmune disorders, the president's personal physician, Dr. Burton Lee, received numerous letters reporting cases of pets suffering from lupus whose owners have Graves' disease.)

There is increasing evidence that links infection, specifically infection by retroviruses, with Graves' disease. The possible link between a retrovirus and Graves' disease can be measured through the level of antibodies in the patient's system.[18] It turned out that both the Bushes had significant levels of antibodies to the virus in their systems. These findings were never made public, however, perhaps because these results did not provide clear-cut proof that the virus was the direct cause of their condition. The medical evidence does strongly suggest, though, that in the cases of the president and Mrs. Bush, infection by a virus contributed to the Graves' disease.

Former president George Bush's case illustrates how difficult it is to prove that stress was a factor in triggering the condition. Did infection by a retrovirus cause Bush's Graves' disease, or did it result from stress generated by the Gulf crisis? Perhaps the most likely scenario is that it was a combination of the two.

Stress Management

Stress management should become a central part of any strategy for treating thyroid patients. Persons who have suffered thyroid imbalances are always on the brink of falling into an escalation cycle. Some need counseling and psychotherapy; others need antidepressants and antianxiety medications. But everyone benefits from thyroid-balance and relaxation techniques, which will help avoid the overwhelming stress that kicks off the cycle. Your brain has to show your thyroid and your immune system that it is in control.

The effect of stress on thyroid disease is not limited to triggering the disease and contributing to the prediagnosis escalation cycle described earlier. Stress can hurt you at all phases of treatment, including when thyroid hormone levels have returned to normal. For instance, patients with Graves' disease who have been successfully treated with a several-month course of an antithyroid medication (methimazole or propylthiouracil) may experience a remission of their disease and no longer require medications to maintain normal thyroid levels. Although the autoimmune disease can become dormant as a result of the treatment—and the physician and patient hope that it will remain dormant indefinitely—the condition will never go away. In such patients, stress and difficulties coping with stress can easily result in flare-ups of overactive thyroid, even after many years of remission. A report presented in 1995 at the Eleventh International Thyroid Congress in Toronto showed that, in patients with Graves' disease, stress could promote a relapse of overactive thyroid.[19]

Stress undoubtedly increases the severity of the autoimmune attack upon the thyroid gland, even when the patient has been stabilized through adequate treatment. In one study of a large number of women whose glands contained dormant Graves' disease, researchers noted that many of the subjects became hyperthyroid during periods of stress. Once the stress went away, the functioning of the gland returned to normal.[20]

Persons who have experienced a thyroid imbalance may continue to suffer adverse effects even after their thyroid levels have returned to normal. Patients who do not feel the same as they used to, despite normal blood levels, are often those who have experienced lengthy cycles of stress-imbalance-stress. These longtime sufferers often describe symptoms similar to those who were affected by an enormous trauma, such as being the victim of a crime or a combatant in war. For this reason, physicians consider the aftermath of thyroid imbalance a form of post–traumatic stress syndrome.

This sounds serious—and it is. Beyond the suffering the patient experiences before diagnosis and into the midst of the cycle, the healing must continue even after the disorder has been corrected. It is essential for friends and loved ones to understand that the thyroid patient may remain vulnerable to the effects of stress for some time. For these longtime sufferers, stress management is one of the most crucial steps toward recovery. Their brain chemistry has been altered, and their ability to cope with stresses, even small ones, has become precarious. They need to assume control again.

After the patient has fallen into a destructive cycle, it is possible to interrupt the spiral by boosting the effects of medication and easing the lingering mental symptoms that have not diminished over time. The combination of support—proper treatment, stress management, and tender loving care—will halt the patient's anguish at the source.

"I'm stressed out." "I can't cope with the pressure." Although statements like these are tossed around lightly, it is important to pay attention to these feelings, in addition to avoiding and managing stress. It is even more important for those who have a thyroid hormone imbalance, have had an autoimmune disease, or have a genetic predisposition to this type of disorder. Like the species that must live in water to breathe, these sufferers must consciously avoid and manage stress or they will get caught up in the vicious cycle characteristic of thyroid hormone imbalance.

Doctors diagnose thyroid disease more frequently than ever before. Many attribute this to wider availability of testing or improvements in technology, both of which have enabled us to conduct more sensitive diagnostic tests. It may also be because contemporary life brings greater stress and makes more demands on us. In 1930, Dr. Eli Moschowitz, in a review concerning psychiatric manifestations of Graves' disease, warned the medical community that "those influences that tend toward conflict and sensitization of the individual will breed Graves' disease" and suggested that Graves' disease was a "social disease and a product of higher civilizations."[21]

If increasing stress is at the root of the rise in thyroid disease, then people with thyroid problems must learn ways to cope better with stress. Relaxation techniques such as meditation, yoga, or tai chi can help prevent thyroid imbalance, especially if you have a family history of thyroid disease or other autoimmune conditions. Practicing stress management is essential for women who have reached menopause or have just delivered a baby, for those holding demanding jobs, and for people caring for demanding households.

There is no single best technique for stress management. The choice of a technique depends on whether you have other health conditions and on whether you can perform physical exercise. It could be deep-breathing exercises with meditation, sitting still while listening to soothing music, or mindful exercise such as yoga or tai chi. The ancient practice of tai chi has been shown to improve mood and emotions,[22] and could be one of the most efficient ways to preserve a healthy mind, immune system, and thyroid. For people with no physical impairment, I recommend tai chi most often.

Relaxing your mind while exercising will boost your brain chemistry and make you feel in control again.

With thyroid conditions, the mind-body connection is not just part of the disorder; it is part of the treatment as well. The thyroid is the annex to the brain—the gland with which and through which the brain communicates. For this reason, it is very responsive to techniques that work on the body through the mind. As soon as you're diagnosed, you should begin working on your own to break your cycle of symptoms. You should expect your physician to control the thyroid hormone imbalance properly, but you as a patient must address your own stress issues. You must take responsibility for your healing regimen and become actively involved in getting yourself well.

Important Points to Remember

- Stress and an inability to handle stress can precipitate the onset of a thyroid imbalance.
- Thyroid imbalance, in turn, impairs your ability to deal with stress and makes you perceive trivial or annoying matters as more significant.
- The stress-illness-stress escalation cycle is a pattern commonly experienced by thyroid patients. The key is to recognize the cycle and halt it by obtaining diagnosis and rapid treatment.
- If you have been diagnosed with a thyroid imbalance, stress management techniques should be part of your treatment program to maintain optimal physical and emotional wellness. If you are genetically predisposed to a thyroid imbalance, stress management techniques may prevent the onset of an imbalance.
- Hashimoto's thyroiditis and Graves' disease are the leading causes of thyroid imbalance. Both conditions represent reactions of the immune system to the thyroid gland. Your genes account for half the predisposition to having these conditions. The effect of the environment, including infections and stress, is far from negligible.

3

HYPOTHYROIDISM:

When the Thyroid Is Underactive

An enemy from within may ultimately have defeated Napoleon, one of history's greatest military leaders. Historians have noted that between 1804, when he was crowned emperor of the French, and his abdication in 1814, Napoleon experienced a steady mental deterioration that transformed him from an incisive, rapid decision maker to a lethargic, hesitant man. He became unable to control his temper and lost such attributes as self-discipline, common sense, and the ability to work for long hours. His minister of marine, Denise Decres, declared, "The Emperor is mad and will destroy us all."

What led some historians to conclude that the root of this dramatic deterioration was a severely underactive thyroid were the many changes to Napoleon's physical appearance that coincided with the alterations in his personality.[1] Napoleon gained a significant amount of weight. His face became round and his neck thicker. His long, straggly hair became sparse and fine. His hands became covered with fatty tissue and were described as "pudgy." Napoleon also suffered constantly from constipation and itchy skin, symptoms of an underactive thyroid. He changed from an impressively fit and vital leader to a prematurely aged man at forty-six, appearing completely worn out.

Obviously, doctors of Napoleon's time did not recognize hypothyroidism as a medical condition. Until fairly recently, similar scenarios of gradual deterioration to extreme levels of illness, ultimately leading to an inability to function, were common among severely hypothyroid patients, simply because doctors did not have accurate means by which to diagnose hypothyroidism. In fact, prior to the 1970s, when sophisticated testing to diagnose thyroid imbalance became available, underactive thyroid was believed to be a rare condition. Physicians often recognized it only after pronounced changes in a person's physical appearance and mental behavior had become evident. The diagnosis was often overlooked until patients needed to be hospitalized because of the effects of very severe hypothyroidism, including coma and insanity.[2] In some cases, the mental state of hypothyroid patients deteriorated to the extent that they became psychotic.[3] In 1949, Dr. R. Asher described his patients as having "myxedematous madness."[4] It turned out, however, that an underactive thyroid is one of the most common medical conditions that affect humankind.

In Chapter 2, I explained that the two most common causes of thyroid imbalance, Hashimoto's thyroiditis and Graves' disease, are disorders of the immune system. Hashimoto's thyroiditis is much more prevalent than Graves' disease. It affects 10 percent of the population and is the most common cause of an underactive thyroid. Numerous other conditions may also cause your thyroid to underperform:

- Treatment of an overactive thyroid with radioactive iodine or medications
- Surgical removal of part or all of the gland to treat nodules, goiter, Graves' disease, or cancer
- Transient hypothyroidism due to subacute thyroiditis, a viral illness that causes temporary partial damage to the thyroid gland (see Chapter 4)
- Transient hypothyroidism due to silent thyroiditis, an immune attack on the thyroid gland that also results in temporary damage to the gland (see Chapter 4)
- Previous radiation to the head or neck area
- Impaired blood supply to the thyroid after neck surgery for a non–thyroid-related problem
- Deficiency of the nutrient iodine (a common problem in several parts of the world; rare in the United States)
- Drug interactions (such as those from amiodarone, lithium, interferon, and interleukin-2)
- Absence or poor development of the gland (congenital hypothyroidism, childhood hypothyroidism)
- Genetic defects of enzymes that are essential for the manufacture of thyroid hormone
- Disorders of the hypothalamus or pituitary gland

Signs of Hypothyroidism

As thyroid hormone levels decrease, the functioning of most organs is affected. The person may begin to experience a multitude of physical symptoms, including:

- General tiredness
- Weight gain

heavy periods
muscle weakness

- Aches and pains in joints and muscles
- Muscle cramps
- Constipation
- Thickened skin
- Dry and pale skin
- Brittle hair
- Hair loss, including loss of eyebrow hair
- Feeling cold even in warm temperatures
- Milky discharge from the breast (gallactorrhea)

The more severe the deficiency of thyroid hormone, the worse these symptoms become—and you may begin to experience other symptoms. Your voice may become hoarse, deep, husky, and slow; your speech may become thick; your face may become puffy; and even your hearing abilities lessen. Your skin, especially on the palms of the hands, may become yellowish due to a buildup of the nutrient carotene in the blood. (The process that normally converts carotene into vitamin A in the body is slowed by hypothyroidism. In fact, if you are taking vitamin supplements containing beta carotene, yellow palms could be an early clue that you have an underactive thyroid.) Also, your feet may swell and you may become short of breath even with minimal exercise. Your heart rate decreases, and your blood pressure may become high or low. It is estimated that high blood pressure occurs in as many as 21 percent of people with an underactive thyroid.[5]

Other important effects of an underactive thyroid on your health are those caused by high cholesterol. An underactive thyroid causes or worsens hypercholesterolemia, which could result in coronary artery disease (hardening of the arteries in the heart). Research has shown that 20 percent of women older than forty with high cholesterol levels have underactive thyroids.[6] An underactive thyroid lowers your defense against infections. Often, as you become hypothyroid, you become more vulnerable to fungal and viral infections and your reproductive function is affected. Heavy menstrual bleeding or even cessation of menstruation is not uncommon in severely hypothyroid women.

Many persons with severe hypothyroidism complain of numbness and a sensation of pins and needles in their hands or feet. These symptoms may indicate a hypothyroid-induced neuropathy, a degenerative nerve condition. Some studies have shown that more than 50 percent of severely hypothyroid patients have damage to their peripheral nerves and some suffer from the pins-and-needles sensation.[7] Another nerve-related condition that can occur in severe hypothyroidism is carpal tunnel syndrome, which is due to compression of the median nerve in the wrist. It causes tingling in your fingers and often resolves with thyroid hormone treatment.[8] Other neurological and muscle problems that can occur as a result of severe hypothyroidism include:

- Myopathy, a disorder of muscle tissue that can cause muscle weakness and result in high levels of creatine phosphokinase (CPK), a blood marker for muscle disease
- A delay in relaxation of the muscle following contraction
- An excessive increase in the bulk of muscles (in children)
- Seizures

With severe hypothyroidism, you can also experience muscle coordination problems, which can prevent you from carrying out your usual daily activities. As a result of being unable to coordinate voluntary muscular movements (ataxia), you may experience loss of equilibrium, unsteadiness on the feet, lack of coordination of hands and feet, and trembling.

Other physical symptoms that may indicate severe hypothyroidism—and that can lead to misdiagnosis—include gastrointestinal and respiratory symptoms such as:

- Decreased movement of the gastrointestinal tract, causing severe constipation
- Intestinal obstruction and, rarely, perforation (only in very severe hypothyroidism)
- Sleep apnea, a temporary cessation of breathing during sleep
- Impaired control of respiration in the brain
- Pleural effusion, an accumulation of fluid between the layers of the membrane that lines the lungs and chest cavity

The physical effects of hypothyroidism vary from person to person. In fact, you may experience symptoms related to only one organ. One patient may experience heart problems, whereas another may experience joint and muscle pain. The patient and physician may focus primarily on the physical symptoms while either overlooking the mental effects or attributing them to the physical suffering. A person with severe hypothyroidism who is not taking medication can slip into a state of myxedema coma, often triggered by exposure to cold, by medications that cause sedation of the brain, or by illnesses such as severe infection or stroke. A person in a myxedema coma has a very low temperature (hypothermia), may develop low blood sugar (hypoglycemia), and often needs a respirator. This condition is dangerous and can lead to death.

Mental Effects of an Underactive Thyroid

Likewise, the mental effects of hypothyroidism vary from person to person, even among those with the same severity of hypothyroidism. Alex may develop severe depression as a result of hypothyroidism, whereas Julia may have only mild, barely perceptible depression, and Bill may exhibit a significant number of anxiety symptoms. The reason for these differences stems from the fact that each person may be predisposed to a different type of response, depending on personality and the existence of either a borderline or a masked, previously unrecognized mental symptom. Environmental and socioeconomic factors may also account for individual differences in the effects of thyroid dysfunction. An underactive thyroid can cause any of the following mental symptoms:

- Depression
- Mental sluggishness
- Increased sleepiness
- Forgetfulness
- Emotional instability
- Loss of ambition
- Decreased ability to pay attention and focus
- Decreased interest
- Slowing of thought and speech
- Irritability
- Fear of open or public spaces (agoraphobia)
- Audiovisual hallucinations and paranoid delusions (rare, only in very severe hypothyroidism)
- Dementia (usually in long-standing severe hypothyroidism)
- Manic behavior

Contrary to common belief, hypothyroidism does not necessarily mean that the thyroid gland has completely stopped functioning. The deficiency could actually range from a minimal amount to a more significant loss, depending on the damage to the gland. Although the physical symptoms become more pronounced in severe cases of underactive thyroid, disturbances to mood and emotions are likely to occur even when the thyroid hormone deficit is considered minimal.

Today we have the tools to catch and treat even the mildest cases of hypothyroidism. Technological advances have enabled us to realize that hypothyroidism is a common condition. While severe hypothyroidism, representing the extreme end of the spectrum, affects 1.5 to 2 percent of the general population, low-grade hypothyroidism affects 5 to 7 percent of the population.[9] There are also people with seemingly normal blood test results whose thyroid is actually deficient (see Chapter 14). If one includes the patients with normal blood tests, the frequency of low-grade hypothyroidism may reach 10 percent of the population.

Although many persons may have mild cases of hypothyroidism that remain stable throughout their lifetimes, some patients may experience a worsening of thyroid hormone deficit over time. Nearly 2 to 3 percent of people suffering from low-grade hypothyroidism progress to more severe hypothyroidism each year.[10]

Despite physicians' increased awareness of how common hypothyroidism is in the general population and the existence of precise testing of thyroid levels, many people still slip into the dark hole of hypothyroidism. If you suffer from any of the physical or mental symptoms described earlier in this chapter, have your doctor request a TSH (thyroid-stimulating hormone) test, which is the most sensitive test for detecting a thyroid imbalance due to a dysfunctioning gland.

Let's take a closer look at how the principal mental and emotional symptoms of an underactive thyroid play out in real life.

"EXHAUSTED AND OVERWHELMED"

Regardless of whether a person's hypothyroidism is mild, moderate, or severe, the most common—and most noticeable—symptom of an underactive thyroid is fatigue. This tiredness typically has a physical component (from the slower metabolism) and a mental component (linked to depression). Depression and loss of brain power are the most common mental effects of an underactive thyroid. In Chapter 5, I will detail how hypothyroidism can either cause depression or be a major contributing factor to it, including low-grade depression, chronic minor depression, or in extreme cases major depression. Undoubtedly, fatigue is a universal symptom of depression, regardless of the type of depression. Hypothyroidism will also make you sleep more than you used to.

Increased sleep is, in fact, viewed as a major symptom of an underactive thyroid. Hypothyroid individuals who sleep more than they formerly did often attribute the increased sleepiness to just being tired when, in fact, it could be related to depression. In many hypothyroid patients, tiredness and sleeping more than usual are expressions of lack of enthusiasm and loss of interest in doing things, even customary, pleasurable activities. When the deficiency of thyroid hormone worsens, the mental slowing and the depression become compounded by the slowing of your body. And this may make you feel as if you are drowning in a hole. Patients suffering from an underactive thyroid may also experience significant anxiety symptoms and a wide range of cognitive impairments.

CRIPPLING ANXIETY

In my clinical experience, anxiety is a much more common symptom of hypothyroidism than physicians generally acknowledge. Because anxiety and panic attacks are typical symptoms of hyperthyroidism, some patients with an underactive thyroid may become confused when they experience these symptoms yet are told they are hypothyroid. Anxiety can have a crippling effect on a person with an underactive thyroid accompanied by tiredness and depression.

Although in many people the anxiety is related to the depression itself, in other people anxiety symptoms are prominent with little or no depression. Even then, however, the thyroid hormone deficit and its effect on brain chemical transmitters result in anxiety. The fact that an underactive thyroid alters a person's mechanisms for coping with stress and lowers self-esteem may account for the prominence of anxiety as a symptom. Also, fears and self-doubt are often compounded by the awareness of defects in memory and concentration.

Hypothyroid people, especially women, often begin to feel they don't "look nice" and may be worried about being seen in public. Their anxiety may grow worse with the advent of other physical symptoms such as headaches, muscle cramps, pains, aches, and hair loss. Not knowing the cause of these symptoms increases their worries.

Marie, a twenty-nine-year-old nurse, had struggled through college with many of the effects of undiagnosed hypothyroidism. Because she suffered from so many symptoms of anxiety, a psychiatrist most likely would have diagnosed her condition as a generalized anxiety syndrome. She was extremely tired and depressed for almost two years before her thyroid problem was diagnosed. She suffered anxiety from having attempted to overcome her physical symptoms, as well as difficulties with memory and concentration, which hurt her performance in a very competitive school environment.

She explained:

I started getting really tired my first year in college. The exhaustion and the need to sleep for extended hours, after what other people would consider a normal day, would really affect my life. I didn't have the desire to do a lot of partying because I was too tired. I had to drive several hours to the hospital to do my clinical training, so I related the fatigue to all the hours of travel and the stress of work and studies. My hair was falling out. My skin and eyes were dry all the time. I had a lot of generalized aches and pains that I couldn't explain other than just being tired.

I was so afraid that I would not pass my exams, that I would be a failure. I had myself so worked up and anxious that one of my college professors called me and said, "What is going on? You're not yourself." I told her I was fine, but I was just a ball of nerves. She said, "No, you're not yourself. You are normally very calm. Now, you seem to be running on adrenaline." I told her it must just be the anxiety of having to take tests.

An impaired memory and a decreased ability to focus and concentrate aggravated Marie's struggle. Her concerns about being unable to accomplish certain tasks generated more anxiety and unrealistic fears, eventually leading to crippling panic attacks. Four to six weeks after we initiated thyroid hormone treatment for Marie's hypothyroidism, she began to feel much better. Four months later, when her thyroid test results were normal and stable, her depression and anxiety symptoms had greatly improved. Her memory and concentration returned to normal. All her physical symptoms resolved except for the hair loss, which persisted for more than six months after correction of the underactive thyroid.

Clearing the Mental Fog

Although you may be able to describe physical symptoms such as joint pain or muscle cramps in a relatively straightforward manner, when you try expressing in detail a subtle deficit in your cognitive abilities, you immediately realize the extreme difficulty of the task. A few years ago, one patient described the mental effects of hypothyroidism to me as "a brain fog." An underactive thyroid can leave you unable to remember details, names, or even events. As a result of low thyroid levels, your brain loses some of the power it normally has to grasp and process a thought. You may comprehend a concept while reading a book or listening to someone talk; then immediately afterward, you may be unable to fully describe it. The concept becomes blurred in your mind. Often when you try to express a thought, you cannot think of the right word, whereas before, you used to quickly review several words and easily pick the most appropriate one.

Lisa, an undergraduate student who was considering law school, became depressed and experienced many of the symptoms of hypothyroidism. "After my baby was born," she said, "I went into a funk. I was exhausted and blue. Sometimes I would get angry at my two older sons for no reason, which was not typical of me."

When Lisa first came to me, her mental dysfunctions had grown more debilitating, and she was no longer considering law school because of the cognitive impairments she was experiencing. She said:

I have lost the ability to concentrate. I ask a question and forget the answer immediately, and I have to ask again. It is humiliating. I think of one thing and then another, and I can't stay focused long enough to think either thing through. I have tried to hide my memory loss so no one would know how bad it is, but it's gotten to the point where I can't hide it any longer. I become easily confused. Now I am even afraid to drive, because I suddenly get disoriented.

Difficulties with memory and concentration are often symptoms of depression and anxiety disorders as well. But when the patient has an underactive thyroid, impaired cognition is worse and aggravates the anxiety.

Anne, a twenty-four-year-old secretary who had moderate hypothyroidism, had suffered from both depression and symptoms of anxiety for three years. But what made her seek medical help was her worsening memory loss. Her husband had become disabled four years earlier as a result of a car accident, which contributed to her general depression. In her words:

Before diagnosis, I definitely experienced a higher level of anxiety than I ever had before. I would begin ruminating on things and wouldn't be able to let them go for days. I would be worried about trivial things. I know when I am anxious: my heart beats faster, my muscles are tighter, I'm tense, and I snap at people. I thought a lot of that was related to my husband's health.

My anxiety symptoms became worse when I started noticing that I didn't have any memory anymore. It was awful at work. Also, I was not able to focus on anything I was doing. I had a hard time concentrating and could not find my words or express myself. My boss almost fired me, and I was the primary support for my family. After a while, it became really scary. One day there was a new toaster sitting on my dryer. I called my sister and told her thanks for buying me this toaster, and she said, "I didn't buy it." I had bought the toaster, but I had no memory of buying it. Nothing. My daughter will tell me she told me something, and I don't remember. It's kind of a joke. We kept it light, but I was losing my memory. I thought it was stress.

Anne's case illustrates how impairments to memory and other cognitive functions can make hypothyroid patients more anxious. Her awareness of the memory impairment and her inability to perform at work generated more worries and worsened her anxiety symptoms.

Boris Yeltsin's Underactive Thyroid

In June 1991, after the collapse of communism in the Soviet Union, Boris Yeltsin was elected the first president of the new Russia. Over the following five years, the world observed Yeltsin change from a slim and quick-thinking political leader to a slow-walking, slow-speaking president whose political career was compromised by apparently serious health problems.[11]

Toward the end of the summer of 1996, Yeltsin's health had deteriorated to such an extent that even his public appearances were curtailed. Critics and the media charged that Yeltsin was no longer in full control of his own government. In September 1996, Drs. Michael DeBakey and George Noon, cardiovascular surgeons from my institution, visited Yeltsin and recommended multiple bypass heart surgery. However, the surgical procedure was delayed by a few weeks for several reasons, including gastrointestinal bleeding, poor heart function caused by a heart attack in late June or early July, and newly diagnosed hypothyroidism, which needed to be corrected before the operation.[12]

Until September 1996, Yeltsin's hypothyroidism, which had probably affected his health for some time, was undiagnosed. Long-standing, untreated hypothyroidism increases the risk of heart attacks because it can raise cholesterol levels, which, in turn, can lead to coronary artery disease (restricted blood flow to the heart).

Before the diagnosis, Yeltsin was also described as being "slow and stiff in his gestures." His speech was said to be slurred and his behavior "peculiar," and he sometimes disappeared from public view without explanation. Rumors of heavy drinking were widespread.

Yeltsin's weight gain and puffiness developed slowly. Pictures taken of him before his heart operation confirm that his facial puffiness gradually worsened. This could be an indication that his hypothyroidism had been long-standing and went undiagnosed for a long period of time.

It was clear that Yeltsin's hypothyroidism caused a lingering depression, which was noticed by political critics and the news media. He had to cancel several meetings because of tiredness and became "prone to sudden mysterious absences and bouts of unusual behavior."[13] For months prior to Yeltsin's diagnosis, he withdrew from public view. In addition, his alcohol consumption increased.

We can only speculate on the extent to which Yeltsin's hypothyroidism (and quite likely the depressed mood that resulted from it) affected Russia during the past few years. We can also only wonder whether these factors contributed to Yeltsin's loss of control of the government in the summer of 1996. It is quite possible, however, that Yeltsin's complete transformation after his bypass surgery was not due merely to the surgical correction of his heart problem. His turnaround after the treatment of his thyroid condition was spectacular and illustrates how thyroid imbalance could affect the course of history.

Physicians caring for political leaders, particularly those in high government posts, should be alert to the possibility of a thyroid imbalance anytime a change in personality, emotions, or judgment is observed and anytime a leader exhibits poorly explained symptoms.

The Challenge of
Low-Grade Hypothyroidism

Once not discussed or even suspected, low-grade hypothyroidism and its effects on physical and mental health are increasingly pervasive. Numerous studies have now concluded that low-grade hypothyroidism can contribute to high cholesterol levels, infertility, miscarriages, tiredness, and depression. Research has shown that correcting low-grade hypothyroidism will result in a lowering of both total cholesterol and "bad" LDL cholesterol.[14] Preliminary results of a study we are conducting on postmenopausal women are showing that women with hardening of the coronary arteries are more likely to be suffering from low-grade hypothyroidism than are women without heart disease. This association may be due to the effect of this "minor condition" on cholesterol levels. Even to this day, however, many physicians continue to believe that low-grade hypothyroidism has no significance. Some will tell their patients, "The condition isn't serious enough to treat." The most common physical symptoms experienced by patients with low-grade hypothyroidism are fatigue, dry skin, hair loss, and cold intolerance. Some women may experience heavier and longer menstrual periods (menorrhagia) as a result of low-grade hypothyroidism.

In addition to having symptoms of depression or becoming vulnerable to depression (see Chapter 5), patients with low-grade hypothyroidism may experience hysteria, more frequent anxiety, and physical complaints. They may also have some impairment in memory-related abilities. The memory deficit and concentration problems improve with thyroid hormone treatment. In Latin America, it was found that people who lacked iodine in their diets were more likely to have impaired cognition.[15] Too little dietary iodine often compromises the manufacture of normal amounts of thyroid hormone. Cognitive impairments in these people improved after supplementation of iodine in the diet. Another study, conducted in Sweden on older women with low-grade hypothyroidism, showed that the memory scores of 20 percent of these women improved after six months of treatment with thyroid hormone.[16] When sensitive memory tests, such as the Wechsler Memory Scale, were used, researchers have shown that more than 80 percent of people with low-grade hypothyroidism had impaired memory functions.[17] Low-grade hypothyroidism impairs both short-term memory and visual memory.

As a result of low-grade hypothyroidism, you may have difficulty remembering what you just read. Many people with low-grade hypothyroidism may believe that there is nothing wrong with them when in fact they have subtle deficits that can be demonstrated only by sophisticated neuropsychological testing.[18] Patients with low-grade hypothyroidism are also more prone to panic attacks. If you are suffering from any of the symptoms of underactive thyroid I have described or if your cholesterol is high, have your doctor give you a TSH test. If you are a woman aged thirty-five or older, have your doctor test your thyroid every five years. If you have been diagnosed with low-grade hypothyroidism, you will probably require treatment for the rest of your life. In fact, the dose of thyroid hormone required to correct your imbalance is likely to increase as time passes.

The lack of awareness that low-grade hypothyroidism may cause suffering and deficits may lead physicians to ignore subtle thyroid test abnormalities consistent with this condition. If your doctor tells you that your thyroid insufficiency isn't serious enough to warrant treatment, do not accept this. Rather, insist on seeking help from a specialist knowledgeable about thyroid disorders. I worry that many people get tested but do not receive treatment despite the fact that they clearly have low-grade hypothyroidism that is causing symptoms.

Questionnaire:
The Physical Symptoms of Hypothyroidism

As we've seen, mental suffering due to hypothyroidism is not just limited to depression. The effect of thyroid hormone deficit on anxiety levels and thinking patterns produces complex neurobehavioral changes. The physical effects on the mind can also worsen depression, anxiety, and feelings of inadequacy. As hypothyroidism progresses, mental effects intensify, job and relationships are affected, and the person feels as if he or she were drowning.

An easy way to determine the likelihood that you may be suffering from hypothyroidism is to complete the following physical-symptoms questionnaire.

Has your hair become dry, or are you losing your hair?	Yes	No
Have your menstrual periods been heavy in recent months?	Yes	No
Have you been suffering from joint aches and pains?	Yes	No
Are your nails brittle?	Yes	No
Have you been getting muscle cramps?	Yes	No
Have you noticed a continuous weakness in your muscles?	Yes	No
Has your skin been dry?	Yes	No
Have your face and eyes been puffy?	Yes	No
Have you been experiencing cold intolerance?	Yes	No
Have you gained more than five pounds?	Yes	No
Has your skin become coarse?	Yes	No

Have you been constipated?	Yes	No
Have you noticed in recent months a milky discharge from your breasts?	Yes	No
Do you sweat less?	Yes	No
Has your voice become hoarse?	Yes	No
Do your fingers tingle?	Yes	No
Has your hearing gotten worse?	Yes	No
Has your heartbeat been slow?	Yes	No
Have you been experiencing stiffness?	Yes	No
Have you been fatigued?	Yes	No
Have your eyes been dry?	Yes	No
Have you been experiencing shortness of breath during exercise or reduced tolerance to exercise?	Yes	No

If you answered yes to four or more of the preceding questions, you may be hypothyroid. If you answered yes to six or more of the questions, you are probably hypothyroid.

In Chapter 5, you will find questionnaires on the symptoms of depression and anxiety. Remember, even if your answers to the preceding physical-symptoms questionnaire indicate a low probability of hypothyroidism, if your answers to the Chapter 5 questionnaires indicate depression or an anxiety disorder, you still need to have your thyroid tested.

Hypothyroidism and Aging

One of my hypothyroid patients who was in her early twenties remarked that she felt as if she had begun to age at a rapid pace when her thyroid became underactive. This is quite insightful, as a number of the effects of thyroid hormone deficit are analogous to aging. As you age, your memory, concentration, and ability to process new information gradually become impaired. Hypothyroidism also causes a reduction in physical exercise, both because of direct effects on muscle function and because of how it impairs mood and emotions, in a way that mirrors how people often tend to become more sedentary with advancing years.

In fact, the normal aging process may be related to some extent to a naturally occurring decrease in thyroid hormone activity in the body. For example, the size of the thyroid gland decreases with age, and its structure and function also deteriorate gradually. The amount of the most active form of thyroid hormone (T3) in tissues decreases, due to an impairment of conversion of T4 to T3 in our body. This explains why the basal metabolic rate, which is highly regulated by thyroid hormone, also decreases with age. By the age of eighty-five, your basal metabolic rate drops to 52 percent of the levels you had at age three. As a result, normal physiological responses requiring thyroid hormone become less efficient. As you get older, you may have a more difficult time regulating your body temperature during extreme heat or cold. As you age, thyroid hormone deficit in your organs also promotes a slowing of the synthesis of essential proteins in your body, a hallmark of the aging process. This natural decline in thyroid hormone activity with age could conceivably contribute to the normal aging process.[19]

Because the effects of thyroid hormone deficit are similar to the effects of aging, the physical symptoms and signs relied on to suspect hypothyroidism in younger people are less useful in the elderly. Both aging and hypothyroidism are associated with decreased mental activity, dry skin, constipation, depression, and an increased incidence of atherosclerosis and high cholesterol. Therefore, unless thyroid testing is done routinely, hypothyroidism may never be uncovered. Quite often, the symptoms of hypothyroidism are attributed to the aging process per se or to other problems.

In one study, only 27 percent of elderly patients suffering from an underactive thyroid had symptoms and signs of hypothyroidism.[20] This means that older people with an underactive thyroid often experience only a limited number of vague symptoms. These symptoms may be mental confusion, weight loss, poor appetite, falling episodes, aches and pains, weakness, muscle stiffness (which may be confused with Parkinsonism), incontinence, and depression. Consequently, hypothyroidism may go unrecognized and become severe over time because of the superficial resemblance to aging itself.

As you get older, you may be more vulnerable to serious mental and emotional problems when the gland becomes minimally underactive. In addition to depression and impaired cognitive abilities, which are quite common among older people afflicted with even minor thyroid hormone deficit, a profound and severe slowing of mental activity can occur if your underactive thyroid is severe enough and is not corrected promptly. This slowing of mental activity may become extreme and lead to dementia. Dementia due to hypothyroidism is caused by disruption in the brain structures that support recent memory, concentration, and problem solving.

Occasionally, family members bring a patient to the hospital or doctor's office because the person has become increasingly withdrawn and has been showing extreme slowing of mental activity. Even today, with the increased awareness of the frequency and effects of thyroid diseases, we continue to see older patients who progress to a state of dementia caused by severe hypothyroidism. Most patients with dementia are unaware of what is happening to them. Because Alzheimer's disease is one of the most common causes of dementia in older people, some patients diagnosed with dementia are thought to have Alzheimer's disease when in fact the main reason could have been long-standing hypothyroidism.

The similarities between dementia caused by Alzheimer's disease and dementia caused by hypothyroidism led scientists to study whether there was an association between Alzheimer's disease and thyroid imbalance. Research has not provided evidence that Hashimoto's thyroiditis or thyroid imbalance are important risk factors for sporadic Alzheimer's disease. One recent study did show, however, that both patients and unaffected relatives of patients with familial Alzheimer's disease have a high frequency of Hashimoto's thyroiditis and hypothyroidism.[21] The association between Hashimoto's thyroiditis and familial Alzheimer's disease appears to be genetically mediated (on chromosome 21, the same chromosome where the gene for Down's syndrome is located). Hypothyroidism may place a person with Alzheimer's disease at a high risk for having more mental and cognitive deficits. Consequently, if you are diagnosed with Alzheimer's disease, your doctor will typically test you for hypothyroidism so that thyroid hormone treatment will slow the cognitive deterioration if you turn out to be hypothyroid. Because the effects of undiagnosed and untreated hypothyroidism can be so serious among the elderly, older people should be screened more often for hypothyroidism.

In Great Britain and the United States, the incidence of hypothyroidism rises abruptly after menopause in women and after the age of sixty in men. Approximately 10 to 15 percent of postmenopausal women have mild, low-grade hypothyroidism, whereas in men the prevalence is 6 percent.[22] Nearly 45 percent of older people have some degree of thyroid gland inflammation characteristic of Hashimoto's thyroiditis. As noted earlier, minor thyroid imbalances often produce greater effects in the elderly than in younger people, and physicians can often achieve spectacular results with adequate treatment, preventing unnecessary suffering to both the person and his or her family. The high frequency of hypothyroidism among older people and the similarities between symptoms of hypothyroidism and changes characteristic of the normal aging process attest to the importance of performing thyroid tests on any older person exhibiting a change in mood, emotions, or behavior.

Congenital Hypothyroidism

Nearly 20 million people worldwide suffer from brain damage caused by hypothyroidism due to iodine deficiency during the critical period of development in the fetus and infancy. When iodine is insufficient in the diet (iodine being essential for the manufacture of thyroid hormone), hypothyroidism and goiter (enlargement of the thyroid) are common effects on the fetus and the newborn. It has been estimated that in areas where nutritional iodine deficiency is common, 10 percent of newborns are hypothyroid. In the United States, iodine deficiency is not a cause of underactive thyroid in newborns. Nevertheless, 1 in 4,000 infants is born with congenital hypothyroidism, a condition often due to the absence or complete undevelopment of the thyroid gland.[23] In some newborns with hypothyroidism, the gland is not in the proper place in the neck. Instead, it is somewhere between its normal location and the base of the tongue, a condition called "ectopic thyroid." Congenital hypothyroidism due to a pituitary defect causing a deficiency in the pituitary hormone TSH is much less common and occurs in 1 in 100,000 newborns. In rare instances, hypothyroidism due to a pituitary deficiency or defective TSH is a familial and genetically transmissible disorder.

Because lack of thyroid hormone during the fetal stage and from birth to age two to three results in brain damage and mental retardation, systematic screening for congenital hypothyroidism has been implemented in the United States and many other countries. Ideally, the diagnosis is made during the first few days of life. The sooner thyroid hormone treatment is initiated, the better the mental outcome for such babies. For instance, the average IQ of infants diagnosed between three and six months is only 19. Infants who are diagnosed late experience permanent learning disabilities, poor scholastic achievement, and difficulties integrating themselves into society. However, congenitally hypothyroid children who are started on treatment early and receive adequate treatment have a normal IQ and satisfactory school performance when they are subsequently evaluated at the age of five to ten years. Ultimately, the intellectual and cognitive abilities of these children also depend on whether they take the necessary medications. If your infant suffers from congenital hypothyroidism and is taking thyroid hormone daily, you should know that soy-based formula interferes with the absorption of thyroid hormone in the intestines.[24] The dose of thyroid hormone must often be increased for infants fed with soy-based formulas.

Genetic factors seem to play a role in the occurrence of congenital hypothyroidism, with many families having had several cases. Black infants are affected less frequently than white ones. A recent population study in Atlanta showed that infants with Down's syndrome are thirty-five times more likely to have congenital hypothyroidism than other infants.[25] Without screening, 70 percent of infants are diagnosed within the first year, but at the cost of irreversible brain damage. One of the consequences of thyroid hormone deficit is deafness, also a symptom in patients with Pendred syndrome.[26] Pendred syndrome, which is transmitted genetically and is defined by a genetic defect in the manufacture of thyroid hormone and deafness, accounts for nearly 7 percent of all cases of childhood deafness.

Because the symptoms of hypothyroidism in the newborn may be minimal and do not necessarily point to the thyroid, the thyroid is routinely tested in the first six days of life. The screening is done by measuring TSH and/or T4 in blood from a heel prick collected on filter paper. Although screening should ideally include both T4 and TSH, because of cost considerations medical authorities unfortunately choose only one of the two methods. If the TSH method is used, the physician may overlook a case of hypothalamic or pituitary hypothyroidism (also known as central hypothyroidism) since, in this condition, TSH may be normal. This is what happened in the recently publicized case of a California infant who was properly diagnosed only six months after birth. The infant now suffers from irreversible brain damage, which could have been prevented if T4 levels had been measured.[27]

The other important limitation of TSH screening is that some newborns with defective thyroid glands have a delayed rise in TSH. In these babies, the test results are normal at the time of screening but become abnormal weeks after birth.

If a T4 test is used as the primary screening method, central hypothyroidism is detected easily, but the pediatrician may miss low-grade hypothyroidism due to a defective thyroid. In such babies, the underactive thyroid will worsen over time and result in brain damage. Low-grade hypothyroidism at birth is often due to abnormal positioning of the thyroid gland, which is also the most common cause of congenital hypothyroidism.

Because the T4 levels of many infants fall in the wide gray zone between low and normal that necessitates retesting, many medical centers choose TSH over T4 for screening purposes. Most countries use TSH for screening. One way to avoid misdiagnosis and unnecessary worrying is to make sure that, on initial screening, the TSH level is less than 20 milli–international units per liter. If it is higher, discuss with the pediatrician testing the T4 level and retesting TSH later. Symptoms that should alert you that your infant might have congenital hypothyroidism include persistent neonatal jaundice, poor feeding, bluish skin color, weak muscle tone, swelling of the tongue, lethargy, constipation, and slow growth. If the TSH level was checked as the screening test and your infant is showing any unusual behavior, have the pediatrician test the baby's T4 level and rerun the TSH test.

MOST COMMON CAUSES OF CONGENITAL HYPOTHYROIDISM
- Abnormally located thyroid gland (ectopic thyroid)
- Poorly developed or undeveloped thyroid gland
- Inborn error of thyroid hormone manufacture
- Hypothalamic or pituitary deficiency
- Transient hypothyroidism of the newborn
- Ingestion by the mother of drugs that inhibit the production of fetal thyroid hormone (antithyroid drugs)

CAUSES OF CONGENITAL HYPOTHYROIDISM IN PREMATURE BABIES WITH LOW T4 AND LOW/NORMAL TSH

- Iodine deficiency
- Iodine excess
- Antibodies from the mother crossing the placenta and affecting the fetus's thyroid

Important Points to Remember

- The most common symptom of an underactive thyroid is fatigue. This fatigue is both physical and mental and often precedes other typical symptoms of depression and physical symptoms of thyroid hormone deficit.
- Anxiety symptoms—including excessive worrying and panic attacks—are common when the thyroid is underactive. Because these symptoms are also typical of an overactive thyroid, they often give rise to confusion.
- Regardless of its severity, hypothyroidism often causes cognitive problems such as poor memory, difficulties processing information, and lack of focus. Such mental fog generates a vicious cycle of low self-esteem and increased anxiety.
- As indicated by blood test results, about 5 to 7 percent of the population has low-grade hypothyroidism. That figure might be as high as 10 percent if we include people with normal blood test results who still suffer from a thyroid deficiency.
- Low-grade hypothyroidism increases the risk of depression and can worsen depression. It also affects cognition.
- An underactive thyroid results in a form of accelerated aging. It can also cause brain damage and slow brain functioning.
- If a severely underactive thyroid remains untreated for a long time, the damage may be so dramatic that it can cause dementia.

4

HYPERTHYROIDISM:

When the Thyroid Is Overactive

Common sense might suggest that if too little thyroid hormone can cause you to sink into a state of clinical depression and rob you of your ability to function as before, too much thyroid hormone would make you feel happy, perky, and on top of the world. This assumption, however, is only partially correct. When the brain is flooded with too much thyroid hormone, some people do experience a lasting elation. Thoughts race through the mind. Activities crowd the day.

Several years ago, my neighbor Nancy had the reputation of being overly friendly. She incessantly helped others with their chores and knew almost everyone in the condominium complex where we lived. She initiated conversations with everyone and constantly came up with new ideas and projects. It never occurred to anyone, including me, that what animated Nancy with this incredible energy and enthusiasm was an overactive thyroid.

Talking to a retired woman one day, Nancy mentioned that her electric bill was outrageous because she always felt hot and had to use air-conditioning most of the time. When I got close to Nancy, I noticed the shakiness in her hands and the stare in her eyes, symptoms of an overactive thyroid.

It turned out that Nancy's mildly manic (or "hypomanic") behavior was not her original nature. Nancy had, in fact, been a somewhat reserved person before she decided to move from Dallas to Houston to study and join her boyfriend. Nancy also suffered from many physical symptoms. She had lost weight despite eating more, her menstrual periods had become scanty, she had some acne on her face, her bowel movements had become increasingly frequent, she was losing some hair, and she had a rapid heartbeat—but to her all these symptoms were trivial. Her brain and body were animated by extraordinary energy and elation. Nancy did not even consider that something might be wrong with her; she simply thought that she had become happier after joining her boyfriend in Houston.

Hyperthyroid patients may have an energy, optimism, and self-confidence that are not characteristic of someone who needs medical or psychiatric help.[1] Even when these personality traits appear suddenly and unexpectedly, they are usually considered positive. The person has lost weight. He or she has a positive attitude about life, is overactive, and expends effort far beyond his or her strength. Not surprisingly, mildly manic hyperthyroid patients can go for years without being diagnosed. They may not even seek medical help unless the symptoms become severe and disturbing.

Fred, a thirty-one-year-old construction worker, was hypomanic for four years as the result of an overactive thyroid. He was viewed as a superman on the job. He told me:

> One time, three tornadoes came through, and nine thousand roofs in the area had to be redone. I was driving a truck by myself every day and throwing three hundred squares of shingles up on a roof. A square of shingles weighs 220 pounds, so that's over 6,000 pounds in a day. Several employees were hired who went out on the road with me for one day but quit. Then, after I would finish roofing, I would go work another part-time job.
>
> Later, when we bought a farm, I fenced in ten acres in about three days. Never thought twice about it.

The tremendous physical energy Fred experienced reflects only a small part of the surge in mental power. It is almost purely a case of mind over matter. The brain is set at a fast pace, similar to what happens to people taking stimulant drugs. As this extraordinary feeling of power animates the brain, hyperthyroid individuals may experience significant anxiety and frustration, primarily because they cannot do everything they considered doing. As Fred described it:

> I would ask you a question, and before you could finish answering, I could already tell what you were talking about and be going on to something else. The number of things I could keep up with at one time was phenomenal. I could watch TV, listen to a conversation, eat, and be doing half a dozen other things and keep track of them all like I was intimately involved in every single one of them.

Being hypomanic, Fred dismissed his physical symptoms as insignificant. His bowel movements had become more frequent, but a physician told him he had irritable bowel syndrome. His hands were shaking almost continuously, and he was feeling hot all the time, but he got used to it. Fred had

Graves' disease, the common form of hyperthyroidism that is caused by an immune disorder. After his symptoms had continued for four years, Fred finally sought medical help—but only when he began experiencing muscle weakness and shortness of breath due to heart failure, caused by his overactive thyroid.

Signs of Hyperthyroidism

The physical symptoms of hyperthyroidism include cardiovascular effects such as a rapid heartbeat and high blood pressure. Weight loss, increased appetite, sweating, hair loss, and heat intolerance are other common symptoms of thyroid hormone excess and are related to its effects on metabolism. In women, menstrual periods may become scanty, lasting only one or two days, or even disappear. The effects of excess thyroid hormone are evident on various organs of the body. Although a complete list of these effects would include dozens of symptoms, the following are the most common:

GENERAL
Weight loss (or less commonly, weight gain)
Fatigue
Shakiness
Feeling hot and becoming intolerant of warm and hot temperatures
Restlessness
Increased thirst
Hair loss
Anemia
Eye irritation

SKIN
Increased sweating
Warm, moist hands
Itching
Hives
Brittle nails

HEART
Rapid heartbeat, palpitations
Shortness of breath
Chest pain

GASTROINTESTINAL
Trembling of the tongue
Increased hunger and food consumption
Increased frequency of bowel movements

MUSCLE
Weakness
Decreased muscle mass

REPRODUCTIVE
Irregular menstrual periods
Cessation of menstrual periods
Decreased fertility

Among the most dreaded complications of an overactive thyroid are the cardiac effects. An overactive thyroid can cause irregular heartbeat and even damage to the heart muscle[2]—damage that, in some patients, can result in heart failure, which may or may not improve after the overactive thyroid is diagnosed and treated. Some patients with Graves' disease may be found to have mitral valve prolapse, a slight deformity that causes a characteristic heart murmur physicians can hear through a stethoscope. Most people with mitral valve prolapse experience no symptoms, but for some, it can cause chest pain and rapid or irregular heartbeat.

An excess of thyroid hormone makes bone lose some of its mineral content. Women, more so than men, who have had an overactive thyroid for a long time can even develop osteoporosis (thinning of the bone), which could predispose them to bone fractures. The greater vulnerability of women stems from the fact that they are more naturally prone to suffer from bone loss and osteoporosis than men. Research has shown, however, that once the overactive thyroid is corrected, some mineral buildup occurs in bone within the next two years.[3] Nevertheless, even after the overactive thyroid is corrected, you might have lost significant bone density. To determine whether you have lost bone density as a result of thyroid hormone excess, it is wise to have your doctor order a bone density test a year or two after your overactive thyroid has been corrected. Another test that would tell you whether you are at higher risk for having more bone loss in the future is urine dipyridoline, which is a marker for exaggerated resorption (dissolution) of bone. Test results indicating reduced bone density and an increased risk of bone fractures call for treatment, which may include estrogens, calcium supplements, and at times even medications, such as alendronate (Fosamax®) or nasal calcitonin. Exercise is also crucial for maintaining bone density.

Breast enlargement occurs in nearly a third of men suffering from over-activity of the thyroid. This enlargement, which doctors call gynecomastia, may be minor or significant enough to be troublesome. It is the result of too much estrogen—a consequence of the overactive thyroid. If you are a man who has experienced weight loss, anxiety, shakiness, heat intolerance, or other symptoms of an overactive thyroid, and you begin to feel enlargement and tenderness in your breast area, you need to mention it to your doctor and have your thyroid tested. For women, there may be some relationship between thyroid disease and breast cancer. Research has shown that women with breast cancer may be at slightly increased risk for thyroid problems, including autoimmune thyroid disease.[4] However, it is probably a cancer-genetic predisposition that makes people with breast cancer more suscep-tible to autoimmune thyroid disorders. This increased risk, however, is not unequivocally established.

As with hypothyroidism, the severity of physical and emotional symp-toms experienced by hyperthyroid patients does not always correspond to how elevated the thyroid hormone levels are. One study that carefully mea-sured the severity of symptoms among patients with Graves' disease using a rating scale system found that symptoms may be mild in people whose thy-roid hormone levels are high.[5] The same study found that the severity of depression and anxiety does not correspond to the degree of elevation of thyroid hormone levels.

If an overactive thyroid remains untreated, the occurrence of severe ill-ness can make the person slip into a thyroid storm, a dreadful condition characterized by mental deterioration, high fever, extreme agitation, and at times heart failure and jaundice.

Mental Effects of Hyperthyroidism

The mental effects of excess thyroid hormone are often described merely as *nervousness* and *hyperactivity*, terms that hide a deeper layer of mental and behavioral instability. In fact, in the mind of many physicians, the term *ner-vousness* connotes a physical effect (motor restlessness and the need to move around) rather than a mental effect.

Doctors frequently fail to emphasize the wide array of mental effects likely to occur in a hyperthyroid patient. The mental symptoms of hyperthy-roidism may precede, or even be more prominent than, the physical symp-toms. In fact, hyperthyroidism can precipitate or cause virtually any form of psychiatric condition,[6] although admittedly, psychosis triggered by Graves' disease is an exceptional occurrence nowadays. Anxiety and panicky feelings may be the earliest and most noticeable symptoms of hyperthyroidism. As time passes, the expression of these symptoms changes with the appearance of other symptoms. The most common mental effects that we see in hyperthyroid patients are:

- Anxiety
- Nocturnal anxiety
- Panic attacks
- Depression
- Excessive concerns about physical symptoms, real or imaginary
- Emotional withdrawal
- Disorganized thinking
- Guilt feelings
- Loss of emotional control
- Unusual degree of irritability
- Intense emotional swings
- Episodes of erratic behavior
- Paranoia
- Aggression

FROM FEELING ELATED TO LOSING TOUCH WITH REALITY

The elation experienced by Nancy and Fred is rarely a stable state characterized by self-confidence and unabated happiness. Although I have seen some patients with an overactive thyroid who stayed in a stable state of elation for months or even years without experiencing the downside of depression, the majority do experience periods of short-lived depression, such as in manic-depression. From a state of mild elation, or hypomania, patients can easily flip into an exaggerated form of elation (that is, mania) in which they lose touch with reality and begin exhibiting abnormal behavior.

Several of my patients have used the analogy that the elation of hyperthyroidism is like being on potent mind-altering drugs. Although your brain is more alert and animated by excessive thinking, your thought processes are disturbed by an inability to focus. You begin to find it hard to think something through in a way that would ultimately make any sense. Your eyes become glassy and your mind unfocused, which prevents sensible conversations. People may think that a hyperthyroid person is on cocaine. The speedy mind also becomes compromised by loss of memory. Impaired cognition coupled with rapid thinking may result in a flow of inconsistent and irrational statements and decisions.

The shift from an elated mood to the severe elation characteristic of mania brings with it confusion, poor judgment, impaired cognition, and abnormal behavior. In severe cases, hallucinations enter the picture. This is when the patient is viewed as "abnormal." The transition from hypomanic to manic behavior may be gradual or abrupt; its onset may occur soon after the beginning of hyperthyroidism or be delayed until long afterward.

Medical literature overflows with cases of acute confusion, "schizophrenia-like" psychoses, and paranoia among individuals with Graves' disease. Such descriptions are reminiscent of severe cases of mania or manic-depression. In some persons, unabated, advanced mania promotes criminal or paranoid ideas, distorted thoughts, and even hallucinations and auditory delusions. In the immediately pre–World War II to post–World War II era, many people with an overactive thyroid exhibited such profound disruptions of behavior that they were considered to have severe psychiatric illnesses.

According to some reports, up to 20 percent of patients with an over-active thyroid had psychotic symptoms.[7] Today, the increased awareness of thyroid disease and more sensitive thyroid testing have allowed earlier diag-nosis. Therefore, the number of patients who reach advanced stages of psy-chosis due to hyperthyroidism has been significantly reduced. As a result, we rarely see people becoming delirious or reaching a state in which they hear imaginary sounds or see delusionary visions, or exhibit bizarre behavior.

Nevertheless, hypomania caused by an overactive thyroid can evolve into mania and abnormal behavior. Consider Connie, a thirty-four-year-old housewife who began to exhibit mild mania three months after she gave birth. For the first eight months, she felt in full control. In fact, like Fred, her mental capabilities were enhanced to such a point that she felt no one could have told that her behavior was abnormal.

"My mind was very occupied and full all the time," she said. "I could lit-erally go around the clock, even while I slept. I could balance my checkbook in my sleep and wake up in the morning and it would be right. I volunteered for all sorts of positions—clerk for the PTO, room mother at school, assis-tant at church."

Several months into her hypomanic trip, however, Connie's cognitive ability became impaired. She had difficulty focusing on any particular thought. Her memory was "halfway gone." The evident confusion that set in changed her from a self-confident person to a disorganized and anxious one. Friends began to view Connie as inefficient, disorganized, maybe even "abnormal." She said:

After a few months, things weren't clear anymore. No longer was I getting the itemized lists in my brain where things were precise. Now they were getting confused, and I couldn't keep up with them. It got to the point where I didn't want to even look at the bills. I just avoided anything that had to do with con-centration. I felt like I was losing touch with reality. I felt like a balloon that was about to pop.

It was worse when I tried to sleep. My mind was so full that I had a lot of sleeping problems. I would watch TV until there was nothing else on, and then I would try to go to bed, but I wouldn't be able to fall asleep until about the time my husband would go to work, like five A.M. And then I would sleep, but it was never a comfortable sleep: it would be overwhelmed with thoughts. My mind was like a computer with no more capacity. It was like there was so much up there, I couldn't decipher one thought.

The anxiety was getting worse because I wanted to hold on to reality. I didn't want to lose anything. So I tried keeping everything in my head, but I just couldn't.

I came to a point where I was worrying about my kids, about my marriage, about the bills. But my worrying was abstract because, at the same time, I could not concentrate on the things I was really worried about.

As her symptoms progressed, forgetfulness, confusion, and loss of a sense of reality led to irrational behavior. Connie became unable to handle basic tasks, such as taking care of her children.

One year after the beginning of her hypomania, Connie deteriorated to such an extent that her husband became convinced she needed psychiatric help. In Connie's words:

He kept saying, "If you don't get help and find out what's wrong, you are going to have to go into a hospital. Something is wrong. This is not normal." That word *normal* came up several times. I remember getting quite upset about it. Then it came to a point where I thought getting hospitalized was a good idea. The anxiety that I had, the frustration, the way my husband saw me not knowing which end was up, whether I was coming or going, forgetting to pick up the kids, made him think I was truly becoming crazy.

Connie's self-esteem gradually slipped. She changed from having a normal amount of security and self-esteem, and being able to undertake any activity, to being unable to do anything right. Amazingly, it took her a year and a half to go see her husband's doctor, who diagnosed her with Graves' disease. As in most patients with Graves' disease, the nature and pattern of Connie's symptoms changed. Initially, Connie had clear-cut hypomania for the first few months, during which her mind was creative, fast, and organized. Later, she was on the verge of becoming truly psychotic. If she had not been diagnosed in time, Connie could have reached a truly confusional state, with delirium and hallucinations. Connie's husband was amazed when he observed his wife regaining her sanity as her overactive thyroid was treated. In most patients, the manic or abnormal behavior improves or even resolves after the imbalance is corrected.[8]

UNCONTROLLABLE ANGER

The emotional responses to what you see or experience take place in the limbic system of the brain, where thyroid hormone plays an important role in regulating the perception of your environment and the way you respond to it emotionally. Whether people exhibit mild mania, depression, or anxiety, the excess thyroid hormone reaching the brain typically causes exaggerated emotional responses to what they see and experience. These responses are expressed as emotional withdrawal (often a component of a depressive state) or, conversely, as loss of emotional control. They become impatient and may inappropriately laugh or cry about matters that would barely affect them under normal circumstances. They often become easily irritated over trivial issues, which may trigger anger or even aggression and violence.

This emotional instability makes such people feel as if they were sitting in a rocking chair on the edge of a cliff, teetering back and forth between being in control and out of control. Most individuals with an overactive thyroid feel their anger levels build up, and then they snap at anyone who comes along. It is indeed a sad place to be in. You don't understand what is making you this way, and if you don't like your behavior, you may think that you have become a bad person.

Mary Lou, a thirty-five-year-old schoolteacher, was referred to me by her gynecologist, who had diagnosed her with Graves' disease. Mary Lou no longer had menstrual periods and was suffering from heat intolerance and a rapid heartbeat, symptoms that had been attributed to early menopause. In my first encounter with Mary Lou, she described the familiar symptoms of impatience and intolerance. Later, she told me:

> Everybody and everything bothered me. I was losing my patience more easily. I had always been very good dealing with people and calming them, but after a while it was, "Mary Lou, you have to calm down. You're not handling this well." Things that would frustrate me would prompt me to react immediately. In some cases, I would have a lot of patience with people initially, and then, when they would go on and on, I would interrupt and ask them to get to the point quickly.
>
> I had a very short fuse with my children, which was odd. I was known to most people as a very patient person. I teach Sunday school, and I couldn't do that anymore. I didn't even have enough patience to read the lesson and to teach it. My co-teacher said I needed help. She told me that I had been teaching Sunday school too long and needed a break. That's the way she put it.
>
> I felt the worst about my oldest son. Being a teenager, he couldn't do anything to satisfy me. If I said, "Take out the trash," he didn't take it out fast enough. If I said, "Put away your clothes," he didn't fold them fast enough. Everything that happened was surrounded by the word *fast*. It was like my

mind no longer controlled my emotions. My emotions were in total control of my mind.

Some of my patients have described the loss of control and altered behavior related to hyperthyroidism as "Graves' madness" because they felt their acts and behaviors were typical of craziness. People may become belligerent and domineering, or have spells of anger and irritability interspersed with intermittent free-floating anxiety, leading to irrational behavior and inappropriate decisions.

WAVES OF ANXIETY

Undoubtedly, the most common mental effect of an overactive thyroid is anxiety. The anxiety due to hyperthyroidism, however, is seldom a pure form of anxiety disorder. It is an exaggerated form in which the increased worrying and overall feeling of insecurity and instability are worsened by mood swings, anger, an inability to focus, and foggy memory. Often, these mental effects exacerbate each other, resulting in a tumultuous mental state. Along with the insidious intrusion of anxiety, panic attacks are another form of anxiety disorder that often appears.

The rising tide of thyroid hormone in the blood and the flooding of brain cells with thyroid hormone often produce unusual feelings. You feel as if you were going to suffocate or your soul were about to leave you. Your heart starts beating very fast. Your palms become sweaty, and you may break out in a generalized sweat. The inability to control your body takes over. You have not passed out but feel you are about to. You may get dizzy. The world around you looks strange, almost unrecognizable.

You also feel frightened—a feeling that actually begins at the peak of despair. After the sense of despair plateaus and wanes gradually, you feel drained—not just tired, but literally exhausted. Then you try to rationalize and understand what happened—to your body, to your mind, and to you. The first time this sensation strikes, you might recognize it as a panic attack. You want to pick up the phone and call a friend, your spouse, or a relative and share these feelings. Now that the anxiety attack has resolved, you are exhausted, wanting only to rest and understand what just happened to you.

A few days later, in the same unpredictable fashion as the previous time, another wave of anxiety attacks you. You panic and try to fight it. In the process, your symptoms get worse and worse. You desperately try to figure out what is wrong with you, feeling that your life is out of control and no longer your own, until finally all you feel is exhaustion. This lasts only a couple of hours, and life resumes its course.

Quite often you are embarrassed by these feelings or even frightened to discuss them with the people closest to you. Having panic attacks induces a constant fear. Because these episodes come and go unpredictably, you worry that you might experience the next one when you are closing a business deal or talking with people at a dinner party. Between these attacks, you may be seized by a chronic, constant anxiety. You tend to worry about the most trivial things—things that never bothered you before. While you should be concentrating on a task at work, your brain goes on automatic pilot. It drifts off the task you are performing, and gradually the worries and anxiety worsen and take over your mind so that your concentration is sporadic and you cannot remember what you are supposed to be doing. This irritates and upsets you. You don't understand why you are reacting this way. As anxiety builds up, you, your closest friend, or your spouse notices that you are becoming a different person.

Your moods swing and are no longer stable. In the morning, you may be happy and outgoing, making plans and excited about new projects. Two hours later, you become angry, irritable, even sad. You may be at work and this wave of sadness will drain your energy and your desire to function normally and be productive. You want to be by yourself. You have difficulty controlling your anger, and you may respond to someone in a nasty way. The waves of anxiety, constant worries, and mood swings build up, affect and reinforce one another, and slowly transform your personality.

I began to see Linda for a second opinion two years after she was diagnosed with Graves' disease. She was in great despair and had almost given up on the possibility of leading a normal life again. Approximately two years before the diagnosis was made, she was thirty-six and working in a stable job as a secretary. As a result of downsizing at her company, however, her workload had doubled. She always felt behind and unable to accomplish her assigned tasks. Her stress level mounted and she began to worry about the financial repercussions if she were to lose her job. She then began noticing changes in her health.

"I started experiencing symptoms of nervousness, irritability, and increased anger," Linda said. "I was losing weight but didn't really pay attention to that. The symptoms progressed and became more intense as the months passed. I was attributing the way I was feeling to nerves, stress, and emotional reactions to things in my life, especially to my job situation."

For the first three to four months, the predominant symptoms revolved around anxiety:

It was a disabling anxiety. I felt like I couldn't breathe, and I would become very dizzy and disoriented. The world did not look real to me any longer. It was like a disorienting feeling. I was having heart palpitations and was short of breath. It was embarrassing to be in a public place, so I would retreat somewhere to try and stop the feeling. The anxiety would occur randomly. I soon developed a fear of anticipating it happening in grocery stores, the post office, the office, in almost any setting. I had no control. I didn't know when it would happen. There was no connection or any way I could logically tie it together. The wave would come on maybe three or four times a day, lasting no more than ten to fifteen minutes of intensity, and wane off over an hour. Then I would be drained and exhausted. I knew it was not a realistic reaction, that I had nothing to fear. But it's hard to correlate your brain to your body.

Linda began to exhibit a fear of crowded or confined places (agoraphobia), although such circumstances had never frightened her before. People with agoraphobia have difficulty traveling away from home because unfamiliar places, which they perceive as unsafe, trigger panic attacks.

Four to five months later, Linda began to experience other symptoms in addition to her recurrent panic attacks:

It felt like a furnace burning inside my body, and the temperature was not adjustable. No matter how cold my external environment was, I was raging inside with heat. There were days I would open the freezer door and put my head in to get relief from the heat intolerance.

I was going through a lot of symptoms that I was dismissing and trying to ignore. I was eating many times a day, and after I finished a meal, I had frequent bowel movements, almost immediately. Then I started having nausea and lightheadedness. I lost hair from all over my head. I had terrible night sweats. My eyes had begun to bulge. At first, they just seemed larger. The people around me did not notice it. I had a dry, gritty feeling in my eyes. Nobody could figure it out. I went to an ophthalmologist, who didn't pick it up and attributed it to allergies.

The tremors began about the same time. I felt I was shaking all over my body, and more so in my hands. It was difficult even to squeeze toothpaste onto a toothbrush. I had to steady my arms. I would drop things. I couldn't polish my fingernails. I couldn't read my own handwriting. Anything that required any dexterity at all was lost to me. I was very short of breath. It would wind me going up a short staircase. I had a lot of muscle weakness in my arms and legs. I couldn't get up from a squatting position. My legs were so weak, I had difficulty even climbing the stairs.

When I finally decided something had to happen, I was afraid I had muscular dystrophy. The muscle weakness was what made me go to the doctor.

The muscular effects of hyperthyroidism can cause weakness so severe that patients have difficulty walking, which often leads doctors to suspect a neurological condition. Patients with muscle weakness due to hyperthyroidism have been confined to wheelchairs until the hyperthyroidism was diagnosed and treated. Linda was so disturbed by her muscle weakness that she rushed to see a physician, who referred her to a neurologist. Although extensive neurological testing was done, the results came back normal, and her Graves' disease remained undiagnosed.

In addition to Linda's anxiety feelings, which were heightened when her muscle weakness became quite pronounced, her moods changed frequently. Sometimes, she was exhilarated; other times, she exhibited symptoms of depression.

Finally, a chance encounter gave Linda the clue she so desperately needed:

> After a full year of symptoms, I went to a party. A total stranger noted my glassy eyes and my nervousness. She asked me if I had a thyroid condition. That was the breakthrough. She told me she had Graves' disease herself and that I appeared to have the same thing. I was shocked and relieved. I knew a little bit about it because President Bush and his wife had recently been diagnosed with it. I saw an endocrinologist two days later who confirmed the diagnosis and started me on treatment.

DEPRESSION

The occurrence of depression in hyperthyroidism may seem paradoxical because depression has been linked primarily with an *under*active thyroid. It is rare, however, for hyperthyroidism to cause clinical depression that warrants admission to a psychiatric ward.[9] In some, antidepressants may aggravate the situation and only the use of antithyroid drugs to normalize thyroid function dispels the depression. It is not clearly understood whether such individuals become depressed because of a predisposition to depression or because of the overwhelming preexisting stress generated by the hyperthyroidism.[10] One doctor described a patient who developed depression during both hyperthyroidism and hypothyroidism,[11] leading the doctor to conclude that the person's underlying makeup is important in determining the effect. In general, though, the depression caused by an overactive thyroid is not constant; rather, the patient typically experiences frequent recurring bouts of depression.

However, I have seen a few patients who experienced a clear-cut, persistent depressive state when they were hyperthyroid.

Alicia was one of them. She was affected with hyperthyroidism six months after she had a baby. Because her husband was a student, Alicia had to work overtime to support her family. She and her physician initially attributed her depression and anxiety to working too much. She said:

> At first, I had headaches to the point where the upper left part of my face would feel numb. My physician told me I had migraine headaches. I became with-

drawn. I was tired, lost interest in everything, and started having suicidal thoughts. I felt I did too much. I would go to bed and sleep from six to ten, get up for an hour and eat dinner, and go back to sleep until the next morning and still be exhausted.

I had a lot of guilt feelings and lost interest in regular activities. I could not cope with problems. If I had a problem with my husband or child, I would overreact. I would break down in tears. I was very irritable and became intolerant of my child. At work, I had a lot of anxiety if I didn't get things done and off my desk.

Many of Alicia's symptoms satisfied the criteria for depression. Although the depression can be mild, as in Alicia's case, occasionally a hyperthyroid person may slip into a major depression. In fact, major depressive disorders accompanied by generalized anxiety disorders are much more common in patients with hyperthyroidism than in the general population.

PHYSICAL AND MENTAL EXHAUSTION

Physicians and patients often associate tiredness with hypothyroidism and hyperactivity with hyperthyroidism. Yet in a significant number of patients suffering from thyroid hormone excess, tiredness and exhaustion may be the initial and most prominent symptom. As in hypothyroidism, the tiredness in hyperthyroidism is both physical and mental.

In some patients, tiredness can be extreme. One middle-aged woman who was suffering from hyperthyroidism said, "You feel you're dragging yourself through the day. I remember standing at the supermarket waiting at the checkout counter. A friend came up behind me and carefully bumped me to get my attention. I was so exhausted that I didn't even react to it. I turned around and just looked at her."

Suzanne, a twenty-four-year-old salesperson in a clothing store who had always been energetic and enthusiastic, began complaining of tiredness three months before her wedding date. She blamed her symptoms on doing too much as well as stress from her wedding preparations. Her symptoms were in fact due to hyperthyroidism. She was diagnosed with Graves' disease one year after she got married.

Here's how she described the beginning of her symptoms:

I was really tired. I'd sleep ten hours a night and still be tired at work. On my days off, I would lie on the sofa. It wasn't a lack of exercise because at my job I am walking all the time. That was the most annoying thing. It wasn't like a good fatigue but just a constant irritant. Not like after you've done a hard day's work. I would wake up and feel better in the morning, and then three hours later I would be tired again. My heart rate was increasing. It was kind of scary. I would turn up the air conditioner, and my fiancé would be freezing. I was so hot. I was sweating, and I only had the sheet on me. I had hot and cold flashes. Whatever I did, it didn't really help.

When I would have headaches, I wouldn't even be able to think clearly. I wouldn't even be able to speak clearly. I felt like my vision changed. I just thought I was getting older and didn't have as much enthusiasm or energy. I started a walking program, but it did not help me to increase the energy. It would make me even more tired, and I couldn't understand why. That is when I would have the heart palpitations because I would push myself.

I withdrew from people. I was too tired to open my mouth and waste my breath to talk to them.

As illustrated by the cases described above, each individual may experience a different pattern of mental effects, although the majority of patients exhibit anxiety and intellectual deficit. These differences in mental suffering stem not only from the wide range of severity of hyperthyroidism but also from differences in personality makeup. Some people with quite high thyroid hormone levels experience few or no mental effects. In contrast, some people with marginal or low-grade hyperthyroidism (discussed in the next section) suffer a great deal from anxiety, tiredness, depression, and mood swings.

Low-Grade Hyperthyroidism

Recently, doctors have become more aware of the wide range of physical and mental effects of low-grade hyperthyroidism. This condition is defined as thyroid hormone excess that has not yet resulted in abnormally high thyroid hormone levels but has caused TSH levels to become low. Low-grade hyperthyroidism often results from an overactive thyroid gland due to Graves' disease or to thyroid lumps that produce excessive amounts of thyroid hormone. It may also result from taking too much thyroid hormone.

Low-grade hyperthyroidism can cause symptoms of depression, rapid heartbeat, weight loss, heat intolerance, increased appetite, increased sweating, and trembling of the fingers. It is likely to make a person more irritable and anxious.[12] This minimal thyroid hormone excess can also result in bone loss over time, particularly in postmenopausal women.[13] Although minimal thyroid hormone excess can also affect the bone of premenopausal women, this negative effect on the bone is counterbalanced by estrogens. Low-grade hyperthyroidism may provoke heart rhythm problems in older patients. In addition, it can affect the normal functioning of the heart[14] and lower your cardiovascular fitness.

Hyperthyroid People at Work

Job performance is frequently affected by an overactive thyroid. In extreme cases, patients even become mentally and emotionally disabled. Often they resign from their jobs or are fired because they could not cope with the demands. When they seek other job opportunities, they are frequently unsuccessful because of their appearance, cognitive impairment, or inability to handle themselves well during interviews (displaying erratic behavior or a short temper, for example). Let's look at how the mental effects of hyperthyroidism can interfere with one's job.

At twenty-nine, Amy had been working at a paper company for five years. Although her job performance had been excellent, when Amy became hyperthyroid, she got irritable and could not maintain a good working relationship with other employees. "Everything bothered me at work. I worked in the sales office, but I handled a situation on the retail floor badly, and the owner of the company heard part of the story. He came back and yelled at me in front of a whole group of people. I couldn't take it. I couldn't erase it from my mind. I wasn't getting paid enough money to deal with the public humiliation. It was so stressful, I decided to leave."

Another patient, Sabrina, who was a department store assistant manager, was terminated from her position because she couldn't cope with the demands of her work. Sabrina says:

My boss kept asking me, "Why aren't you working?" I was trying to express to him how sick I was. Finally, they asked me to leave. I spent several months job hunting to no avail.

I was shaking and looking wild-eyed. I had dropped sixteen pounds. I was probably looking a little emaciated. People probably thought I was a drug addict or an alcoholic because I was antsy and nervous. I felt insult added to injury when no one hired me or called me back. I was sensitive about my nervous behavior and mannerisms. I was aware I was talking very fast. I had to be very careful and monitor how quickly I spoke. Yet I didn't realize just how fast I was talking. People couldn't even understand me.

Several months prior to the diagnosis, I had to move back to my mother's house because I could not afford to pay rent. It was becoming difficult even to go out and look for a job. The fatigue was more overwhelming than the need to look for a job. There was a lot of guilt. With my background and my experience, I felt I should be hired. The fact that I was not hired compounded everything. Even when I was diagnosed, I thought it was the beginning of getting out of this vicious circle. But it took some time after my thyroid was regulated to find a suitable job.

Questionnaire:
The Physical Symptoms of Hyperthyroidism

An easy way to determine the likelihood that you may be suffering from hyperthyroidism is to complete the following questionnaire.

Have your nails been brittle or separating from the nail bed?	Yes	No
Has your skin been unusually warm?	Yes	No
Have you been sweating more than usual?	Yes	No
Have you been experiencing hair loss?	Yes	No
Have you become intolerant of heat?	Yes	No
Have your menstrual periods become scanty?	Yes	No
Have you been unusually hungry?	Yes	No
Have you been experiencing diarrhea or increasingly frequent bowel movements?	Yes	No
Do your fingers shake constantly?	Yes	No
Has your heartbeat been rapid at rest?	Yes	No
Have you lost more than five pounds without changing your dietary and exercise habits?	Yes	No
Do you get short of breath with exertion, or has your tolerance to exercise been reduced?	Yes	No
Have you been experiencing generalized muscle weakness?	Yes	No
Are your palms sweaty?	Yes	No

If you answered yes to four or more of the preceding questions, you may be hyperthyroid. If you answered yes to six or more of the questions, you are probably hyperthyroid.

Other Hyperthyroid Conditions

Even though Graves' disease accounts for 70 percent of the cases of overactive thyroid that are routinely diagnosed, you need to make sure that your overactive thyroid is not the result of another thyroid disorder that can be easily confused with Graves' disease. For instance, some patients have an overactive thyroid because one or more lumps (called nodules) within the thyroid gland become autonomous. These autonomous nodules take over the function of the entire gland but produce more thyroid hormone than the body normally requires. This condition, which is common in older people, is called simple toxic nodule or multinodular toxic goiter, depending on whether the gland has one nodule or whether several of the hyperfunctioning nodules begin to grow independently from the rest of the gland.

To confirm these disorders, your doctor will order a nuclear thyroid scan and uptake. The nuclear medicine doctor will have you ingest a tiny amount of radioactive iodine, which will be readily picked up by the thyroid gland and can be detected when the thyroid area is scanned. Six and twenty-four hours after you ingest the radioactive iodine, a counting probe placed over your neck will detect the radioactivity present in your thyroid. High scores on this radioactive iodine uptake test tell your physician that your thyroid is overworking and producing excess levels of thyroid hormone. The pictures taken of your thyroid (scan) will show the nodule(s).

Doctors can treat simple toxic nodules and multinodular goiters by administering radioactive iodine to destroy the overactive areas or by performing surgery aimed at removing the portion of the gland that contains the toxic nodules. Medications are not an option, as they are for patients with Graves' disease.

An excess of thyroid hormone may also result from silent thyroiditis and subacute thyroiditis, two conditions that cause a temporary destruction of thyroid cells that leak too much of the preformed thyroid hormone into the bloodstream while the cells are being destroyed. These conditions are easily confused with Graves' disease.

Silent thyroiditis is the result of what is believed to be a transient immune attack on the thyroid gland that produces hyperthyroidism. The hyperthyroidism is often mild and lasts only a few weeks, although in some cases, it can go on for as long as three months.

After resolution of the inflammation and (temporary) destruction of the thyroid gland, you may become hypothyroid for a few weeks because the damage to the thyroid renders the gland unable to meet the usual demands of the system. After a few weeks of hypothyroidism, however, the thyroid repairs itself, leading to regeneration of a normally functioning gland. If you consult your physician during the initial period, when your thyroid levels are still high, it is sometimes difficult to tell whether you have silent thyroiditis or Graves' disease. A radioactive iodine uptake count will differentiate between the two conditions, however. Typically, a high count indicates the overactivity characteristic of Graves' disease, and a low uptake indicates the temporary destruction characteristic of silent thyroiditis.

A similar scenario occurs when the cause of your hyperthyroidism is subacute thyroiditis. This is a viral infection of the gland that results in temporary destruction followed by transient hypothyroidism and then recovery. This condition is often more easily diagnosed because you are likely to suffer from fever and pain in your neck area that may spread to one or both ears. Many viruses can cause subacute thyroiditis, including those that have been tied to the common cold, mumps, and measles. The key test to confirm that your hyperthyroidism is caused by subacute thyroiditis is the radioactive iodine uptake count, which will be low in subacute thyroiditis and high in Graves' disease.

Prior to the infection of the gland, you may experience a sore throat, pains, aches, headaches, fever, and a cough. During the hot phase, most physicians prescribe anti-inflammatory nonsteroidal drugs and a beta-blocker. Some people may need cortisone if the inflammation is severe and the pain excruciating. At times, the gland may remain inflamed for several months even after thyroid levels have returned to normal. Taking cortisone may then be the solution. Even though the majority of people who experience subacute thyroiditis regain normal thyroid function down the road, some patients may remain permanently hypothyroid. The message here is that you need to have your thyroid hormone levels rechecked six months later to make sure they have returned to normal and have stayed normal.

The accompanying table summarizes the diagnostic characteristics of the most common causes of hyperthyroidism.

CAUSES OF HYPERTHYROIDISM

	TSH	Thyroid Hormone Levels	Radioactive Iodine Uptake
Graves' disease	Low	High	High
Single toxic nodule	Low	High	High
Multinodular toxic goiter	Low	High	High
Silent thyroiditis	Low	High	Low
Subacute thyroiditis (viral)	Low	High	Low
TSH excess*	Normal/high	High	High

*Such as from a tumor in the pituitary gland or a dysregulation of the pituitary cells that manufacture TSH.

Hyperthyroidism in Older People

Hyperthyroidism is quite common in older people, affecting approximately 1.5 percent of men and 1.9 percent of women older than sixty.[15] The effects of hyperthyroidism on older persons are often different from those experienced by younger people. With respect to physical symptoms, thyroid enlargement, intolerance to heat, increased perspiration, and increased appetite are not as common in older people. Heart problems, however, such as atrial fibrillation, as well as weight loss and reduced appetite, increase in frequency with aging.[16] In addition, constipation (a symptom typical of hypothyroidism), depression, and decrease in muscle mass leading to weakness are quite common. Muscle weakness due to hyperthyroidism may predispose older patients to fall and further injure themselves. The falling is frequently attributed to other illnesses before the correct diagnosis is made.

Because the consequences of hyperthyroidism in older people are general and are so similar to many other health problems, even hospital physicians often diagnose the condition incorrectly. In one study of hospitalized hyperthyroid patients, the diagnosis was suspected in only one-third of the patients.[17] For those who require hospitalization, psychiatric diagnosis is the most common reason for admission, with debility and cardiac failure with atrial fibrillation also accounting for a large number of admissions.

The differences in symptoms are not only physical. The first adverse effect of hyperthyroidism in older people may be mental changes, which are frequently overlooked and attributed to aging. Instead of being overactive, hyperdynamic, and overwhelmed by anxiety and irritability or exhibiting mania, older people often experience withdrawal and depression. The effect of thyroid hormone excess on the minds of older people may be quite significant and manifests frequently as dementia, confusion, and apathy. They may even experience delirium. Increased nervousness, a common symptom in younger people, is seen in less than 20 percent of older patients.[18]

Older people often suffer from what doctors call "apathetic hyperthyroidism," characterized by depression, apathy, and intellectual stupor. Patients with apathetic hyperthyroidism show exhaustion, a slowing of physical and mental activity, and an expressionless face. Because this appearance and change in personality are usually ascribed to aging,[19] the disease frequently goes undiagnosed for a long time.

Hospitals' use of certain X-ray procedures, such as cardiac catheterization and intravenous pyelogram, to visualize the heart, urinary tract, or other bodily organs may trigger hyperthyroidism from the iodine that is administered to provide sufficient contrast. An older person admitted to the hospital for evaluation of a cardiac or kidney condition may return home and display an altered state of mind or even delirium within a few days. Often, the family is alarmed by the new, unexplained symptoms.

How an excess of thyroid hormone affects the brain depends on age and perhaps personality. Overactive thyroid has many faces. It may affect the mind in different ways. The end result is often a mixture of anxiety, emotional and behavioral changes, mood swings, anger, poor stress-coping mechanisms, impaired cognitive ability, inability to cope with job demands, and family problems. One patient described all these effects lumped together as "a monster inside me." Fortunately, you have many options at your disposal to help you tame this monster.

Important Points to Remember

- If you have been experiencing weight loss, jitteriness, tremors, increased sweating, or palpitations, you could be suffering from an overactive thyroid. But these are physical symptoms. While you are hyperthyroid, it is not unusual to become hypomanic and talkative and to feel as if you were on top of the world.
- Depression, waves of anger, and lethargy could be symptoms of an overactive thyroid; mood swings and loss of touch with reality are also typical.
- If you are experiencing episodic panic attacks characterized by feeling out of control and a rapid heartbeat, you may have an overactive thyroid. Describe these symptoms in detail to your doctor.
- Although Graves' disease accounts for 70 percent of cases of hyperthyroidism, there are other causes, too, including a transient hyperthyroidism due to temporary destruction of thyroid cells.
- As you get older, the symptoms of overactive thyroid are not necessarily the same as in younger people. With aging, an overactive thyroid tends to produce more depression, lethargy, muscle weakness, and heart symptoms.

5

THYROID IMBALANCE, DEPRESSION, ANXIETY, AND MOOD SWINGS

Your brain is unique. It creates your individual talents, perceptions, and moods. Yet its individuality presents some challenges to physicians and brain researchers when they try to figure out how the brain, body, and mind work together to generate specific mental states. For example, exact measurements or even precise definitions of what constitutes normal mental health continue to elude scientists. In the recent past, some doctors may have defined normal mental health merely as the absence of overt mental diseases such as manic-depression or schizophrenia. Today, most doctors have come to recognize that millions of people have various, more subtle forms of depression and anxiety.

More often than not, thyroid imbalance gives rise to mental and emotional symptoms of mild depression, intermittent rage disorder, mild attention deficit disorder, or other "minor syndromes"—conditions that cause suffering but are not pronounced enough to meet the psychiatric criteria of a mental condition. People with these conditions will find that their symptoms are magnified when a thyroid imbalance occurs. For a minority of patients, such magnified symptoms may cause them to slip into a more pronounced mental illness, but for most thyroid patients, the mental effects of thyroid disease—such as fatigue, low mood and mood swings, and lack of mental clarity—cause great suffering without being "psychiatric."

Just as severe hypothyroidism is much less common than low-grade hypothyroidism, low-grade and borderline depression are much more common than easily diagnosed major depression.

Low-Grade Depression:
Thyroid Shadow Syndrome

It is a common misconception that depression means mere sadness. The feeling of sadness is a normal response to the occurrence of a distressing event or to a disappointment in life. Although you may feel down and sad when depressed, sadness is not always a symptom of depression. In depression, a person's feelings are disconnected from all that surrounds that person, so that he or she may be neither sad nor happy. This disconnection causes a blunting of excitement about life in general. Although, when asked whether he or she is depressed, the typical response is, "No, I don't feel I'm depressed. I'm not sad," this person may in fact be suffering from the characteristic symptoms of depression.

An easy way to determine the likelihood that you may be suffering from depression is to complete the following questionnaire. If you answer a question with "No," proceed to the next question; if you answer with "Yes," score the severity of your symptoms (1 = mild, 2 = moderate, 3 = severe) before proceeding to the next question.

Are you tired all the time?	Yes	No	_____
Have you lost interest in activities that you used to enjoy?	Yes	No	_____
Are you in a sad mood more or less constantly?	Yes	No	_____
Are you often irritable, and do you get angry over trivial matters?	Yes	No	_____
Do you experience crying spells?	Yes	No	_____
Do you have feelings of worthlessness?	Yes	No	_____
Do you often experience a sense of guilt about things or have you become too critical of yourself?	Yes	No	_____
Has your appetite increased, and/or have you gained weight?	Yes	No	_____
Has your appetite decreased, and/or have you lost weight?	Yes	No	_____
Do you have difficulty remembering things and/or concentrating on normal activities?	Yes	No	_____
Do you have trouble making decisions, or do you feel inefficient?	Yes	No	_____
Do you have trouble sleeping through the night?	Yes	No	_____

Do you sleep more than 8 hours (either going to bed
   too early or sleeping late)?   Yes No _____
Do you wish you were dead?   Yes No _____
Have you become very sensitive to criticism or
   rejection?   Yes No _____

TOTAL SEVERITY SCORE   _____

If you answered yes to three or more of the preceding questions, you may be depressed; if you answered yes to five or more of the questions, you are probably depressed.

Now add the scores for each symptom to obtain your total severity score, the meaning of which is explained in the accompanying table. The total severity score will be useful later in assessing your response to treatment.

DEPRESSION/ANXIETY SEVERITY

Total Severity Score	Severity of Symptoms
15 or less	Mild
15–25	Moderate
25 or more	Severe

In addition to the feelings of disconnection and fatigue, the main symptoms of depression are changes in appetite, sleep disturbances, lack of interest in enjoyable activities, and problems with memory and concentration.

In general, as thyroid hormone begins to decrease, changes in a person's mental energy are barely recognizable. Gradually, subtle changes occur, and the person begins to slow down and often "loses steam" in the afternoon. The fatigue itself precipitates a growing concern that there might be something terribly wrong somewhere in the body. The lack of energy may result in a great deal of frustration, a sense of no longer being able to function as the person has done in the past. This, in turn, produces feelings of guilt, inadequacy, and lower self-esteem. Even if a hypothyroid person's symptoms do not fully satisfy the criteria for depression, he or she may be experiencing a low-grade depression (a chronic, even milder form of depression than dysthymia) that is manifested primarily as fatigue and lack of enthusiasm.

Dawn, an educational consultant who conducts seminars all over the

United States, began to notice a lack of energy a year before she sought medical attention. She said:

> I would hit three in the afternoon and be ready to go to bed. That was terribly frustrating, since previously I had had such a high energy level. I felt that people would think I was inadequate, that I was giving up, when it wasn't me who was giving up, it was my body. I waged a constant battle within myself to keep up with things at work and try to live a normal existence. I felt that I was dancing as fast as I could and going nowhere. At lunchtime and during afternoon breaks, I would find a quiet place and take a quick nap to try to recoup. I would eat a piece of chocolate to give me a boost, but nothing helped.

I diagnosed Dawn with a moderately underactive thyroid. Although, when I asked, she did mention several other symptoms of hypothyroidism, what was affecting Dawn the most was the deficiency in energy. She attributed almost every other symptom that she exhibited to her tiredness, yet Dawn was suffering from borderline depression as a result of her underactive thyroid. At times, she was experiencing unexplained anger, increased appetite, and cravings. She was also deeply affected when someone was critical of her and when she perceived that someone was rejecting her.

A thirty-nine-year-old surgeon's wife, Nina, repeatedly told her busy husband, "I am tired. I feel that there must be something wrong with my body." His reply was always the same: "You are trying to do too much with all these social activities. Just slow down."

Nina didn't think it was stress or too much activity. Rather, she was convinced that something was physically wrong with her. Her energy level was low. She was sleepier than she felt she should be and could not control her weight gain. In her words:

> I wanted to go to sleep at seven in the evening. I was feeling down. I was not that type of person before. I could not concentrate, and I could not work. I had anxiety. Often, for no reason, when I was by myself, I would cry. Many times I was not happy even though I felt I had to be happy. I was forgetful, which would really upset me. I also had problems concentrating on things and became very bad with names. I didn't care to do much, and I withdrew.
>
> I thought to myself, what could be wrong? I knew that weight problems were related to thyroid disorders, so I went to see an experienced endocrinologist. He said, "Don't worry. This is nothing. I don't want to put you on medication."

A year later, because her symptoms had persisted, Nina came to see me. After she told me about her suffering, she said, "I know a problem exists, and there has to be a reason." I asked Nina whether she had told the first endocrinologist about all the problems besides the tiredness. "I don't think so, because he didn't ask me. I was disappointed when he said the levels were borderline normal. I didn't believe it. That's why I thought I had to see somebody else."

Nina's blood test showed low-grade hypothyroidism. She was also suffering from a case of low-grade depression. I started Nina on thyroid hormone treatment, and she showed dramatic improvement. Her tiredness and the intermittent sadness and anger went away. Nina was suffering from a "shadow syndrome" caused by a minute deficit of thyroid hormone in her system and her brain. Getting on the medicine restored Nina's energy and made her other symptoms disappear. Slowly but surely, she saw her body starting to cooperate with her again instead of being her enemy.

Many people like Dawn and Nina suffer needlessly from low-grade hypothyroidism. Research conducted on women has recently shown that even those who have low-grade hypothyroidism *but no symptoms of mood disorders* show evidence of improvement in objective scores that test levels of depression, hysteria, and obsessive-compulsive behavior when they are treated with thyroid hormone.[1] This illustrates that even those who suffer from low-grade hypothyroidism may not necessarily sense the effect of the thyroid hormone deficit. They might be attributing the way they feel to just "being themselves."

Because the majority of patients with low-grade depression do not seek psychiatric help, establishing the frequency of hypothyroidism in people suffering from low-grade depression is a real challenge for researchers. I expect that a minor thyroid imbalance occurs in a significant percentage of people suffering from low-grade depression, however. In a recent study conducted in the German state of Bavaria, ultrasound exams showed an enlarged thyroid gland in 86 percent of patients suffering from chronic depression, but in only 25 percent of people not suffering from depression.[2]

Let's look at how even a minute thyroid hormone imbalance could be responsible for lowering mood.

Thyroid Hormone: Serotonin's Cousin

The explosive advances in the knowledge of brain chemistry and its effects on mood began in the early 1960s. Within the past decade, doctors have recognized that serotonin imbalance is an important factor in causing depression. Acceptance of the idea that most psychiatric conditions can be attributed to a chemical imbalance in the brain opened the door to drastic changes in the way doctors explain and treat mental disorders. This new era of biological psychiatry, or *biopsychiatry*, witnessed a convergence of psychiatry and medicine, fields previously separated by rigid boundaries. A psychiatric illness now tends to be viewed in much the same manner as a physical illness.

In the early days of biopsychiatry, neuroscientists believed that each mental disorder was associated with a corresponding brain chemical imbalance. This assumption led psychiatrists to hope that they could diagnose a psychiatric condition by measuring the levels of specific bodily chemicals or their by-products in the blood or urine. But brain chemistry is not so simple. Most often, multiple imbalances of chemicals—such as serotonin, noradrenaline, and others, including those we are concerned with here, the thyroid hormones—are responsible for mental symptoms.

Scientists now consider thyroid hormone one of the major "players" in brain chemistry disorders. And as with any brain chemical disorder, until treated correctly, thyroid hormone imbalance has serious effects on the patient's emotions and behavior.

Once the important thyroid hormones, T3 and T4, are released into your bloodstream, they enter cells of organs and play an important role in regulating major functions in the body. Adequate amounts of thyroid hormone are also required throughout your life if your brain is to function normally. Most of your cognitive abilities—such as concentration, memory, and attention span—as well as mood and emotions depend on normal thyroid hormone levels. Mounting evidence suggests that T3, the most potent form of thyroid hormone, is a bona fide brain chemical. It is found in the junctions of nerve (synapse) cells that allow these cells to communicate with one another.[3] This thyroid hormone also regulates the levels and actions of serotonin, noradrenaline, and GABA (gamma-aminobutyric acid), now accepted as the main chemical transmitters implicated in both depression and some anxiety disorders. Maintaining normal serotonin and noradrenaline levels in the brain depends to a great extent on whether the correct amount of T3 is available. Extensive animal and human research has led scientists to conclude that serotonin levels in the brain decrease if T3 is not delivered in the right amount.[4] Also, a deficit of T3 in the brain is likely to result in noradrenaline's working inefficiently as a chemical transmitter,[5] and noradrenaline deficiency or inefficiency is, in some people, the chemical reason for depression.[6]

Findings that T3 is very highly concentrated near the junction between brain cells strongly support the concept of T3 as a brain chemical transmitter that is essential for maintaining normal mood and behavior. This is the location where chemical transmitters such as noradrenaline are released to relay messages from one brain cell to another. The potent thyroid hormone T3 is found in greater quantities in the limbic system, a region of the brain that regulates mood, emotions, and perception of happy and sad events. The resemblance of thyroid hormone to other important brain chemicals is also striking:

the amino acid tyrosine is an essential constituent both of thyroid hormone and of the brain chemicals noradrenaline and dopamine.

Beating the Blues

My wife and I once attended the symphony with a colleague, Jim, and his wife, Lorraine, whom I hadn't seen in several years. Upon being reintroduced to Lorraine, I was surprised to see that she now had a slightly enlarged thyroid gland, or goiter. Even though she used to be an avid devotee of the symphony, she was clearly not enjoying herself that evening. She had a hard time smiling and appeared isolated, disconnected from her friends, hardly paying attention to our conversations or the music. During the intermission, when my wife and Lorraine went off by themselves, I mentioned to Jim that I was surprised to see how much Lorraine had changed. I also suggested that she appeared to have thyroid disease.

Jim seemed relieved at the opportunity to talk to someone and confessed that his wife had completely changed three or four years earlier. She gained weight, was often very tired and sleepy, and became overly sensitive to criticism. Lorraine didn't seem to enjoy many things that used to bring her great pleasure, such as cooking and the symphony. Her relationships with Jim and their children were really suffering. She had undergone counseling for six or eight months, thinking her problems were psychological, but no real changes resulted. Several physicians said she was simply "stressed" and told her to learn to relax. A holistic doctor administered herbs, which, like everything else, did not seem to help. Obviously, these physicians had failed to pay attention to Lorraine's enlarged thyroid gland. Lorraine became pretty discouraged about going to doctors for help and seemed resigned to this as her new way of life.

A week later, Jim convinced Lorraine to try one more time. She came in to see me and tested positive for hypothyroidism. After three months of treatment, Lorraine dramatically improved. She started to enjoy life again and regained control over her weight. In retrospect, Lorraine was suffering from a case of hypothyroidism with symptoms of atypical depression that resolved with thyroid hormone treatment.

Atypical depression is a common form of chronic depression experienced by people with an underactive thyroid. Such patients can be cheered up temporarily by positive events, but the recovery tends to be brief. The patients often slip back into a depressive state a few hours or days later. The symptoms may be mild to severe. In this type of depression, the patients become sensitive to rejection and criticism and develop a tendency to overeat, especially carbohydrates, and to oversleep. Overeating and oversleeping are important characteristics of atypical depression. They help psychiatrists distinguish this quite common type of depression from major depression, which causes the person to suffer from insomnia and loss of appetite.[7] Some patients with atypical depression experience anxiety attacks and severe lethargy, which may impede their normal functioning. The depression and fatigue are frequently worse in the evening. The patients may appear introverted and gloomy.

People with atypical depression often remain undiagnosed because their suffering rarely reaches the severity of major depression and is easier to hide. They may not consider themselves depressed; at times they may not realize that anything is wrong with them; and suicidal thoughts are unusual.

Hypothyroidism can also cause the person to suffer from dysthymic depression, or "chronic blues," another common form of chronic depression. It is perhaps also the most common type of depression experienced by people with normal thyroid function. It affects at least 6 percent of the general population during their lifetimes. Patients afflicted with dysthymia are depressed more often than not. They feel down but are able to function. People with this form of chronic depression also tend to oversleep; their appetite may be either increased or decreased, however. They frequently become used to the way they feel and may not even recognize that they have a problem. Dysthymic people do not go through well-defined periods of depression but remain more or less depressed constantly: it is a lingering type of depression.

The accepted diagnostic criterion for dysthymia requires that at least two symptoms—change in appetite, insomnia, fatigue, low self-esteem, poor concentration, indecision, and feelings of hopelessness—in conjunction with depressed mood be present for most of the time over at least two years.[8] Although two years of suffering may be acceptable as a psychiatric criterion, that doesn't mean you should suffer unnecessarily for two years before being diagnosed and treated. This is especially true if the cause of your depression is a thyroid imbalance.

As you can see, atypical depression and dysthymia share many features. They are chronic, lingering forms of depression that do not lead to suicidal thoughts. The fatigue in atypical depression, however, is in general much more severe. Further, although overeating is characteristic of atypical depression, loss of appetite can be seen in many patients suffering from dysthymia.

Erica, a forty-year-old teacher, was suffering from dysthymia along with other physical symptoms of hypothyroidism for two years. She said:

> I became so tired. I would lie down and sleep for hours just to get my energy back. I would take naps in the afternoon after school. I would go to bed early. It was like a stress relief. I loved to sleep. I never got enough.
>
> I wasn't suicidal, but I was very depressed. I took one day at a time. I didn't

talk to anyone. I kept to myself. I rarely visited family. When I came home from work, I immediately went to sleep. I lost my appetite and kept losing weight. I worried about paying bills. I always had to write things down or I would forget.

I wondered where my life was going. I was afraid of the future. Urged by my sister, I began to see a psychologist, but this was not helping.

One day, Erica saw her general practitioner for a sore throat. The doctor noticed a goiter and suspected hypothyroidism. Erica tested positive for hypothyroidism, and her depression completely resolved with thyroid hormone treatment. A few months later, Erica said, "Thyroid treatment has helped me cope with the depression and stress. I am more alert. I am not as depressed. I am able to really talk to my therapist frankly and follow her suggestions."

Erica's dysthymia was in large part caused by an underactive thyroid. People with thyroid imbalance who suffer from dysthymia often continue to try to function despite their tiredness and other symptoms and attribute the tiredness to stress, work, or too many activities. Gradually, they feel overwhelmed and start perceiving that what they are doing is more than they can handle. Yet this can be corrected, and they can feel like their old selves again if treated promptly and properly. The key is to think thyroid and to have your doctor order the appropriate thyroid test.

Major Depression and Thyroid Imbalance

Although hypothyroidism in general causes either low-grade depression or chronic minor depression of the atypical type, or dysthymia, it also places people with these minor, lingering forms of depression at a high risk for slipping into major depression—the most extreme and most dreaded form of depression. In many cases, a minimal thyroid imbalance is enough to trigger a vicious cycle that ultimately leads to major depression. When hypothyroidism is not immediately addressed and lingers untreated for years, minor depression can evolve into major depression, which can lead to a severe feeling of disconnection and even suicidal thoughts. In such patients, the extreme tiredness associated with hypothyroidism and depression is part of a never-ending vicious cycle that drains them and ultimately leads to deeper depression.

Christina, a thirty-four-year-old receptionist, suffered from gradually worsening depression. She described her two years of suffering before doctors diagnosed her with hypothyroidism: "I would come home from work really, really tired. I didn't want to do anything. I had no motivation to go out and spend time with my friends. It was a struggle to work around the yard and to do all the daily chores like cooking and taxiing kids. For the past two years, I have gone to bed by 9:00 or 9:30. It is a joke in my family that the kids stay up later than I do."

As the months passed, Christina felt as if she had become disconnected from the world and was no longer able to sleep. She quit her job and one day tried to kill herself by taking an overdose of painkillers. "I just wanted to escape and die," she said.

Before she became severely depressed, Christina had been in a state of minor, lingering depression. Because doctors failed to diagnose and treat her hypothyroidism, however, she progressed from minor depression to full-blown major depression. Her struggle with the extreme tiredness was a signal that more serious depression was evolving.

In major depression, a patient becomes quite disconnected from his or her surroundings and meets whatever happens with extreme indifference. The feelings of disconnection and tiredness are worse in the morning. The person typically suffers from insomnia and may wake up several hours early and have difficulty falling back to sleep. Other characteristics are loss of appetite, disinterest in eating, weight loss, and difficulty concentrating. People suffering from major depression often have the feeling that life is not worth living. They blame themselves and feel that they do not deserve help. Often they begin to think about death and suicide. Major depression can occur unexpectedly at any age and gradually worsens over a period of months. In some cases, the patient may be out of touch with reality and have hallucinations (major depression with psychotic features).

Researchers who screened severely depressed patients for thyroid disease found that up to 15 percent of them have an underactive thyroid.[9] But the striking finding was that their underactive thyroid was often low-grade rather than severe.

A study also demonstrated that nearly 20 percent of patients hospitalized because of severe depression had Hashimoto's thyroiditis.[10] The fact that a significant number of people, particularly women, being treated for major depression have low-grade hypothyroidism is best explained by the fact that a minor deficiency of thyroid hormone in the brain makes the person more vulnerable to slipping into major depression. In fact, women with low-grade hypothyroidism who are not currently suffering from major depression often experienced one or more episodes of depression in the preceding years.

In one study that compared the psychiatric history of sixteen women who had low-grade hypothyroidism to the psychiatric history of fifteen women with normal thyroid function, none of the women in either group was suffering from major depression at the time of the study.[11] The researchers found, however, that 56 percent of the women with low-grade hypothyroidism had a major depression episode at least once in their lives, compared to only 20 percent in the group with normal thyroid function. The study also showed that most episodes of depression had occurred in the preceding five years in the patients with low-grade hypothyroidism. This illustrates that low-grade hypothyroidism may make a woman more vulnerable to major depression when stresses occur in her life. Correcting low-grade hypothyroidism in such women should be viewed as a way to prevent the occurrence of major depression.

Scientists have been intrigued for years by the fact that a tiny thyroid hormone deficit in the brain (such as results from a minimally failing thyroid gland) can precipitate major depression. Stress, depressing events, and threats to livelihood are perceived and integrated in the brain, and messages are immediately transmitted to the thyroid gland so that the gland can adjust its function and increase the production of thyroid hormone.[12] The increased production of thyroid hormone triggered by these threatening events will help maintain an adequate brain chemistry that allows you to deal better with the stress, depressing event, or threat to your livelihood.

Even in low-grade depression, serotonin levels in the brain tend to decrease. The brain transmits the decrease in serotonin levels, however, to the pituitary. The message prompts the pituitary to produce more TSH so that the thyroid gland manufactures and releases more thyroid hormone. This thyroid adjustment works to bring serotonin levels back to normal so that mood does not deteriorate further. Thyroid hormone in the brain has the ability to enhance the production of serotonin in brain cells (see the accompanying diagram illustrating the role of thyroid hormones in preventing depression). But if the thyroid is failing and is unable to rescue brain chemistry or provide the extra thyroid hormone needed, serotonin levels will

THE ROLE OF THYROID HORMONES
IN THE PREVENTION OF DEPRESSION

Brain	Low serotonin	Increased serotonin
	↓ (+)	↑
Hypothalamus	TRH		
	↓ (+)		
Pituitary gland	TSH		(+)
	↓ (+)		
Thyroid gland	Thyroid hormones	____|

continue to fall, and depression escalates. This explains how a dysfunctioning gland could deprive a person of a primary defense mechanism against major depression. The increased vulnerability to major depression in patients with a previous history of major depression was elegantly illustrated in a study that assessed the severity of mood disturbances occurring in people who became hypothyroid after the surgical removal of their thyroid gland. The study showed that patients who previously suffered from major depression had the most severe symptoms when they became hypothyroid.[13]

Consider the case of Sara, aged twenty-nine. She had been engaged for six months, was extremely happy and excited, and had just begun preparing for her wedding. She was a sales manager in a big department store, and the demands of her job were overwhelming because the Christmas season was approaching. She began feeling tired in the afternoon. When she went home, all she wanted to do was to sit down, watch TV, and then go to bed.

Sara also began to lose interest in going out with her fiancé. As the stress of preparing for the wedding and the demands of her job increased, she became easily irritated, had crying spells, and became angry about trivial matters. Gradually, the relationship deteriorated, and ultimately, the wedding was canceled. Sara did not share any of her feelings with anyone at that point. She attributed all of this to stress, the demands of her job, and her inability to cope with all these things at the same time.

Over a few weeks, Sara slipped into a state of major depression. When her sister came for a visit at Christmas, she insisted that Sara see a psychiatrist. Sara agreed, partly because she had experienced severe depression four years previously and had a strong family history of depression.

Sara tried several antidepressants, but none of them seemed to work. Unable to function any longer, she stopped eating, lost a lot of weight, and was nearly fired from her job.

"I had problems with memory," she said. "I could not remember orders or where I placed papers. I would not return phone calls to customers." This made Sara feel even worse, and she started having suicidal thoughts. When finally another psychiatrist tested her thyroid, she was found to have low-grade hypothyroidism. As a result of thyroid hormone treatment added to the antidepressant, her memory improved, and she began eating again. Her original perky, happy personality reemerged. Her energy level increased, her performance at work improved, and her moodiness and anger disappeared.

In Sara's case, the job- or wedding-related stress and the genetic predisposition toward depression could have been what originally triggered the depression. But hypothyroidism made her more vulnerable to slipping into a state of major depression. When her brain needed a little extra T3 to prevent serotonin from falling further during the stress of the approaching Christmas season and her wedding, her thyroid gland was unable to do its job, and a complex sequence of brain chemistry imbalance led to major depression.

Diagnosing and treating a thyroid hormone imbalance may help prevent you from slipping into major depression. But if you are already suffering from depression, as in Sara's case, you must have your thyroid hormone imbalance diagnosed and treated. If the thyroid imbalance is not corrected, the depression will not be helped by conventional antidepressants. Research has shown that 52 percent of patients who suffer from major depression—and do not respond to antidepressants—have hypothyroidism.[14] Once doctors add thyroid hormone treatment to the antidepressant, the depression often resolves. Hypothyroidism also accounts for nonresponse to antidepressants in a significant percentage of people suffering from chronic minor depression. Yet in a recently published book that provides numerous accounts of depressed people who were being treated with antidepressants, none of those patients mentioned that his or her thyroid had been tested—and many of them did not fully respond to the antidepressants.[15]

If you are suffering from depression or have recently experienced depression, you should be tested for a thyroid imbalance, especially if you are experiencing other unexplained symptoms. A TSH measurement is the first test that doctors should run to assess thyroid function. At times, an accurate evaluation of thyroid function requires a thyrotropin-releasing hormone stimulation test if the TSH level is normal, particularly if it is in the upper range of normal. (Thyrotropin-releasing hormone, or TRH, is produced by the hypothalamus and normally regulates pituitary TSH secretion. See Chapter 14 for more information on this and other thyroid tests.) TRH stimulation testing consists of injecting TRH into a vein and measuring TSH in the blood every fifteen minutes for one hour. An exaggerated increase in TSH response to TRH usually indicates low-grade hypothyroidism even though the basal TSH level is normal. In about half of the patients who are both depressed and hypothyroid, the hypothyroidism is detected by TRH testing.[16]

Clearing the Depression

If you are suffering from depression and test positive for hypothyroidism, in general, you can expect the depression to clear once you correct the thyroid imbalance. The depression, in some cases, may not fully respond to thyroid hormone treatment alone. The depression may have taken on a life of its own and require additional treatment, particularly if the underactive thyroid had been undiagnosed for a long time.

Generally speaking, if you have a dysthymia, an atypical depression, or a low-grade lingering type of depression and your doctor diagnoses an underactive thyroid, your doctor should treat the underactive thyroid first for at least three months. If the depression does not fully resolve despite adequate thyroid hormone treatment, your doctor will add an antidepressant, such as a selective serotonin reuptake inhibitor (SSRI), for six to twelve months. Another option will be to use the combination T4/T3 treatment (discussed in Chapter 17). However, if you have major depression and hypothyroidism, you must immediately begin treatment with both thyroid hormone and an antidepressant. If you are still suffering from symptoms of depression after three months of treatment with thyroid hormone and an antidepressant, the T4/T3 combination treatment may be the solution.

After your thyroid is well regulated and the depression has fully resolved, your doctor will probably consider stopping the conventional antidepressant after twelve months. If, despite normal thyroid levels, depression recurs after you stop the antidepressant, then antidepressant treatment should be resumed.

Anxiety Disorders and Thyroid Imbalance

As is the case with depression, anxiety disorders can be triggered or worsened by a thyroid imbalance. According to a survey by the National Institute of Mental Health, 10 percent of the adult American population suffered from an anxiety disorder in the preceding six months.[17] It is estimated that 27 percent of adults suffer from an anxiety disorder during their lifetimes.[18] At any one time, nearly 15 million Americans suffer from an anxiety disorder. Undoubtedly, thyroid imbalance accounts for some of this anguish. One study even demonstrated that thyroid disorders are very common among family members of patients suffering from an anxiety disorder.[19] Also, in some people anxiety seems to predispose them to the occurrence of an overactive thyroid.[20]

Two types of anxiety disorders often occur as a result of a thyroid imbalance:

1. Generalized anxiety disorder, defined as excessive, exaggerated, and unrealistic worrying about trivial matters for at least six months
2. Panic disorders, characterized by attacks of abnormal physiological responses accompanied by extreme fear, causing physical symptoms

Less common anxiety disorders that have been noted to occur as a result of thyroid imbalance include:

- Social phobias
- Specific phobias
- Obsessive-compulsive disorder
- Post–traumatic stress disorder (see Chapter 2)

In addition to excessive and unrealistic worrying, the most typical symptoms of a generalized anxiety disorder are restlessness, feeling superalert and on edge, fatigue, difficulty concentrating (which may be expressed in extreme cases as an inability to think or process information), irritability, muscle tension, and difficulty falling or staying asleep.

As is the case with depression, the severity of anxiety disorders varies. Many people with mild generalized anxiety disorders become used to the way they feel: the mental and emotional struggles can become a way of life, and they may not even suspect that something is wrong. Other people, in contrast, are overwhelmed by the symptoms. Many seek medical help and may go from physician to physician trying to find a reason for their suffering.

Although, as noted earlier, it is commonly assumed that anxiety accompanies an overactive thyroid and depression accompanies an underactive thyroid, in fact, hypothyroidism frequently causes significant anxiety and even panic attacks. Abnormal noradrenaline levels in the brain may be the basis not only for depression but also for anxiety disorders such as panic attacks. A decrease in serotonin and an increase in noradrenaline activity in certain parts of the brain, coupled with an increase in the activity or the sensitivity of the body's respiratory center, cause the mental and physical symptoms of panic disorders.[21] Noradrenaline firing in the midbrain is the main reason for the physical effects on the heart and respiratory system experienced during a panic attack. The physiological responses accompanying a panic attack are real and are generated by the autonomic nervous system. An overactive thyroid causes noradrenaline activity to increase, which results in symptoms of anxiety and panic attacks. An underactive thyroid is likely to cause the levels of GABA, an antianxiety brain chemical, to decrease. This also contributes to the occurrence of anxiety during hypothyroidism-caused depression.

Panic Attacks

As explained in Chapter 1, the physical symptoms of a thyroid imbalance are similar to those resulting from an anxiety attack. Thus, a physician evaluating a patient with a thyroid disorder may believe that what the patient is experiencing results from an anxiety disorder rather than a thyroid imbalance.

Among the most common symptoms of a panic attack are:

- Pounding heart
- Accelerated heart rate
- Sweating
- Trembling or shaking
- Sensation of shortness of breath
- Feeling of choking
- Chest pain or discomfort
- Nausea
- Feeling of dizziness, light-headedness, unsteadiness, or faintness
- Feeling of unreality or feeling disconnected from oneself
- Fear of losing control
- Fear of dying
- Numbness or tingling sensation
- Chills or hot flashes

When patients experience their first panic attack, they often go to a hospital emergency room. Because the rapid heartbeat, difficulty breathing, dizziness, and other symptoms may resemble a heart attack or other heart problem, people suffering from panic attacks, including those with a thyroid imbalance, may undergo repeated and costly cardiac and neurological evaluations. Whether a person needs to have more than one panic attack to fulfill the criteria for a panic disorder is debatable. A person who has had only one panic attack will fear having another one. It has been estimated that nearly 30 percent of the American population experience at least one panic attack in their lifetime.[22]

Too often, doctors imply that a patient's symptoms are not real or are "in your head." For someone who has just experienced a rapidly beating heart, tingling in the hands and feet, and dizziness or nausea, this is not helpful.

When panic attacks recur, people enter a vicious cycle of anticipatory anxiety—excessive worrying about when the next attack will occur. They may also become afraid to be in a place or situation from which they cannot exit quickly because of the fear that a medical catastrophe or death might happen at any time. The vicious cycle of attacks and fear of attacks becomes debilitating and leads sufferers to see physician after physician, specialist after specialist. They continue to receive the same answer: "There's nothing physically wrong with you!"—which further perplexes the patients, who know their symptoms are real.

An easy way to determine the likelihood that you may be suffering from an anxiety disorder is to complete the following questionnaire. If you answer a question with "No," proceed to the next question; if you answer with "Yes," score the severity of your symptoms (1 = mild, 2 = moderate, 3 = severe) before proceeding to the next question.

Have you intermittently been having difficulty breathing calmly?	Yes	No	_____
Do you experience feelings that something bad is going to happen?	Yes	No	_____
Do you feel tense all the time?	Yes	No	_____
Do you feel at times as if your arms and legs shake for no obvious reason?	Yes	No	_____
Do you often feel restless and unable to sit still?	Yes	No	_____
Have you had trouble falling asleep, or have you been waking up restless in the middle of the night?	Yes	No	_____
Have you been worrying excessively over trivial matters?	Yes	No	_____
Do you often feel as if you have to do things right now?	Yes	No	_____
Have you been experiencing spells of pounding heart, rapid heartbeat, and sweating?	Yes	No	_____
Have you been experiencing spells of shakiness, shortness of breath, and feelings of choking?	Yes	No	_____
Have you been experiencing spells of chest pain, nausea, light-headedness, and unsteadiness?	Yes	No	_____
Have you been experiencing spells when the world feels unreal?	Yes	No	_____
Have you been excessively afraid of dying?	Yes	No	_____
Have you been getting unexplained numbness, tingling, chills, or hot flashes?	Yes	No	_____
TOTAL SEVERITY SCORE			_____

If you answered yes to three or more of the preceding questions, you may be suffering from an anxiety disorder. If you answered yes to five or more of the questions, you are probably suffering from an anxiety disorder.

Now add the scores for each symptom to obtain your total severity score, the meaning of which was explained earlier in the chapter, in the "Depression/Anxiety Severity" table. The total severity score will be useful later in assessing your response to treatment.

Mood Swing Disorders
and Thyroid Imbalance

From birth, all human beings have mood swings that occur during the day as well as over periods of weeks and months. These swings, however, are confined to a normal range, and we adjust to them. In the normal upswing, trivial news or events may make you unusually happy. If the same events or news occurred in the normal downswing, you would experience much less happiness. Similarly, bad news or a minimal disenchantment could make you very sad if it happened during the normal downswing but might not have much effect during the normal upswing. These are "healthy" mood swings.

With mood, as with most biological variables, there is a gray zone between normal and abnormal. Biopsychiatrists see "abnormal" mood swings as being due to defects in regulatory biochemical mechanisms that normally maintain mood swings within an acceptable range. The confinement of mood within what is considered to be a normal range is tightly regulated by several brain chemicals, including serotonin and noradrenaline.

A balance of thyroid hormone in the brain is also crucial for maintaining mood stability. If you suffer from a deficit or an excess of thyroid hormone resulting from a dysfunctioning gland, you may even experience clear-cut manic-depression. For patients with an underactive thyroid, even those with low-grade hypothyroidism, depressive moods can occur unexpectedly during the day and last for hours. More severe hypothyroidism has even been blamed for causing manic-depression, with poor judgment and hallucinations. Doctors always wonder, however, whether such patients might not have preexisting minor forms of manic-depression, which have become more severe as a result of the thyroid imbalance.

Hyperthyroidism can also cause mood swings in a person who does not have a preexisting mood disorder. In some people, an overactive thyroid can result in an elated mood called "hypomania" or "mania," depending on whether the elation is moderate (hypomania involves no major behavioral disturbances) or severe (mania is associated with irrational behavior). In some patients, the thyroid condition may not be diagnosed until several years after the onset of the mood swing disorder that it caused.

By and large, if you are suffering from manic-depression you have a much higher chance of having a thyroid disorder. Psychiatrists have recognized for quite a few years that hypothyroidism is much more common in patients with manic-depression than in the general population.[23] Although the reason for this thyroid inefficiency is not always clear, one factor is that patients suffering from manic-depression are often treated with the chemical element lithium. One of the first substances recognized as a mood stabilizer, lithium has since been shown to decrease thyroid activity.

A recent study conducted on a large number of psychiatric patients in the Netherlands showed a clear association between rapid-cycling bipolar (mood swing) disorder and autoimmune thyroid disease.[24] The reasons for this link require further research. Women seem predisposed to mood swing disorders and depression when they suffer from an immune attack to the thyroid even when they are not treated with lithium. Is the immune system in these patients producing substances that affect the limbic system and alter mood and emotions, or do some thyroid antibodies cross the blood/brain barrier and affect the limbic system? Perhaps it is not only the thyroid imbalance but immune factors as well that contribute to the manic-depression.

Doctors diagnose many patients with mood swing disorders only when the thyroid condition is recognized because of how the superimposed thyroid imbalance affects mood swings. Psychiatrists and thyroid specialists who fail to consider these effects may find it difficult to obtain optimal results treating their patients.

The most common reshaping of a mood swing disorder resulting from hypothyroidism is the precipitation of severe depression and the blunting of the upswings. When hypothyroidism is superimposed on top of a mood swing disorder, the person's depression may be more pronounced and he or she may simultaneously lose touch with reality. This is frequently the point at which the individual or his or her family seeks help from a psychiatrist.

Thyroid imbalances have another important effect on the kind of mood swings a patient has. Approximately 10 to 15 percent of persons suffering from manic-depression have rapid cycling, in which episodes of depression alternating with mania occur rather frequently—more than four cycles per year. Patients whose manic-depression involves infrequent swings may change to a rapid-cycling pattern when they become hypothyroid. Although mood swing disorders occur about equally often in men and women, rapid cycling is more common in women. This is related to some extent to the coexistence of hypothyroidism. In fact, about half of the patients with rapid cycling who fail to respond to conventional treatment for bipolar disorder are hypothyroid. Some patients with mild mood swing disorders, in whom the elation and the depression are not drastic enough to be noticed when their thyroid function is normal, become more manic-depressive (having a clear-cut bipolar disorder) when they have a severe thyroid imbalance.

BEWARE OF TEENAGE BEHAVIOR

Frequently, manic-depression starts at a young age, as do Hashimoto's thyroiditis and hypothyroidism. A teenager who begins to show mood instability leading to behavioral changes may frequently be thought to have "age-related issues" or be suspected of having drug problems. Leslie, the daughter of a woman afflicted with manic-depression and hypothyroidism, exhibited drastic changes in behavior. Her mother explained:

> When everything started showing up, it showed up as attitude problems. Until it got severe, being twelve, starting her periods, and going into the teenage years were the ways it was explained. A teenager with manic-depression may be sleeping a lot, but so do many teenagers. She was being a problem in school. The teachers sent notes that she was having outbursts and that this was totally out of character.
>
> It was like an alien had entered her body. She cried every day. She started doing irrational things that she would never have done in the past. She took acid. I could see her—if it continued—reaching suicide before she reached health.

With thyroid hormone treatment and lithium, Leslie experienced a major improvement in her energy level, attitude, and concentration. Her mood stabilized. Since then, her mother made sure she took the thyroid medication every day and became compulsive about testing her thyroid quite often (maybe too often), fearing that a thyroid imbalance would trigger the rapid cycling again.

THYROID IMBALANCE AND
THE MILD MOOD SWINGS OF CYCLOTHYMIA

Cyclothymia, a long-standing condition characterized by periods of mild depression alternating with periods of slightly elated mood, often begins in late adolescence. The change in mood may be quite rapid, involving a shift from an upswing to a downswing every few days. At times, one type of mood lasts longer than the other. Frequently, the more noticeable swings are the downswings, which may be described by some as intermittently depressive moods. If you are suffering from cyclothymia, an underactive thyroid may make you experience a blunting of the upswings that results in chronic low-grade depression. Or it may make you shift continually from a happy to a depressed mood.

An overactive thyroid could also make the swings in mood more apparent and more severe. Even if you have never suffered from cyclothymia, thyroid imbalance can cause patterns of mood swings similar to those of cyclothymia.

Evelyn, aged thirty-seven, had been diagnosed with hypothyroidism fifteen years previously. She had been doing well on a stable dose of thyroid hormone and never had mood problems in the past. Then, two years ago, her general practitioner inadvertently reduced her thyroid hormone dose by half. As a result, she became hypothyroid. She also began experiencing noticeable mood swings, similar to the pattern of cyclothymia. As Evelyn described it:

> For three or four days, I could make decisions quickly. The self-confidence was there. I didn't let anybody else tell me I couldn't do something. I felt like I was on top of the world. I'd do various creative projects and activities.
>
> Three days of that, then I didn't want to do anything. I'd find it very difficult to come up with an idea for what to make for dinner. When I played bridge, I couldn't concentrate and my play would slip.

Three months after Evelyn's thyroid treatment was adjusted, her mood swings went away.

For most patients with mood swing disorders, treatments to stabilize mood do not work well when the brain is not receiving normal levels of thyroid hormones. Therefore, a mood swing patient who is also hypothyroid may be more difficult to treat. This may be due to depression causing the patient to neglect to take his or her medications. Family members of mood swing patients ought to make sure that thyroid medications are taken regularly to avoid difficult cycles. During depression, alcohol abuse may add to the pattern of self-neglect. To make matters worse, alcohol has a greater effect on a hypothyroid brain.

An End to Needless Suffering

In this chapter, we've seen how new discoveries are helping us understand thyroid disease better—especially how thyroid hormone balance affects the brain. As a result of these advances, endocrinologists and neuroscientists are focusing more on thyroid hormone because it is such an important component of brain chemistry. Unfortunately, because thyroid imbalances can go unrecognized, people experiencing psychiatric problems may not be receiving the appropriate treatment.

Endocrinology's impressive progress in finding remedies for psychic pain is overshadowed by the use—and perhaps the overuse—of antidepressants as primary solutions to brain chemistry imbalances. Yet the science of endocrinology is reaching a promising new frontier, one that begins at the border where we can resolve the effect of thyroid hormone imbalance on the mind and emotions.

Physicians stand on the verge of a breakthrough to a more complete understanding of the processes that thyroid hormones set in motion. Psychopharmacology and endocrinology are drawing closer together as disciplines, and nowhere is this more important than in the treatment of the thyroid, our annex to the brain. Thyroid hormone may even be the serotonin of the next millennium.

Important Points to Remember

- The mental and emotional consequences of a thyroid imbalance may include serious conditions such as manic-depression. More often than not, however, the symptoms are more subtle and typical of borderline or shadow syndromes, such as mild depression.
- A thyroid imbalance, in turn, magnifies the symptoms of people with mild mood disorders and emotional problems.
- Even if a hypothyroid person's symptoms do not satisfy the full criteria for depression, he or she may be experiencing borderline depression that is manifested primarily as fatigue.
- Women who have low-grade hypothyroidism, even without obvious symptoms of depression, may achieve mood benefits from taking thyroid hormone.
- Scientists now recognize thyroid hormone as a major brain biochemical that, like serotonin, has prominent effects on moods, emotions, and behavior.
- If you are suffering from depression or have had depression in the recent past, you should be tested for a thyroid imbalance, especially if you are currently experiencing other symptoms of thyroid imbalance.

6

MEDICINE FROM THE BODY:

Thyroid Hormone as an Antidepressant

Biopsychiatrists often say that the first drugs shown to alleviate depression by altering brain chemistry were lithium and imipramine, the first tricyclic antidepressant. (Developed in the mid-1950s, tricyclics were hailed for being able to "normalize" mood without causing euphoria.) In a way, however, thyroid hormone pills are one of the oldest medications known to treat depression.

In 1890, Spanish doctors implanted a sheep's thyroid gland beneath the skin of a thirty-six-year-old woman suffering from severe hypothyroidism. They noted an immediate improvement in her symptoms and appearance. This experiment inspired Dr. George Murray to extract a fluid from sheep thyroid glands the following year. He achieved spectacular results by injecting this fluid into a severely hypothyroid patient.[1]

The discovery that extracts of animal thyroid could reverse the physical and mental effects of an underactive thyroid was the first major breakthrough in the history of thyroid disease. Patients who had been institutionalized due to extreme symptoms, such as a form of madness from severe hypothyroidism, regained their sanity when they took extracts. Suddenly, underactive thyroid—once a fatal condition—became controllable, allowing afflicted people to lead normal lives.

Subsequently, the production of desiccated (dried) extract of thyroid in the form of tablets provided a more standardized form of thyroid hormone replacement for hypothyroid patients. Desiccated thyroid, commercialized as Armour thyroid, is obtained from animal thyroids. It contains both thyroxine (T4) and its by-product triiodothyronine (T3). Until the early 1970s, Armour thyroid was the most widely used thyroid hormone pill.

Even though doctors continue to prescribe the natural Armour thyroid (primarily because it contains the two principal forms of the hormone), most doctors now prefer to treat an underactive thyroid with a synthetic form of T4 (thyroxine).[2] This form of the hormone stays active longer in the body, which converts a portion of T4 into the more potent T3. Although synthetic T3 became available in the 1950s, doctors did not find it useful in treating hypothyroidism because T3 caused blood levels of thyroid hormone to fluctuate too much, and it was active in the system for a much shorter period than the synthetic thyroxine pills.

Over the years, however, many psychiatrists have used T3 in conjunction with conventional antidepressants to treat patients with major depression who failed to respond well to the antidepressants alone.[3] Even depressed patients treated with electroshock therapy appeared to have benefited from taking T3. When given T3, these patients need fewer electroshock sessions, thus helping to avoid the cognitive impairment that may result from this treatment.

In the 1990s, we are witnessing a surge in interest among psychiatrists in using and reassessing T3 as a medication to treat depression in conjunction with conventional antidepressants such as the selective serotonin reuptake inhibitors (SSRIs) like Prozac and Zoloft®.

Norma was among the first of my patients to find in T3 the solution for depression. A forty-five-year-old lawyer, Norma is divorced and shares custody of two adolescent boys. According to Norma, when she first became ill, her boys were the only reason she got out of bed at all. Norma had changed from an expansive, high-energy woman with a vibrant intellect into a listless and somewhat desperate person. Three years before I met her, Norma had gone into severe clinical depression with no apparent precipitating incident. Although her psychiatrist had treated her with conventional antidepressants, she was still exhausted and suffering from mental anguish.

Norma's relentless search for a way to get back to normal led her to insist that she be tested for a thyroid imbalance. Norma was convinced that her thyroid was the key to her illness. A well-read woman, she was familiar with the similarities between a thyroid imbalance and the symptoms of fatigue and lack of joy that plagued her. But thyroid hormone testing showed that her thyroid gland was in working order and was not at the root of her persistent symptoms.

Despite the fact that Norma's blood tests were normal, I prescribed synthetic T3 (Cytomel) in addition to Prozac, which she had been taking for the past six months. For the first time in three years, Norma regained her former sense of self. The helpless feelings, exhaustion, and sense of isolation resolved.

There was nothing wrong with Norma's endocrine system. Her symptoms were due to a mix-up in her brain's use of such biochemicals as serotonin, noradrenaline, and also thyroid hormone. Although Norma's thyroid was fine, the mechanism that distributes the hormone through her brain and transports it to where it is needed was deficient. That's why she required chemical assistance with thyroid medication.

Thyroid Hormone's Role
in ADHD and Depression

Thyroxine (T4), the main thyroid hormone produced by the thyroid, is a small molecule that contains four iodine atoms. In the cells of many organs (including the brain), a well-regulated process causes thyroxine to lose iodine, generating the much more potent thyroid hormone T3. In the brain, probably more so than in any other organ, T3 rather than T4 appears to be the critical form of the hormone that regulates cell functions. Because the amount of T3 present in the brain must remain in an optimal range to keep the mind functioning properly, fluctuations in the crucial process of converting T4 to T3 will inevitably affect the mind.

The thyroid system is one of the body's most tightly and precisely regulated systems. Minute changes in the way thyroid hormone is delivered to or dispersed in the brain can have drastic effects on mood, emotions, attention, and thinking. A problem with the delivery of T3 can cause disorders ranging from depression to attention deficit in people with normally functioning thyroids. Neuroscientists are teaching us the wide range of ways in which T3 regulates brain function and the brain chemistry syndromes that are likely to result from the alteration of thyroid hormone levels in the brains of people with normally functioning thyroid glands.

For instance, researchers recently discovered a connection between addiction to alcohol and thyroid imbalance in the brain. Free University of Berlin researcher Andreas Baumgartner conducted an experiment involving rats and alcohol.[4] He found that the animals that had slower inactivation of T3 in the amygdala—an area of the brain that plays a major role in emotions, sensory perceptions, and "reward memory"—exhibited greater behavioral dependence on alcohol. In essence, it is possible that, like rats, humans are more prone to alcoholism if that region of the brain produces more T3 from T4. High levels of T3 in some regions of the brain induced by chronic alcoholism could be part of the reason for the psychological and physical symptoms that chronic alcoholics often experience, such as irritability, aggression, sweating, and trembling. In the field of psychothyroidology, another breakthrough is the discovery that an imbalance of thyroid hormone in the brain can be responsible for attention deficit hyperactivity disorder (ADHD).

Cynthia, twenty-five years old, was referred to me by a family practitioner because of elevated thyroid hormone levels and a slightly high TSH.

She had been changing jobs on a regular basis because she was never able to concentrate well enough or stay still while working.

Cynthia had been suffering from attention deficit hyperactivity disorder since childhood, but doctors never made the connection between her attention deficit and the thyroid. She says:

> When I was younger, the teacher would be talking, and I would be off looking at the acoustic ceiling and getting totally lost. Then I would go back, and everybody would be flipping the page, and I would be trying to catch up. In class, I tried to listen to the teacher, but I couldn't understand why I didn't get it. I understood what she was saying, but I couldn't catch on. We had a comprehensive exam in English, and I tested low even though I read pretty well.
>
> Even now, I read two paragraphs and may not even remember what I read because I would be thinking of something else simultaneously. I cannot concentrate on what happens at work or what I'm going to fix for dinner. I'll be driving and not remember having driven to a certain point. I'm aware of the cars around me, but I'm not really thinking about my surroundings. At the same time I feel hyper. I can't keep my feet still. I have a lot of energy. All up and about.

Cynthia's condition turned out to be related to a familial, genetically mediated brain thyroid hormone imbalance called "syndrome of thyroid hormone resistance." In these patients, a genetic defect causes thyroid hormone to work less efficiently in the brain, pituitary, and other organs.[5] Therefore, despite high blood levels of thyroid hormone, the brain may in fact be deficient in the hormone, resulting in attention deficit.

Relatives of children with ADHD seem to be at much higher risk for having the disorder as well. Some relatives have been noted to be antisocial or depressed, perhaps as a result of how inefficiently T3 works in their brains. Adults afflicted with this condition tend to have high anxiety levels and often become drug addicts.

Because the pituitary becomes desensitized to thyroid hormone (does not sense correctly the amount of thyroid hormone in the bloodstream), higher TSH levels result, causing the thyroid gland to produce more thyroid hormone. Paradoxically, despite high levels of thyroid hormone, many of these patients exhibit symptoms of underactive thyroid function and frequently experience hyperactivity as well.

In patients suffering from generalized resistance to thyroid hormone, thyroid hormone levels could affect other chemical transmitters such as noradrenaline, which is considered to be one of the culprits in ADHD. In such patients, the behavioral symptoms, such as distractibility and restlessness, may improve with T3 treatment. Thyroid hormone treatment could be used alone or in conjunction with other medications to regulate the noradrenaline levels in the brain. A chemical analogue of T3, triiodothyroacetic acid, has recently been shown to be effective in treating the disorder.[6]

In Chapter 5 we saw that thyroid hormone is essential for the chemical noradrenaline to work as a transmitter and perform its function in the brain. In fact, the highest levels of T3 produced in the brain are present in areas that are richest in noradrenaline.[7] This striking overlap in brain regions between thyroid hormone and noradrenaline explains why, if the body is not producing enough T3 or if it is not delivering it to the brain in the right amount, you require supplemental T3 in order for noradrenaline to work effectively.

In many patients suffering from depression, the initial problem may be a low level or an abnormal distribution of T3 in the brain even though the thyroid gland produces adequate levels of thyroid hormone. The reason for this may be a lower conversion of T4 to T3 or an inability of T3 to produce its effects on brain functions efficiently. Research has also concluded that depressed patients have reduced levels of a protein called transthyretin, which normally carries T4 from the bloodstream into the brain.[8] Treatment with T3 can circumvent these delivery and conversion problems to enhance brain T3 content and thus resolve depression.

This is probably what happened to Anita. She is one of many patients I've treated who did not respond to a conventional antidepressant at first but then showed an almost miraculous response when T3 was added. A few months later, when her depression had resolved, I stopped her Zoloft but continued the T3 treatment. Her depression did not return while she was taking synthetic T3 alone. In her case, which is not necessarily the case of everyone suffering from depression, the primary source of the depression was probably an inability to generate sufficient amounts of T3. For this reason, T3 by itself eventually led to a long-term stability in mood.

Even if the primary brain chemistry problem is decreased noradrenaline or serotonin levels rather than T3, T3 levels in the brain decline as well, due to complex brain chemistry interactions. Therefore, depressed people with low noradrenaline or serotonin levels also have a low T3 content in certain regions of the brain. In essence, patients suffering depression due to either low noradrenaline or low serotonin levels in brain cells have brain hypothyroidism even though blood thyroid hormone levels are normal. To some extent, the depression caused by low serotonin or low adrenaline could be at least partly the result of low T3 levels in brain cells. In fact, antidepressants work to some extent by restoring normal T3 levels.[9]

For instance, the SSRI fluoxetine (Prozac) increases the conversion of T4 to T3 in brain cells and therefore ensure the availability of T3 in the brain. This, in turn, will raise serotonin. Other pharmaceutical treatments of depression (lithium, carbamazepine, and desipramine), and even some nonpharmaceutical ones like sleep deprivation, seem to produce some of their effects by increasing T3 levels in the brain and restoring normal serotonin levels.

The accompanying diagram illustrates the role of T3 in the maintenance of normal brain chemistry and shows how T3 treatment can help antidepressants become fully effective.

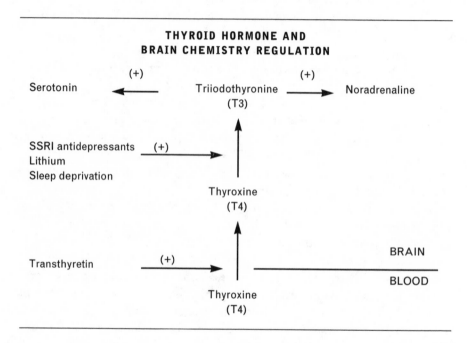

**THYROID HORMONE AND
BRAIN CHEMISTRY REGULATION**

Recent research suggests that those patients with slightly higher T4 and lower TSH levels are more likely to respond to the addition of T3 to an antidepressant.[10] These changes are consistent with some deficit of T3 in the brain. In Chapter 5, we saw how depression, whether due to low serotonin or decreased manufacture of T3, will cause the hypothalamus and pituitary to stimulate the thyroid to produce more hormone. Decreased availability of T3 in the brain causes an activation of the thyroid system, which is designed to correct the deficit of T3. But often this activation is not sufficient, and T3 levels in the brain remain suboptimal. Once a patient receives T3, the symptoms of depression resolve, T4 goes back down, and TSH goes back up to normal.

Consider the case of Melissa. She tried several antidepressants, but none of them cured her depression. It was only when T3 was added to her treatment that the depression resolved. Most likely this resistance to the antidepressant medication was caused by the persistence of low T3 levels in the brain. After she divorced her husband, Melissa said:

> My mind had a dullness. I didn't really experience life. I was dealing with the children and the tremendous amount of financial worries. I went into a depression. Sometimes I couldn't get out of bed. I went to counseling. But gradually I was not able to cope with anything. I tried to commit suicide.
>
> They first put me on Prozac, which gave me relief for a few weeks. It took a lot of inhibitions away. The second month, I started noticing the depression coming back. Then the psychiatrist thought I would do well on the tricyclic antidepressant Anafranil, and in some ways that drug was very pleasant. Things weren't quite as stressful. All the sexual function was back. I ate slower. Then the depression came back.

Melissa's depression improved and temporarily resolved in the first few months of Anafranil treatment. But the symptoms returned, possibly because of the persistence of low T3 levels. When synthetic T3 was added, at 5 micrograms three times a day, Melissa's depression went away.

"The thyroid pill was a miracle for me," she said. "Now I am like a new person. When I started on thyroid hormone, I started having energy. In the mornings, I would feel good when I got up. A lot of my self-esteem came back. I was sleeping better. The anxiety went down. The mood swings were better."

The Best Way to Use T3 in Treating Depression

Norma and Melissa are among the millions of patients suffering either clinical depression or mood swing disorders who can benefit from treatment with thyroid hormone. Research has shown that antidepressants do not work in nearly a third of patients diagnosed with depression.[11] Half of those who fail to respond to tricyclic antidepressants, for instance, improve when the potent thyroid hormone T3 is added to the antidepressant medication.

Augmenting or potentiating the action of antidepressants is not the only way T3 can be useful. Thyroid hormone treatment also accelerates the action of antidepressants. In most patients, it takes several weeks for an antidepressant to begin showing an effect on the depression. When T3 is added to the antidepressant from the outset, the antidepressant may begin to relieve the symptoms sooner. We don't know why this accelerating effect of T3 is seen only in women.

T3's effectiveness in boosting the efficacy of antidepressants in controlling depression is similar to that of lithium.[12] The patient's symptoms often respond to the addition of T3 within a few days. Therefore, if no beneficial effect has been noted within three to four weeks, T3 treatment should be stopped.

Taking T3 along with the more modern antidepressant drugs—such as the SSRIs Prozac, Zoloft, and Paxil®—seems to benefit patients who have failed to respond using these medications alone.[13] The effects of taking T3 along with the SSRIs have not been as well studied as T3 and the tricyclics. Nevertheless, several psychiatrists have shared with me their positive experiences with adding T3 to the SSRI antidepressants. Taking T3 along with an antidepressant does not work for all patients, however. One of the reasons may be the way psychiatrists administer T3 treatment, both in their clinical practices and in their research in this field. Researchers have yet to develop clear guidelines for how and when to use a combination of conventional antidepressants and T3.

In contrast to T4, T3 (Cytomel®) stays in your system for a much shorter period. Cytomel comes in 5, 25, and 50 microgram tablets. Taking a single dose of 25 micrograms of T3 in the morning, for instance, causes T3 levels to increase above the normal range for a few hours. A marked drop follows by midafternoon, resulting in wide fluctuations in the blood and perhaps to a lesser extent in brain cells. Since fluctuating T3 levels may reduce the effectiveness of the medication, I have found that dividing the total dose into two or three small doses is more effective and safer. The regimen I often prescribe is 5 micrograms three times a day (seven A.M., noon, and five P.M.), to be taken five hours apart. This is what I call "the rule of five." In severe depression, I prescribe a higher dose, such as 10 micrograms three times daily. Weeks later, with improvements in symptoms, the dose could be lowered to 5 micrograms three times a day. Using T3 treatment in this fashion, I have been surprised to observe its beneficial effects in many patients who had not responded to the SSRI antidepressants or had responded only marginally. Perhaps the secret is to provide steady levels of T3 without the major fluctuations that inevitably result from the high conventional doses given once a day by psychiatrists.

T3 alone prescribed in the way I just described may have great potential as an effective medication to treat depression, but it has not been tried frequently enough to advocate its use as a sole treatment at this time. It would theoretically work as the only medication in depressed patients whose primary chemical imbalance is a low level of T3 in the brain. But research is needed in this field. It surprised me to see that one of the first two studies examining the use of synthetic T3 as an antidepressant assessed patients who were not taking antidepressants.[14] T3 used alone was effective in treating the depression. Surprisingly, too, in several patients the required dose consisted of only 15 to 20 micrograms daily in divided doses—a regimen quite similar to what I advocate for my depressed patients.

Note, however, that no research has been conducted on the use of T3 in combination with other antidepressants such as the atypical antidepressants and monoamine oxidase inhibitors. Many psychiatrists are, however, currently combining T3 treatment with these antidepressants and are obtaining good results in some patients.

Treating Manic-Depression
with Thyroid Hormone

The discovery in the 1940s that lithium could control manic-depression marked a watershed moment in psychiatry. Until that time, doctors believed that only psychotherapy could help manic-depressive patients. Now the options available to treat mood swing disorders have been expanded to include thyroid hormone treatment.

If you or a close relative suffers from manic-depression, you probably know that this can be a devastating disorder. But it is important to keep in mind that the thyroid could be the problem and the solution for this condition.

Because the severity of mood swings varies from one person to another, often only severely disturbing up- or downswings are noticed and lead to a psychiatric evaluation. While a bipolar disorder in its severe form (manic-depression) affects nearly 1 percent of the population, 5 percent of us have minor forms that are not disturbing enough to be noticed. Many people suffering from mood swing disorders remain undiagnosed for years. Family members and friends may regard these people as being somewhat different, sensitive, or emotional, or as having an "unstable personality." Hence, people with manic-depression can suffer for many years. Many manic-depressive patients suffer primarily from recurrent depressive episodes lasting weeks or months and very few intermittent manic or hypomanic episodes. Manic-depression can be rapid-cycling, in which the swings may last hours or days, or it may follow the typical bipolar disorder pattern of no more than three or four cycles per year.

Mood swing disorders often start with an episode of depression that ends with a sudden mood upswing, although many patients may have several recurring episodes of depression before experiencing any manic episodes. In many patients, periods of abnormal mood are separated by periods of normal mood lasting months or years. Mood swing disorders often begin earlier in life than major depression. Most patients start having the wide swings in their early twenties. In manic-depressive patients, the depression may be extremely severe, with the risk of suicide. Some patients with mood swing disorders are very lethargic during their depressive period, sleep all the time, and do not experience the insomnia common in major depression.

During periods of elated mood, friends and relatives of manic-depressive individuals may consider the behavior part of their personality. When in a hypomanic state, these individuals are charming and successful in business or any other undertaking. They appear to be very organized, efficient, well adjusted, and able to achieve more than normal people. Hypomanic people have much more energy than usual and are very creative. Quite frequently, the family notices that there is something wrong with them only during the depressive period.

There is now increasing evidence that, in some people, a thyroid hormone imbalance localized in the brain, or an inability of thyroid hormone to work efficiently in certain regions of the brain, may contribute to the disorder. In such patients, the thyroid gland is functioning properly and producing adequate amounts of thyroid hormone, but the abnormality is in the brain. Correcting this abnormality by thyroid hormone treatment can lead to resolution of the mood swings.

As mood varies during the day, the amount of T3 produced in the brain by conversion from T4 also changes. Dr. Angel Campos-Barros, a researcher at the Free University of Berlin, has recently shown that the activity of the enzyme in the brain that converts T4 to T3 is subject to variations during the day.[15] This leads to fluctuations in T3 levels in certain regions of the brain. The increase in conversion of T4 to T3 in brain cells corresponds to periods of increased activity in animals. Variations in T3 levels in the brain during the day and at night could be playing an important role in normal mood swings. Body temperature also fluctuates during the day. The same variations in T3 levels could be related to these temperature fluctuations. People suffering from bipolar disorders tend to have lower temperatures during the day and higher readings at night,[16] possibly as a result of more ample changes in the levels of T3 in the brain.

If you are suffering from a mood swing disturbance called seasonal affective disorder (SAD), you may be having a problem with the delivery of adequate amounts of thyroid hormone in your brain. For some patients, SAD of the depressive type occurs annually, usually in winter or early spring. Research suggests that persons with SAD lack thyroid reserve—a shortage that becomes more pronounced in winter and spring. The seasonal variation in thyroid hormone levels (higher in winter than in summer) suggests a need for more thyroid hormone in the wintertime, when your body tends to generate more heat.[17] People unable to meet these demands may have a seasonal deficit in thyroid hormone in the brain that could account for seasonal mood abnormalities.

Recently researchers have been able to successfully treat patients suffering from manic-depression with high doses of thyroid hormones. This treatment added to lithium, for example, eliminates the wide mood swings. Lithium may not be effective when used alone.[18]

In rapid-cycling bipolar disorder, T4 adjunctive treatment (up to 500 micrograms) reduces manic and depressive symptoms as well as the number of relapses. Administering thyroid hormone can also reduce the number of cycles manic-depressive patients experience. It may change the pattern of cycling, so that these patients swing from "low" to "manic" fewer than three times a year rather than several times per day, per week, or per month. This suggests that mood swing disorders can be caused at least partly by low brain thyroid hormone levels or an inability of thyroid hormone to work efficiently in certain parts of the brain. As I explained in Chapter 5, thyroid hormone imbalance plays such a significant role in the brains of patients with manic-depression that, when their thyroid gland starts to fail, leading to minimal shortages of thyroid hormone, they begin to experience a worsening of the manic-depressive seesawing.

Many physicians and patients have wondered, however, whether high doses of thyroxine would cause harmful effects on other organs, particularly the heart and bones. Recently, a study assessed bone density in ten premenopausal women receiving high doses of levothyroxine for the treatment of manic-depression.[19] The patients exhibited no significant bone loss compared to control subjects and seemed to experience no adverse effects when given high doses of levothyroxine. This observation may imply that patients with mood swing disorders are somewhat resistant to thyroid hormone. Nevertheless, I think we need more research in this field.

At this time, I usually recommend T3 rather than levothyroxine for patients who require further treatment for manic-depression. It is clear that T3 should not be administered in doses higher than 25 to 30 micrograms a day, because if you combine the total daily production of thyroid hormone (including T4 and T3), this amount is equivalent to 25 to 30 micrograms of T3 per day in an average person. If higher doses are given, there is a risk of having too much thyroid hormone in the system.

Let me give a quick example of how T3 can help a patient with manic depression. Priscilla, aged forty-eight, had been diagnosed with manic-depression five years previously. She had tried several medications but in recent months had been taking valproic acid, an anticonvulsive medication also effective in treating manic-depression. Despite maximum doses of the drug, however, she had continued to frequently relapse into depression.

Priscilla's condition had been noticeable as far back as her teens. She had a tremendous drive and desire to do wonderful things. Her creativity flowed constantly. She had great ideas and liked to accomplish things. Her inability to bring some of these ideas to fruition was due to the fact that she would intermittently get into a depressed state and become unable to carry out her plans. Priscilla, like many bipolar patients, struggled with this discontinuity, in which periods of creativity and artistic sensitivity are typically interrupted by depressive episodes.

Priscilla described the struggle she had been enduring most of her life:

> During the depressive period, I would become more withdrawn and agitated at the same time. The depression came about very insidiously. Unless you know that you have a bipolar disorder, which I did not know most of my life, you are ignorant about what is going on. It is slow and sneaky, and before you know it, you are overwhelmed with anxiety and depression and a feeling of hopelessness.

Her sister said, "It was absolutely tragic to see what happened to Priscilla. There came a point in time when I simply said to my family that I couldn't stand by and watch Priscilla live like this. She was deteriorating in front of our eyes, and if we didn't intervene and do something to help her, we were going to lose her."

Priscilla's treatment with valproic acid helped somewhat, but the dreadful depressive periods, albeit of shorter duration, inevitably continued to haunt her. It was not until she started taking T3 in an appropriate amount that Priscilla's mood became stable and she felt better than ever. Priscilla has now been receiving thyroid hormone for three years, during which she has not experienced a single relapse of severe depression.

If you have suffered from rapid-cycling manic-depression and have not improved with conventional medications such as lithium or valproic acid, discuss with your psychiatrist the addition of thyroid hormone treatment. It may reduce the frequency of your mood cycles, and stabilize your mood for a long period of time.

T3 Treatment for Depression Must Be Carefully Monitored

The dose of T3 used to treat depression varies considerably from one psychiatrist to another. Regardless of the dose used, careful follow-up of patients and regular thyroid testing are important to avoid the serious physical and mental effects of thyroid hormone excess. Such thyroid monitoring, however, is not always done.

If a high dose of thyroid hormone is given to a patient with a psychiatric condition, hyperthyroidism may occur. Not only does the depression fail to improve, but further mental suffering is likely. The following example is of a manic-depressive patient who was followed by her psychiatrist for two years, during which she experienced tremendous mental suffering as a result of an unchecked thyroid hormone excess—an excess that her psychiatrist virtually ignored.

Natalie was thirty-seven when I first saw her for her thyroid condition. She had been diagnosed with manic-depression three years earlier, was treated with lithium, and was then prescribed T3 (Cytomel) at a dose of 50 micrograms daily. Her psychiatrist failed to do a regular follow-up, however. The excess thyroid hormone resulting from the Cytomel led to hyperthyroidism, which, in turn, caused Natalie's manic-depression to deteriorate significantly.

During her first visit to my office, Natalie said, "Initially, I noticed an increase in my energy level, but only for a short time. Then I reached a plateau. Later, the Cytomel made me progressively more sick. It was masked by the exaggerated symptoms that happen to someone on lithium, so it was deceptive and insidious. I developed such a sense of hopelessness."

When I tested Natalie, I found that her thyroid levels were very high. After she stopped the Cytomel, her thyroid levels returned to normal. She said, "It took me sixteen weeks to reach a point where I was beginning to get my thoughts back together—to be able to assess my situation rationally and reasonably. For the first time, I looked at things in terms of how I was going to make things better. That was monumental."

The Barnes and Wilson Treatment Methods

In the 1950s, it was recognized that symptoms such as fatigue, headaches, irritability, menstrual irregularities, muscle aches and pains, lethargy, and emotional instability in women could be interpreted in different ways by different doctors.[20] Based on these symptoms, an endocrinologist might diagnose hypothyroidism, whereas a psychiatrist might diagnose depression or melancholia.

The late Broda O. Barnes, M.D., Ph.D., in his book *Hypothyroidism: The Unsuspected Illness*,[21] advocated thyroid hormone treatment for people suffering from various symptoms of an underactive thyroid such as headaches, fatigue, infections, skin conditions, infertility, arthritis, and weight problems. Barnes suggested that the way to diagnose hypothyroidism and to monitor treatment is to take the patient's basal temperature. This approach was based on research he published in the early 1940s showing that hypothyroidism is associated with low basal temperature and that many people with low basal temperature and symptoms of hypothyroidism improved with thyroid hormone treatment.[22]

Some patients treated according to the Barnes method with natural thyroid hormone do indeed respond to the treatment and do indeed have hypothyroidism (see Chapter 14). Thus, a number of physicians began to advocate thyroid hormone as a treatment for patients suffering from tiredness, depression, or other nonspecific complaints accompanied by a low basal temperature—without thyroid testing. They believe that low basal temperature is always an indication of low thyroid. A low temperature, however, could merely be an indication that the patient's metabolism is slower than normal. It could also be seen in patients with depression, post–traumatic stress syndrome, eating disorders such as anorexia nervosa, and renal failure. If the symptoms improve or resolve with thyroid hormone treatment, it could in many cases be due to the antidepressant effect of the medication rather than the correction of hypothyroidism.

A depressed person's body temperature is slightly higher at night than that of a nondepressed person, but during the day, the body temperature is a little lower than that of a nondepressed person. Because depression impairs thermal regulation, utilizing body temperature as the only indicator of a thyroid hormone deficiency is clearly inappropriate. Also, a decrease in temperature is not sensitive enough to diagnose hypothyroidism. Only profound, severe hypothyroidism causes low temperature. Increasingly, though, doctors who use the Barnes method for diagnosing hypothyroidism are monitoring their patients with blood tests. Ideally, the use of body temperature to diagnose and monitor treatment of hypothyroidism should be abandoned.

In recent years, other doctors have advocated the use of thyroid hormone to treat symptoms that follow a major stress, attributing them to low levels of T3 in our bodies. These doctors also use basal temperature as an indication of low thyroid levels in organs and to monitor thyroid hormone treatment.

For instance, Dr. E. Denis Wilson, in his book *Wilson's Syndrome: The Miracle of Feeling Well*, described a particular syndrome as a cluster of debilitating symptoms brought on especially by significant physical or emotional stress that can persist even after the stress has passed.[23] Wilson attributed this persistence to maladaptive slowing of the metabolism, characterized by a body temperature that runs, on average, below normal, and thyroid blood tests that are often in the normal range. Curiously, many of the symptoms he referred to—fatigue, depression, headaches, migraines, premenstrual syndrome (PMS), anxiety, panic attacks, irritability, hair loss, decreased motivation and ambition, inappropriate weight gain, decreased memory and concentration, insomnia, and intolerance to heat and cold—are symptoms of depression. He also included irritable bowel syndrome, delayed healing after surgery, and even asthma.

Wilson postulated that this suffering results from a deficit in the activity of the enzyme that converts T4 to T3 brought on by physical or mental stress. He hypothesized that a decrease of T3 in the organs causes a slowing of the metabolism, reflected by a drop in temperature.

Wilson also postulated that the decrease in the enzyme responsible for the conversion of T4 to T3 and the reduction in metabolism occurring as a result of the stress do not return to normal after the stress has passed. Therefore, despite normal thyroid levels in the blood, hypothyroidism remains as a residual effect of post–traumatic stress syndrome. In his book, Wilson recommended treating patients having this constellation of symptoms with a high dose of T3 and monitoring and adjusting the T3 dose based on basal temperature, rather than on thyroid testing.

The logical explanation for Wilson's observations is that, during and following stressful events, a person may begin to suffer from depression (resulting in low brain T3 levels because of impaired conversion of T4 to T3). This could persist for a long time after the stressful period, leading to a brain deficit of thyroid hormone. Therefore, "Wilson's syndrome" is merely a combination of the symptoms of depression and/or post–traumatic stress syndrome following major stresses.

Several symptoms—such as migraines, PMS, panic attacks, night sweats, and mood swings—may be closely related to thyroid hormone deficit in the brain rather than in the other organs. Furthermore, in these patients, there seems to be no scientific basis for true hypothyroidism in organs other than the brain. The mechanisms that tightly regulate the thyroid hormone level in the brain are quite different from those in other organs. Even if some of the patients diagnosed as having Wilson's syndrome are truly hypothyroid, they should not be treated with such high doses of thyroid hormone as to make them hyperthyroid.

Treating patients indiscriminately with high doses of T3, failing to do thyroid testing, and adjusting the dose only according to basal body temperature is unacceptable even for thyroid specialists who have developed an expertise in the interaction between the brain and the thyroid. T3 therapy for either depression or post–traumatic stress syndrome should be carefully monitored by both thyroid function testing and clinical assessment.

Kathleen, a thirty-seven-year-old nurse, was referred to me by a friend of hers. Her amazing story illustrates how the mislabeling of suffering and inappropriate use of thyroid hormone can result in further suffering. When I saw Kathleen for the first time, she brought with her a pile of temperature charts and a sheet outlining a complicated protocol of thyroid hormone treatment based on checking basal temperature that was given to her by a physician three months previously. The doctor had diagnosed Kathleen with Wilson's syndrome and told her to take T3 (Cytomel) three times a day. She was to adjust the Cytomel dose according to temperature readings taken three times a day. As long as her average daily temperature was lower than 97.8 degrees Fahrenheit, she was to increase her dose of Cytomel. She was guided during treatment by a manual for Wilson's syndrome.

Before she began having symptoms, Kathleen was experiencing tremendous stress at home dealing with a chronically ill husband and serious financial difficulties. Although her symptoms fit the description of Wilson's syndrome, they were all symptoms of depression as well. When given a very high amount of T3, Kathleen became severely hyperthyroid, which resulted in severe anxiety symptoms, hypomanic behavior, and irregular heartbeat.

I urge doctors who treat hypothyroidism and depression to monitor their patients with thyroid testing and not use doses of thyroid hormone that exceed what the body and brain need to function properly.

Important Points to Remember

- If you are suffering from depression, mood swing disorders, alcoholism, or attention deficit disorder, the root of the problem may be a thyroid hormone imbalance or a disturbance in the way thyroid hormone works in some parts of your brain.
- Increasing evidence indicates that T3, the most active form of thyroid hormone, is an effective antidepressant, when used in conjunction with a conventional antidepressant.
- If you have been suffering from depression but your antidepressant has not fully worked for you, adding 5 micrograms of synthetic T3 three times a day may resolve the depression.
- If you are about to start taking an antidepressant, you may want to consider adding 5 or 10 micrograms of T3 three times a day. This is likely to speed up the effects of the antidepressant. Remember that it usually takes two to three weeks for an antidepressant to start working on the symptoms of depression.
- If you have been combining an antidepressant with T3 and have done very well, discuss with your psychiatrist the possibility of decreasing the dose of the antidepressant.
- If you are taking thyroid hormone to treat the symptoms of depression, do not rely on your basal temperature to tell you whether you are doing well. Have your doctor test your blood levels of thyroid hormone and evaluate your symptoms.

PART II

NO, YOU ARE
NOT MAKING IT UP:

Common Emotional
and Physical Interactions

7

WEIGHT, APPETITE, AND
METABOLISM:

The Thyroid's Actions

Julie, a twenty-four-year-old graduate student, was normally a cheerful, outgoing person. As a result of an underactive thyroid, however, she had started to gain weight, which caused her to become mildly depressed. Her weight problem affected her self-esteem to such an extent that she began to become shy and withdrawn. She said:

> I had to watch everything that went into my mouth, because I was afraid of becoming fatter. But I had a huge appetite, and I ate anyway. I felt guilty about it. I would not go out to eat with anybody except one dear friend. I wouldn't eat in the cafeteria because I didn't want anyone, especially male friends, to see me eating.
>
> I didn't have the energy or enough of a sense of well-being to go out to parties. I felt like I wasn't good enough. I used to like to go out dancing, but I began to think that if I asked any of my male friends to go with me, they'd say no. When guys would call and ask me out, I would say I was busy.

Julie's experience was typical of the vicious cycle of thyroid imbalance, weight problems, and emotional conflicts and serves to demonstrate again the intricacies of the relationship between brain and thyroid. Julie's weight gain resulted from three factors:

1. A slowing of metabolism due to the underactive thyroid
2. A decrease in caloric expenditure from getting less physical exercise, both because Julie was always tired and because she had less tolerance for exercise
3. Depression and anxiety, resulting in overeating and a lowering of

Julie's self-esteem, which prevented her from going out, thereby further reducing her caloric expenditure

These three interrelated factors resulted in a significant weight gain.
Julie herself blamed her depression and reduced self-esteem on her weight
problem, when in fact at the core of her problem was a thyroid imbalance.
When treatment began to address Julie's hypothyroid condition, all three
factors—metabolism, reduced burning of calories, and depression-related
overeating and lowered self-esteem—were resolved. Julie began to lose
weight, her confidence returned and her outlook brightened, and she once
again became more physically active.

Although, as we'll see, not all weight problems can be blamed on
thyroid-related conditions, Julie's battle with weight gain is one faced by
many people, and by women in particular. A study published in the *Journal
of the American Medical Association* in 1994 examined the prevalence
of obesity among adults living in the United States.[1] It found that one-
third of adults between the ages of twenty and seventy-four were overweight during the 1988–91 period. Furthermore, women in each of the race
and ethnic groupings studied—which included non-Hispanic whites, non-
Hispanic African-Americans, and Mexican-Americans—were more likely
to be overweight than men were. The study also showed that half of non-
Hispanic African-American and Mexican-American women were overweight and that women are more frequently overweight today than they
were twenty years ago.

The social and cultural challenges faced by overweight women can be
tremendous, due to the pressures to be slim. Many women claim that they
eat virtually nothing, but they still have weight problems. The reason many
of these women have difficulty losing weight, despite exercise and dieting, is
probably a slow metabolism. The growing awareness that an underactive
thyroid can result in weight gain by slowing metabolism, coupled with
despair over their inability to find a reason for the weight gain and lose the
weight, has led increasing numbers of people to seek medical help and insist
that their thyroids be tested.

Physicians in general and thyroid specialists in particular often deal with
women who are frustrated with their weight problems and believe that a
thyroid condition is causing them. What is even more frustrating to these
women is that many of them turn out not to have a thyroid condition.
Nevertheless, there is no doubt that thyroid disease may be responsible for
frustrating weight problems that, for many women, cannot be corrected
without appropriate treatment of the thyroid condition. Equally important,
though, is the need to take care of the mind as well as the body, before and
even after correction of the imbalance.

Understanding Your Eating Behavior

Appetite, eating behavior, and weight gain are all regulated in certain parts of the brain by the interaction of nerve cells tightly linked to brain cells involved in emotions, mood, and perception of stress. Some of the chemical transmitters in the brain that regulate emotions, mood, and stress are the same chemicals implicated in the complex interactions regulating satiety, food selection, and even taste.[2] The chemical beta-endorphin, one of the body's natural opioid or painkilling substances, creates a rewarding chemical effect in the brain in response to the stimulus of eating. Stress stimulates the release of endorphins, which then affect eating behavior. Naloxone, a molecule that counteracts the effect of opioids in the brain, reduces the binge-eating behavior of bulimic patients.[3]

Other brain chemicals such as the neurotransmitters noradrenaline, GABA (gamma-aminobutyric acid), and serotonin, which are implicated in mood disorders and anxiety, also affect eating behavior.[4] The body's noradrenaline-using system stimulates carbohydrate ingestion and affects how much we eat. While a person is eating, serotonin rises in the brain to a point at which the hypothalamus senses a feeling of satiety, and then it inhibits food intake by reducing the size and duration of meals. Chemical substances that elevate serotonin levels in the brain decrease carbohydrate intake but do not affect the intake of proteins. While noradrenaline increases the desire for fats and carbohydrates, serotonin decreases the desire for both. Changes and interactions among these and many other chemicals and hormones in the brain affect not only your appetite—how frequently you eat and when you end a meal—but also which foods you choose to eat.[5] Frequently, when people are depressed, serotonin levels are low, and as a result, they tend to crave fats and carbohydrates and to consume larger portions of food. An unavailability of serotonin may explain why a depressed person eats to excess without reaching full satisfaction and a feeling of satiety.

Weight gain or loss is so commonly associated with depressed mood that weight changes are typically looked upon as major symptoms of depression. Depressed people, regardless of whether they are hypothyroid, may not admit to overeating. This is because overeating is often the result of an impulse triggered by low serotonin levels in an attempt to ease or relieve the low mood and anxiety. Food is viewed as a way to feel better, to increase comfort. Typically, individuals suffering from serotonin deficiency report an improvement in their mood after consuming carbohydrates.

This link between weight and the serotonin-using system has been further corroborated by the fact that modern antidepressants as well as drugs used for weight control and the treatment of obesity, such as fenfluramine (Pondimin®) and dexfenfluramine (Redux®, which has been withdrawn from the market), work by affecting serotonin availability or activity. Sibu-tramine (Meridia®), the recently approved medication for weight control in obese people, decreases appetite by affecting both serotonin and noradrena-line in the brain.[6] In fact, researchers first tested sibutramine as an antide-pressant before they discovered its impressive effects on weight control.

Dr. Thomas Carew, chairman of psychology at Yale University, has noted that serotonin is "only one of the molecules in the orchestra. But rather than being the trumpet or the cello player, it's the band leader who choreographs the output of the brain."[7] Thyroid hormone in the brain is certainly an important instrument, and its alteration will disturb the har-mony of the orchestra.

How Thyroid Hormone Affects
Both Eating Behavior and Metabolism

Thyroid hormone plays a major role in regulating eating behavior. Certainly it affects and interacts with some of the chemical transmitters involved in eating behavior. For example, an excess or a deficiency of thyroid hormone alters the levels of beta-endorphin, noradrenaline, GABA, and serotonin, the same molecules that regulate eating behavior.[8] Thyroid hormone also has direct effects on appetite centers in the brain. Excess thyroid hormone in the brain, for instance, causes a person to eat more often and to select carbohy-drates rather than other types of food.[9]

The recently discovered hormone leptin, which is produced by fat tissue, appears to be the most important chemical that regulates our metabo-lism. Leptin promotes a reduction in caloric intake and an increase in meta-bolic rate. When you do not eat for a long period of time, leptin levels decrease and lead to changes in the endocrine system that result in slowed metabolism—and thus a tougher time losing weight. Likewise, in people struggling with obesity, leptin does not work efficiently. This results in an increase in caloric intake and in a slowing of metabolism. When the potent thyroid hormone T3 is not delivered in sufficient amounts, leptin becomes inefficient in enhancing metabolism.[10] This inefficiency also increases your cravings. If, on the other hand, you are one of the many people attempting to cope with low metabolism due to inefficient leptin, this inefficiency will make the thyroid hormone in your body less effective at burning calories.

Severe hypothyroidism is often associated with weight gain and an inability to lose weight by dieting. This weight gain is best explained by the slowing of the body's metabolism, so that the breakdown of fat and energy is much lower than normal.[11] Severe hypothyroidism may also result in depression and anxiety, triggering increased caloric intake. Low serotonin in the brain resulting from an underactive thyroid contributes to a craving for carbohydrates and overeating.

The craving for carbohydrates and even the bingeing that thyroid patients may experience explains why some may be temporarily misdiagnosed as having reactive hypoglycemia, a condition characterized by low glucose (sugar) in the blood. (See Chapter 10 for more information on hypoglycemia.)

Often people who are hypothyroid lose control of their eating patterns and cannot follow the nutritional and lifestyle guidelines necessary to alter caloric intake and boost mood. They may no longer be able to schedule meals and snacks or choose mood-enhancing foods. The increased caloric intake coupled with low metabolism may result in significant weight gain, often as much as twenty to thirty pounds. Hypothyroid women who gain weight are often more aware of their weight gain than nonhypothyroid women simply because of their anxiety, depression, and insecurity, all of which are heightened by the added weight.

Frequently, hypothyroidism causes someone who has been exercising regularly to stop due to tiredness, muscle weakness, shortness of breath, and depression. The lack of exercise coupled with an increased appetite, also due to the thyroid condition, may result in rapid and significant weight gain, which can cause profound depression.

Candace is an attractive young woman who had been married for two years when I saw her. She used to be a health-conscious, physically fit person who made going to the gym and exercising part of her daily routine. Her lifestyle gradually began to change when she started feeling tired, sleeping more, and noticing other symptoms of hypothyroidism. When she was hypothyroid, keeping her weight down was a struggle. She told me:

> When I started to gain weight, I didn't want to be around any of my friends. I didn't want to go out dancing or drinking. I didn't want to do anything, mostly because I didn't feel good about the way I looked after gaining so much weight. But I was also becoming inactive as a result of my tiredness. I went to my primary care physician twice because of the weight gain and the fatigue. I figured something had to be wrong.
>
> I was eating a lot more, constantly nibbling. I don't know if it made me feel stronger physically or better mentally. I would start off every day being careful and eating grapefruit, but by the afternoon I would get really tired and break down. I'd start craving something, often a sweet. If I had it, I seemed to enjoy it more than before.
>
> Normally, when I exercise, I find that it helps to suppress my appetite. Almost overnight, I went from running three to six miles per day to not working

out at all. I began to eat more, but not enough to gain thirty pounds. As I gained weight, I became irritable. As a result of the irritability, I ate more and gained more weight. I would sit for hours in the dark and quiet.

I lost control over everything. I'd wake up and say, "I'm going to eat right today." But by the end of the day, I didn't care. While going home, I couldn't make it twenty feet out of my way to stop at a grocery store to buy decent food. I'd stop and get a hamburger, go home to eat it, and then go to sleep. The cycle took complete control of my life.

Lectures on willpower have no effect on people who are suffering like Candace. They simply cannot continue eating a healthy diet and exercising as they used to. Candace's mother said, "We went on Jenny Craig together. The diet worked perfectly for me, but not for her. She kept cheating and didn't have the willpower to do it. She was depressed and crying."

Candace's case illustrates the vicious cycle frequently generated in hypothyroid people—a cycle in which hypothyroidism triggers depression and low self-esteem, which are then coupled with changes in metabolism. The depression contributes substantially to the weight gain, and the weight gain exacerbates the depression. Although these people feel as if their increased eating could not possibly be causing such rapid weight gain, they fail to take into account that they typically become less active physically. In this setting, when doctors diagnose hypothyroidism and administer appropriate treatments, people will lose the weight and the depression. So the vicious cycle can be broken at two levels—by enhancing the metabolism and by alleviating the depression.

Why Weight Problems May Persist
Even after the Thyroid Imbalance Is Corrected

Many women who gain weight when they are hypothyroid don't fall back to their original weight even after their thyroid condition has been corrected with thyroid hormone treatment. Physicians and others often attribute the lingering weight to a lack of effort on the patient's part to reverse the gain. Quite frequently, however, the increased caloric intake that began during hypothyroidism persists as a result of ongoing low mood or anxiety. This, in turn, causes difficulties in coping with the weight problem. The weight problem itself may contribute to perpetuating the low mood. In these women, thyroid hormone treatment has been unable to break the vicious cycle described earlier. Hypothyroidism causes people to become much less physically active, which perpetuates the weight problems. The reduced physical activity has caused the muscle mass to decrease, leaving the person with a slower metabolism than before the onset of the thyroid imbalance.

This is a typical dead end faced by many thyroid patients who may persist in thinking that their thyroid is still not regulated and continues to be responsible for their weight problem. Because of this belief, physicians caring for the thyroid condition face dissatisfied, unhappy patients who feel they are not receiving answers, guidance, or explanations.

This dead end is frequently the result of hidden effects from the thyroid condition, however, and from the fact that thyroid hormone treatment by itself is simply not sufficient. Many patients will need to follow a strict diet and a regular exercise program to return to their ideal weights. The exercise program should aim at not only burning extra calories, but also building up the muscle mass that was lost during the imbalance. At least now their medication will have eliminated their cravings and fatigue, which had prevented them from losing weight before their diagnosis.

In many cases, though, the occurrence of hypothyroidism has triggered marital, familial, or work problems, which may also persist after thyroid treatment. As a result, the environment in which the patient lives may have become—and may remain—more stressful than before the disease's onset. This stress and the depression that may have resulted (although originally caused by the hypothyroidism) may perpetuate the weight gain if they are not addressed.

When their weight gains persist after thyroid treatment, patients often feel very frustrated. Physicians should anticipate this frustration and explain clearly why exercise, diet, and counseling may be necessary, as I recommend above. Yet many do not appreciate or sympathize with the mind-body changes their patients have just undergone and the confusion they may feel in having had to redefine who they really are. Patients often need help and direction in dealing with the stress and the life problems they face. Patients who still don't feel well after their treatments will have difficulty initiating and maintaining a weight-reduction program based on a healthy diet and exercise. Psychological counseling and addressing the underlying psychosocial factors, as well as the use of appetite suppressants and, in severe cases, appropriate anxiety or depression medications, should help them. Mind-body medicine together with diet and exercise can provide significant help in controlling the weight problem.

After hypothyroidism is corrected, some patients will feel appreciably less depressed, others only moderately less depressed, and some hardly any less depressed. Why low moods persist has not been extensively studied. Most likely this continued low mood is linked to lower-than-normal serotonin levels, either because T3 is less available in the brain or because of chronic stress that resulted from the effects of hypothyroidism and continues after treatment. Regardless of the exact reasons, a healthy diet and an exercise program are the keys to recovering fully. (See Chapter 18 for specific diet and exercise information.)

Does a Mildly Underactive
Thyroid Cause Weight Problems?

The most severe weight problems experienced by hypothyroid patients tend to occur in those with a severe deficit of thyroid hormone. Severe hypothyroidism occurs in only 2 percent of the population, however. You may wonder, then, whether thyroid imbalance does indeed contribute significantly to the weight problems that half the population is facing. Clearly, the contribution would be minimal if one considered only the effects of moderate or severe hypothyroidism. However, at least 5 to 7 percent of the population suffers from low-grade hypothyroidism.[12] Researchers have done few well-controlled studies that could help us determine whether low-grade hypothyroidism is responsible for weight problems.

One study conducted on a small number of patients determined that thyroid hormone treatment did not make patients with low-grade hypothyroidism lose weight.[13] This study, however, did not look into the long-term effects of low-grade hypothyroidism on mood and weight. Many doctors treat women who are predisposed to weight gain because of stress, depression, or lack of exercise and also gain weight from low-grade hypothyroidism. In these women, correcting the thyroid condition helps them achieve their desired weight loss only if the other factors have been addressed and their depression has fully lifted with treatment. Therefore, we should not discount low-grade hypothyroidism as an important reason for the weight problems that some women are facing. Weight gain should be a reason for thyroid testing, particularly if you are also suffering from emotional and physical symptoms of hypothyroidism.

When Your Gland Is Overactive

Many women with an overactive thyroid are pleased with the weight loss resulting from their condition. The weight gain that they experience when they begin taking medication to correct the overactive thyroid can be a disappointment. I have seen women who stopped taking their thyroid medication on purpose! If the other symptoms of hyperthyroidism are not so severe, they prefer to continue putting up with these symptoms rather than regain the weight. This is something I try to discourage. If left untreated, excess thyroid hormone in your system can eventually lead to heart problems, bone loss and osteoporosis, and many other debilitating conditions.

This desire to lose weight at any cost applied in the case of Audrey, aged thirty-two, who had had some weight problems most of her life but became slim when she became hyperthyroid. I started her on antithyroid medication and asked her to return for a follow-up with repeat thyroid testing. Displeased with the weight gain after only three weeks of treatment, Audrey stopped taking the medication and returned to see me eight months later, still hyperthyroid.

When I asked her why she had not followed through with her treatment, Audrey replied honestly:

> First, I started going through denial. I started feeling good, a little normal. The underlying fact was, I knew all that weight loss was artificial. I never did a thing to lose the weight. I knew I would start gaining all that weight back. I played along with the idea that it wasn't so bad. I told myself, I don't feel that bad, so I'll just stop taking the medication. The medication started making me gain the weight back. My husband was always on top of me about the medication. "You need to take it every day. You're not supposed to miss it."
>
> We went on vacation, and I purposely left it at home. He found out and made me go to a pharmacy that was able to fill the prescription. I still didn't take it for the two weeks we were there. I had finally gotten into something different than the one-piece bathing suit I had always worn. I had a two-piece and I remember thinking there is no way I'm going to take this medication and gain weight while I'm down here. Even after I came back home from vacation, I had an appointment with you afterward. I thought, Oh, man, if he does lab work, he's going to see I haven't taken it in a while. I was in denial that there wasn't anything badly wrong with me and that the disease was not really so bad because I was looking better.

Prompt treatment of the overactive thyroid is extremely important to halt all the deleterious effects of excess thyroid hormone on the body and mind. While getting their thyroids regulated, patients should adhere to commonsense principles to achieve optimal weight control.

It is not necessarily true that an overactive thyroid always results in weight loss, just as it is a mistake to believe that an underactive thyroid always causes weight gain. In fact, some women with an overactive thyroid gland gain weight instead of losing it.[14] What happens in these cases of hyperthyroidism is that the increased body metabolism, which tends to reduce fat storage, is coupled with increased caloric intake. Hyperthyroid patients often crave food and eat large amounts, much more than they used to, because of thyroid hormone's direct effect on the mechanism for appetite regulation, which is located in the brain. The increased caloric intake is probably a defense mechanism designed to preserve the body's energy when it is flooded with thyroid hormone.

A good example of this can be seen in the case of Jessica, who developed Graves' disease at the age of thirty. Prior to the onset of her thyroid condition, she had always been slim and physically fit. When her thyroid became overactive, in addition to the typical symptoms of hyperthyroidism, she experienced a significant weight gain, which made her quite depressed and increased her irritability. She said:

> I felt exhausted and tired, and I was depressed, with crying spells. There was a definite increase in appetite while I was gaining. I don't know if it was appetite or because I was so exhausted, but I ate more to satisfy myself. It took a while to find the right dosage of medication to make me feel better again. While I was taking the medication, I lost weight because my thyroid was getting better and I made a very special effort. I was extremely careful and managed to lose all the weight. I had to be very strict.

Quite often, the increased fat breakdown and energy loss generated by the excess of thyroid hormone significantly exceed the hyperthyroid patient's caloric intake, and this negative balance will lead to a weight loss. In some people, however, the effect on the appetite center and the increased caloric intake resulting both from the thyroid hormone excess and from the severe anxiety caused by hyperthyroidism or depression could exceed the amount of calories burned as a result of enhanced metabolism. The resulting positive balance will cause weight gain, which can be as significant as the weight gain hypothyroid patients may experience.

Because the weight gain resulting from an overactive thyroid can be as depressing for the hyperthyroid person as for the hypothyroid one, mind-body treatment is important for controlling stress and anxiety.

Hyperthyroid patients are often not warned that, after their condition is corrected, they could begin to gain weight. The weight problem itself could then cause or contribute to significant anxiety and low mood. Frequently, women who have lost weight as a result of hyperthyroidism gain a significant amount of weight when their thyroid condition is treated appropriately and corrected. After correction of hyperthyroidism, their weight may be even greater than it was before they became hyperthyroid. One study showed that nearly half the women treated for hyperthyroidism experienced a significant weight gain after their thyroid function became normal.[15] Although many patients may believe that their thyroid has become underactive and is therefore responsible for the weight gain, the mechanism for the weight gain in this case is entirely different.

There are three primary reasons for the rebound weight gain experienced by hyperthyroid patients when their thyroid condition is regulated:

1. When the body is exposed to too much thyroid hormone, its metabolic activity shifts to a higher level. After normal thyroid function is restored, metabolism returns to a lower level.

2. If the excess thyroid hormone has disturbed the appetite center, the disturbance may persist even after the thyroid function is corrected. This could lead to residual effects, including increased appetite and increased caloric intake.

3. Hyperthyroidism causes a breakdown of energy stores, not only in body fat but also in muscle tissues. Many hyperthyroid patients may experience some loss of muscle mass as a result of their condition. The most significant muscle loss tends to occur in muscles such as the quadriceps and biceps. Once thyroid levels have become normal, the compensatory rebound of building up energy stores will be directed at building up fat rather than muscle. One study showed that correction of hyperthyroidism is spontaneously accompanied by a 20 to 40 percent increase in muscle performance, although the muscle strength remains lower than normal.[16] For this reason, exercise and physical activity aimed at building up muscle mass that was lost during hyperthyroidism will enhance the person's metabolism and help prevent weight gain after hyperthyroidism is corrected.

Controlling Your Weight

With support from your physician, family, and loved ones, you can take steps to counteract the effect of a thyroid condition on your weight once your thyroid imbalance is corrected. In some cases, it may be helpful to take an appetite suppressant such as sibutramine (Meridia) as thyroid levels become normal. However, doctors typically prescribe appetite suppressants only if the body mass index (BMI) is higher than 30. The BMI, which gives doctors a measure of the severity of a weight problem, is calculated by a formula that factors in weight and height. A BMI score in the range of 20 to 26 is considered healthy.

But appetite suppressants are not magic bullets for weight loss. Although sibutramine, for example, enhances satiety, reduces fat intake, and facilitates the burning of calories through its effects on "brown" fat tissue, it has side effects, as do most other appetite suppressants. These side effects, which seem to be rare, include rapid heartbeat and an increase in blood pressure. Using sibutramine for a couple of months, though, may help you start the mind-body program that will enable you to maintain your ideal weight.

Another recently introduced weight-loss medication for overweight people is Orlistat, which works on fat absorption. This medication, however, can cause a deficit in vitamins and may result in diarrhea. Because it might also affect the absorption of your thyroid medication, I do not highly recommend this drug.

To promote weight loss, regular exercise at least four to five days a week, healthy eating habits, and high-fiber products are a better approach for most people than long courses of appetite suppressants. Lifestyle modifications like these can help maintain high serotonin levels without the need to take serotonin-altering medications.

Diet can be especially important. Serotonin is derived in the brain from an essential amino acid, tryptophan. As is true for all amino acids, tryptophan is found only in proteins. Consuming high amounts of most protein foods, however, does not significantly affect brain serotonin levels because other amino acids in the protein compete with tryptophan for passage into the brain. Some complex carbohydrates, however, selectively promote the passage of tryptophan into the brain. Animal research has confirmed that eating a high-complex-carbohydrate meal increases tryptophan and serotonin levels. Therefore, in your diet program, increase your consumption of complex carbohydrates to alleviate depression.

If your depression is significant and persistent, you may find that a serotonin-altering medication such as a selective serotonin reuptake inhibitor (SSRI) will help you with the depression and the weight.

An option that has worked well for some of my patients who repeatedly gain weight despite correction of hypothyroidism is to take thyroid hormone treatment in the form of a T4/T3 combination. Treating these people with synthetic thyroxine alone may not provide all the T3 needed to regain normal metabolism. The full amount of thyroid hormone required to maintain a normal thyroid function can be given primarily in the form of synthetic thyroxine, together with a small amount of T3. Delivering this extra T3 might also help the hormone leptin to increase metabolism. Besides having an effect on peripheral metabolism, T3 treatment may affect the brain chemicals that control eating behavior.

Not long ago, tryptophan pills were commercially available and widely used for the treatment of serotonin-related conditions such as appetite control, depression, anxiety, insomnia, and symptoms of premenstrual syndrome. Unfortunately, in 1989, a contamination problem with tryptophan produced by a Japanese company caused more than three dozen deaths. The federal government responded by banning the sale of all tryptophan supplements, a ban that remains in force today.

To manage food cravings, you may find it helpful to take a tryptophan substitute such as 5-hydroxytryptophan (5-HTP), a related amino acid that has begun to be sold as a nutritional supplement in the past few years. Talk to your doctor about its potential risks and benefits. Also, you should avoid calorie-rich, refined carbohydrates, such as cookies, ice cream, doughnuts, cakes, and pastries. Avoid saturated fat as well. Instead, consume a diet rich in healthy, serotonin-enhancing complex carbohydrates, such as pasta, vegetables, fresh fruits, crackers with no added sugar, whole-grain bread, and low-fat, unsweetened muffins.

Do not rush into a low-calorie diet (800–1,200 calories per day)—such as those promoted by Slim Fast, Jenny Craig, or Nutri/System—or a very-low-calorie diet (less than 800 calories per day), such as those promoted by Optifast and Medifast. When my patients rely exclusively on low-calorie diets to solve their weight problems quickly, they often regain the weight because it is hard to continue such diets indefinitely. Rather, follow a "balanced-deficit diet," which takes into account how many calories you burn a day. A balanced-deficit diet provides approximately 20 percent fewer calories than you would require to maintain your current weight. (You can get an approximate idea of the total calories that would maintain your current weight by multiplying your weight in pounds by fifteen, assuming you have a moderate level of physical activity.) You can follow a balanced-deficit diet just by changing the type of food you eat (avoid foods rich in refined sugar and animal fats) rather than by reducing the amount of food and counting calories (for more details, see Chapter 18). Certainly, the weight loss will be slow. But it is a sure way of achieving your goal if at the same time you take charge of your lifestyle and exercise. Use the "Dietary Guidelines for Americans" published by the U.S. Department of Health and Human Services[17] to guide you on the types of food you should avoid.

Weight problems related to thyroid imbalance are no myth. Although the majority of people concerned about weight problems do not have thyroid disease, some people do have a thyroid imbalance that could either play a primary role or simply be a contributing factor. There is no doubt that people struggling with weight problems should ask themselves the question, "Is it my brain or my thyroid?" Sorting out the answer, with the help of their physicians, will guide them in determining how to obtain help in losing weight and feeling better.

Important Points to Remember

- Thyroid imbalances can cause weight gain or loss by changing body metabolism, by altering dietary and lifestyle factors, and by promoting depression and lowering self-esteem.

- Thyroid hormone interacts in the brain and body with some of the same biochemicals that play key roles in eating behavior, including beta-endorphin, noradrenaline, leptin, and serotonin.
- Some of the physical effects of hypothyroidism—such as tiredness, muscle weakness, shortness of breath, and depression—can derail plans for regular exercise and thereby contribute to rapid and significant weight gain.
- Although some people may welcome the short-term weight-reducing effects of an overactive thyroid, the long-term consequences of untreated hyperthyroidism are dramatic and may include heart problems, bone loss and osteoporosis, and many other debilitating conditions.
- After a thyroid imbalance has been corrected, it is important to follow a healthy diet, get plenty of exercise, and arrange for support from your doctor and family to maintain proper weight.

8

HORMONES OF DESIRE:

The Thyroid and Your Sex Life

When I began my career in the thyroid field, it never crossed my mind that I would play the role of marriage counselor. Most of the time when patients have marital or sexual difficulties as a result of a thyroid imbalance, I refer them to a couples therapist or a sex therapist. Yet sex therapy or couple therapy may not be successful unless I take the initiative to counsel the patient and explain the effects of thyroid imbalance on sexual function. It is indeed the role of the doctor who is treating the thyroid disorder to explain that the thyroid imbalance is the source of these difficulties and guide the couple in resolving their marital problems. The doctor also needs to communicate with the psychotherapist and explain how the thyroid imbalance can generate these problems.

Both hypothyroid and hyperthyroid patients experience changes in their sexuality. Some of the examples discussed in this chapter can shed light on important aspects of how the thyroid affects sexual desire and activity.

Beatrice and Leonard had been married for almost fifteen years and had a daughter. The CEO of a large company, Leonard was quite successful, and the family was wealthy. During most of their marriage, they had a happy, stable relationship. All this changed rather suddenly.

Beatrice's gynecologist referred her to me because he had noted a goiter and a tremor in her hands. Tests showed that Beatrice's thyroid levels were high. In my first encounter with Beatrice, I established that she had Graves' disease, and I started her on treatment. A few days later, I received a call from Leonard, who wanted to discuss some issues with me. He told me his wife had been unfaithful in recent months, and because of this, he was planning to divorce her. He was wondering if by any chance there were a connection between her thyroid condition, hormones, and the changes in personality and sexual desire his wife had experienced during the past year.

At her husband's request, Beatrice returned to my office to explain the situation from her viewpoint. She said:

We got married when I was twenty-five years old. I loved Leonard and was attracted to him, but from the very beginning, I was not all that interested in sex. Even before the marriage, I never really understood what the big deal was about sex. In fact, if I had any problem with my husband, it was because for years I was not very interested in sex. I'm sure that after our child was born, what little of me had been there for him was probably totally taken away. I had a lot of guilt feelings about not being a good wife sexually all the time.

Beatrice recalled that, the previous summer, she had started losing weight, feeling hot, sweating, and at times feeling shaky. Then, gradually, she became more and more interested in having sex with her husband. She said:

Definitely once in the morning, definitely at night before bed, and almost always in the middle of the night. At least three times a day and, if the opportunity arose, four times a day. This was in addition to when I was by myself. It became a constant thing on my mind.

I began to log on to our computer and go into chat rooms on the Internet. At that point, I wasn't thinking I was going to get involved with somebody or experience sexual fantasies, but later I was totally consumed by the possibility of sex. It got to the point where I couldn't wait for my husband to leave the house so I could get on the computer. It would annoy me when he wouldn't leave when he was supposed to.

I was sexually stimulated most of the time. This happened when I was on-line pretty much throughout the day. Most definitely when I was with my husband it happened. I masturbated while talking with people on the computer. In turn, they masturbated when I was talking to them. That whole sick thing went on for a few months.

During the same period of time that all this was going on, my husband and I were partying, drinking, and dancing all the time. I just had energy constantly. I started becoming more aware of myself, more aware of everybody else, and wanting to get out and do things. I was paying less attention to my daughter.

The constant sexual obsessions and the manic behavior led Beatrice to have an affair that almost destroyed her family. One of the men to whom she had been talking on the computer decided to meet her. She described the encounter as follows:

I had talked to him for a number of months on the computer and also on the phone. I told Leonard I was going to spend the night with my cousin. The affair lasted one night, but Leonard found out almost immediately. How come other people can have affairs their whole lives and never get caught while I'm good as gold for fifteen years and get caught from having a one-night stand? Probably Leonard was already suspicious because of my behavior over a period of time. He confronted me about the episode, and I couldn't lie. I said yes, and everything went downhill from there.

Leonard became totally depressed and unsure of himself. Our relationship became like a roller coaster. We'd be okay for a day or two, and then he'd give me a zinger or we'd get into an argument. We started seeing a counselor, but that didn't seem to be helping at all.

After my interview with Beatrice, Leonard called me on the phone. He confirmed that his wife's infidelity had affected him tremendously, and he was having difficulty coping with it. I explained to Leonard that what he and his wife had experienced could be the result of hyperthyroidism's effect on the functioning of the brain. The total transformation of Beatrice's personality—from a fairly nonsexual, stable, supportive, and loving wife and mother to a self-centered person obsessed with sexual thoughts—was due to chemical changes in the brain that were making her a different person.

Although he found my explanations comforting, Leonard remained somewhat skeptical. His doubts persisted even though Beatrice returned to her previous self two to three months later when medication helped correct her hyperthyroidism. She stopped having the sexual fantasies and chatting with strangers on the computer. Beatrice herself could hardly believe that she had really been doing these things. In a subsequent conversation with Leonard, I dissuaded him from thinking that hyperthyroidism had unmasked Beatrice's "true" personality. Hyperthyroidism did not unmask hidden desires and hidden personality. It triggered and changed feelings, drives, and perceptions. Thyroid dysfunction altered the most intimate aspects of Beatrice's life, as it has with many other people.

Thyroid disease can precipitate or contribute to significant sexual problems, which are often a source of frustration between couples and can lead to the deterioration of relationships. Such problems aggravate the emotional chaos that both partners feel when one suffers from a thyroid condition.

Most patients with thyroid disease do not discuss their most intimate acts with their physicians and seldom bring up sexual disturbances, except sometimes to refer vaguely to "changes in my sex life." Sexual issues remain hidden and unexplained, yet they can be responsible for distancing and significant marital problems. Physicians seldom inquire about the sexual difficulties that thyroid patients may be experiencing, nor do they provide explanations or counseling. People who experience sexual difficulties often hide them and do not attribute them to the thyroid disease. In extreme cases, when sexual dysfunction weighs on the relationship and becomes a source of conflict between two partners, the couple may seek psychological counseling. Some people may even seek help from a sex therapist. Yet, for the majority of thyroid patients who experience sexual dysfunction, neither psychotherapy nor sex therapy will help unless the thyroid imbalance has been corrected and both the therapist and the partner have a good understanding of the thyroid disorder and its effects.

How Thyroid Function Governs Sexuality

In the sex act, there are four steps or stages that normally lead to sexual fulfillment or orgasm, each of which is affected by thyroid function. A sexual thought, a touch, or a signal that our brain interprets as erotic causes certain parts of the brain to emit chemical transmitters. These transmitters generate a surge of sexual interest and fantasies, making us willing to become intimate. Brain chemistry stimulates the autonomic nervous system, which will make us experience a range of physical responses: the skin becomes more sensitive, breathing and heart rate become more rapid, blood rushes to the genital organs, and so forth. This phase of excitement (or readiness) varies in duration from one person to another. As stimulation continues, the physical responses generated by the autonomic nervous system intensify, causing lubrication and engorgement of the external genital organs in women. The vaginal opening narrows, the labia swell, and the clitoris pulls in and becomes close to the pubic bone. In men, the autonomic responses cause an erection due to engorgement of the penis with blood.

The brain chemistry involved in sexual arousal and excitement is affected by the level of thyroid hormones. They promote the pleasurable body-mind response that culminates in orgasm. At the time of climax, the brain increases the release into the bloodstream of the hormone oxytocin, which causes the involuntary rhythmic contractions of muscles in the genitals, anus, and uterus. These orgasmic contractions depend on normal thyroid hormone levels. After we reach orgasm, we experience a period of relaxation. In women, the resolution of the lubrication and engorgement may take several hours, whereas, in men, the resolution of the engorgement and return of the penis to a flaccid condition occurs almost immediately after ejaculation.

Thyroid hormone not only has a direct effect on the brain chemistry interactions that lead to the autonomic nervous responses and sexual fulfillment; it also has an effect on the levels of sex hormones. In men, hypothyroidism often causes a decrease in the testosterone (male hormone) level,[1] whereas hyperthyroidism causes a change in the ratio of female to male hormones so that levels of some forms of female hormone become higher than normal.[2] In women, hypothyroidism causes a reduction in estrogen and progesterone levels and can contribute to a cessation of ovulation.[3] The lack of estrogens has significant peripheral effects, not only on the brain but also on the lubrication of genital organs. In a hyperthyroid woman, the concentration of male hormones in the blood rises, and estrogen levels may remain normal or decrease.[4] Thyroid hormone excess may enhance libido in some women because of the increase in androgen levels coupled with the direct effects on brain chemistry. In fact, this same increase in androgen can cause acne, growth of facial hair, and loss of scalp hair due to a shortening of the life of the hair follicle.[5]

The various effects of thyroid hormone on the brain, on the autonomic nervous system, and on sex hormone levels account for the multiple sexual disturbances that thyroid patients often experience. Because thyroid imbalance is much more common in women than men, and its effects on sexual function are quite often more complex, I will focus primarily on women's sexual problems in this chapter.

Hypothyroidism and Low Sexual Energy

When a woman becomes hypothyroid, the decrease in estrogen levels and the effect on the brain of low thyroid hormone levels often lead to lack of interest in sex. The desire gradually declines and may ultimately vanish. The healthy fantasies that existed prior to the occurrence of hypothyroidism occur less and less often. Most hypothyroid women have a tendency to masturbate less than they used to, again reflecting the evaporation of the sex drive.

A woman may not wish to be intimate with her partner or with anyone. In many women, the sexual changes are the predominant symptoms of a thyroid imbalance. They become so significant that a woman often visits her gynecologist to find out what is wrong. Gynecologists frequently attribute the lack of desire for intercourse, coupled with the absence of excitement and lubrication, to either hormonal changes or age.

The frustrations related to sexual dysfunction that hypothyroid women experience stem from an inability to cope with the changes. The effect on self-esteem and the fact that the women may not understand the reason for the changes tend to exacerbate these frustrations. An additional frustration, which may preoccupy women more than the dysfunction itself, is the need to deal with unsatisfied partners. Both partners may conclude that the problems are attributable simply to age, hormones, or stress.

Whereas one male partner may feel rejected and no longer desired, another may be understanding (or at least give the impression that he is). The woman may reassure him that her problem "has nothing to do with him" and that she "is working on it." The hypothyroid woman who describes this situation to her gynecologist may be given estrogen to improve the sexual dysfunction, often to no avail. The frustration and friction between the partners escalate. A friend may advise the woman that, to reduce the conflict, she should just have sex when her partner wants, regardless of whether she is in the mood. Often, however, if a woman isn't aroused, she simply doesn't want to bother with sex.

A good example of this problem is Olivia, who was hypothyroid for at least a couple of years. She told me, "When I was hypothyroid, I didn't want anybody near me." Another hypothyroid woman said, "You need more sleep, your hair is falling out, and you have no sexual drive, which is abnormal for a young married woman. Watching something erotic on TV doesn't do anything for you. You know something is wrong. You don't want to be bothered or touched. You may think to yourself, I know it's my problem. I don't want to tell him no. That's not right for him."

Another factor contributing to sexual problems is that a hypothyroid woman is often exhausted. As soon as she comes home from work, she wants to rest and sleep. The tiredness and other physical symptoms, coupled with the direct and indirect effects of thyroid hormone deficiency, typically result in withdrawal from activity and lack of interest in other people. "I feel miserable," said Anne, who had just been diagnosed with hypothyroidism. "I'm tired. I don't feel good. My body aches. Being intimate is the last thing in the world I want. I want somebody to give me a massage and let me sleep."

Weight gain may lead to a decline in self-esteem and distorted perceptions of body image, further contributing to marked decreases in sexual activity. Melanie had been married for only two years when, as a result of hypothyroidism, she reached the point of seeking excuses not to have sex with her husband. She was quite affected, as are many hypothyroid patients, by her physical appearance. She said, "It is hard to feel sexy about yourself when you look like a toad, you gain all this weight, and you are all bloated. The physical part of it is very detrimental to your psyche. It gets in the way of even being able to enjoy yourself or put yourself in that position."

When a hypothyroid woman engages in a sex act just because she wants to please her partner, some sexual arousal may occur, although it may be blunted compared to before. She may have difficulty reaching a normal state of sexual excitement. A woman who, during foreplay, normally reaches an excitement plateau within ten to twenty minutes may not reach that level when she is hypothyroid even after an hour of foreplay. Many hypothyroid women will continue to work at it, but because they are exhausted and have not reached an adequate level of arousal after such a long period of foreplay, they often give up and interrupt the sex act.

Nicole, who was suffering symptoms of hypothyroidism when she first came to my office, described this problem to me in the following way:

I have never been a really highly sexed person: sex once every week or two was fine with me. In the early years of marriage, we engaged in sex more. Then it was kids and mellowing, so it was probably about once a week. In the last year, I have had no interest. I don't really miss it nor need it. We probably have sex maybe once every two months. It has taken longer to stimulate me. Sometimes I even think, Are you up for all this? It takes longer, and it's more work.

Because thyroid hormones are crucial for the response that women need in order to achieve engorgement of the clitoris and lubrication of the vagina, they may not achieve this state in a normal sex act. The vaginal dryness in particular may cause women to experience pain during sexual intercourse. So in addition to the lack of desire, the pain then becomes another reason for avoiding sex. Fear of pain may also become a source of anxiety, which prevents the woman from relaxing enough to enjoy sex. The pain and the lack of pleasure during intercourse become a significant burden in the mind of a hypothyroid woman, and she often prefers to avoid sexual contact. Women who continue to be sexually active at the insistence of their partners often fail to achieve an orgasm, and if they do, it is short-lived. Multiple orgasms are unlikely, even if they were common before hypothyroidism.

According to a young woman being treated for an underactive thyroid:

Sex is not enjoyable any longer. The dryness in the vagina and the severe pain during intercourse make it a horrible experience. When my thyroid has been under control, I have felt sexier. I have actually desired sex. The pain during intercourse disappeared. When my thyroid is not in control, when it is too low, that is the last thing on my mind. Then sex is like work, and it causes great discomfort.

Many couples face similar problems. Painful intercourse can be a frustrating barrier to a gratifying sex life. Surveys have shown that 15 to 30 percent of all women experience physical discomfort or pain when they engage in sex.[6] Causes may include superabsorbent tampons, allergic reactions to contraceptive foams or creams, and vaginal infections. Often, when a gynecologist finds no obvious vaginal or abdominal abnormality, he or she may merely suggest psychotherapy. Yet the problem has several possible causes, including thyroid imbalance leading to inadequate arousal and lubrication.

Pain or discomfort during intercourse may also be due to lichen sclerosus, an inflammation of the genital skin that can cause extreme itchiness. Recently, one doctor reported that nearly 50 percent of women suffering from this skin condition have a thyroid disorder.[7] Doctors treat lichen sclerosus with hydrocortisone ointment or 2 percent testosterone ointment twice a day for two to three months.

Lichen sclerosus appears as a patchy white lesion on the labial skin (outside the vagina). This lesion at times extends to the area between the legs and up to the anus. If you continue to have discomfort and pain during intercourse after your thyroid imbalance has been corrected with treatment, have your gynecologist look for lichen sclerosus. Another often overlooked reason for the dryness is Sjögren's syndrome, an autoimmune condition that occurs in a large number of thyroid patients, resulting in dryness of the eyes, mouth, and vagina (see Chapter 14).

When Depression Aggravates the Problem

When women are depressed and hypothyroid, they lose any interest in sex and may even develop an aversion to it. Although these women may experience an improvement in many of their symptoms with thyroid hormone treatment, the lack of sexual desire may persist. One patient who continued to have residual depression after correction of hypothyroidism told me, "Since I increased the dose, I don't think I have more arousal. I'm more energetic and less tired. I sleep less. The PMS symptoms are less. I feel less impatient. But when it comes to desiring sex, this has not changed. I still don't have any interest." When a lack of sexual desire persists, it may be due to depression or to a distancing that has developed between the two partners over a period of time.

Dana, aged twenty-eight, who has suffered lingering effects of thyroid imbalance, told me, "Before all this, I remember having the desire to have sex, and we were very active sexually. Now the desire has pretty much gone away, even when I am on the thyroid medication. I do have desire, but it's very seldom and not like it used to be. I like to be with my husband and talk to him. Mainly I want *just* to be close to him without the sex."

The struggle to maintain a loving, caring relationship is common among patients suffering from hypothyroidism. The husband may not understand that, although his wife has lost her desire to engage in sex, she still loves him. If her husband is supportive, the woman may attempt to please him, quite often to no avail. Relationships can be seriously disturbed, however, by the sexual dysfunction resulting from thyroid imbalance. The following case illustrates how sexual dysfunction and some distancing resulting from thyroid imbalance can precipitate a snowball effect and the breakdown of a relationship.

During the first two years of her marriage, Betty had had a happy relationship and was very active sexually. When her thyroid then became underactive and made her tired, exhausted, and withdrawn, however, her sex drive diminished. She told me:

Our intimacy went downhill. He became resentful because I did not give him enough attention. He was also stressed out because of his job situation. I stopped having fantasies, and I was so tired that I didn't care. Sex became an unpleasant chore that was often painful. It felt like all of a sudden we grew apart. I became withdrawn and irritable, and he was trapped in stress because of his job. We were not as close to each other as before.

As the distance between them increased significantly, Betty's husband found excuses to travel out of town. She just wanted to be by herself and became depressed as a result of the hypothyroidism.

"I became a loner," Betty said. "When I came home from work, I went to sleep. When he came back from one of his trips, he announced to me that he had had an affair, and he told me that he had made a mistake in marrying me. He told me he couldn't stand living with me any longer."

Unfortunately for Betty and her husband, it took three years for a doctor to diagnose Betty's hypothyroidism.

Raging Libido and Other Sexual Problems of Hyperthyroid Women

The effects of hyperthyroidism on sex life are more complex and varied. Many hyperthyroid women respond in the same manner as hypothyroid women: they gradually lose interest in sex, both because they are overwhelmed by their chaotic thoughts and because of the indifference to pleasure so characteristic of depression. Some hyperthyroid women may experience greater depression, and the accompanying physical exhaustion and tiredness may cause them to lose interest in sex.

I saw Robin for the first time when she was referred to me for hyperthyroidism. She had been married for three years and had just recently become separated from her husband, who had filed for a divorce. She said:

I had noticed a loss in my sex drive. That was the first thing that happened to me. We had been married for six months, and it was just great. We had great sex. Then, all of a sudden, I had no interest. It took forever to excite me. I would still be able to get excited once I had allowed myself to relax completely. My husband thought that I didn't love him anymore! I tried to explain it wasn't that. I told him I wasn't interested in anybody else. I just had lost the desire. He couldn't understand why, and I couldn't tell him why.

Her husband hired a private investigator, who followed Robin for a month. When the investigator came up with nothing, Robin's husband gave up. Then he met a woman who could give him what he wanted. For months, Robin continued to feel guilty that she hadn't been able to control what was happening to her sexually. Later, when Robin's overactive thyroid was corrected, it took months of counseling and psychotherapy for her to regain a normal sex life.

Julia, another young woman who became hyperthyroid in her first year of marriage, said:

> I think my lack of interest in sex was tied in with the exhaustion. The sexual interest started going when I began having many other symptoms of hyperthyroidism. I would have liked to have somebody else to talk to, especially some other person who had gone through it. When I was diagnosed, my doctor was quite open with me and told me everything that could possibly go wrong except for the sexual effects.

The increased anxiety and mood swings of a hyperthyroid woman often create a distance between her and her partner, and this may cause her to avoid intimacy. Her moodiness and self-esteem problems make communication and focus difficult. She may think about sex and be interested, and she may experience a burst of fantasies and sexual desire, but these feelings can dissipate quickly from a wave of anxiety.

Many hyperthyroid women, however, do not lose their sex drive. Their excitement period is unaffected or may even be shortened. It takes less time for them to achieve a state of lubrication and engorgement, but during sexual intercourse, they may experience tremendous pain, similar to what hypothyroid women would experience. At times, the pain is caused by an involuntary spasm of the outer part of the vagina (vaginismus). The fear of having pain during sexual intercourse may create significant anxiety in hyperthyroid women, who may then attempt to avoid sexual intercourse altogether.

Hyperthyroidism can provoke a mildly manic (hypomanic) state that may continue for a long time. In the hypomanic state, the sex drive may be increased, and there may be an obsession with sexual thoughts. Some women with an overactive thyroid experience too much vaginal lubrication, even before they start showing symptoms of hypomania and raging libido.

This happened to Alexandra, who could not understand why she was experiencing excessive lubrication, even during the day, and initially thought she had a yeast infection. She said:

> I called my gynecologist and told him that I had an excessive amount of mucus, even in the daytime, and I didn't understand it. He did a Pap smear and said everything was clear. I was worried about infections, and he said because it was a clear mucus, nothing was wrong. At that time, I became wet very quickly. To

reach an orgasm, however, it took longer. It was fine for me, but it was very stressful for my husband.

Thyroid hormone excess may have a direct effect on the brain chemicals that regulate sexual interest. As a result of a hypomanic state, increased sexuality may become a hyperthyroid woman's focus—a situation illustrated by the case of Karen, a thirty-eight-year-old housewife who experienced a sudden surge in her sexual interest and fantasies after twelve years of marriage. In her words:

I became extremely involved in my appearance. I was overweight at that point. I began having sexual fantasies. I started reading books that were more erotic. It seemed to happen rather suddenly. I spent hours reading erotic books and lying down fantasizing. My fantasies didn't involve my husband and not even any men I knew, really, just fantasy people—strangers.

At that time, I was home and not working. I engaged in masturbation several times a day. I started having dreams that I was developing relationships with men that I saw on talk shows on TV. I was also experiencing other symptoms of hyperthyroidism. I had a rapid heartbeat, I was feeling hot, and at times, I was shaky. I was talking faster and definitely talking louder.

This hypomanic state induced by thyroid hormone excess is similar to what can be seen in manic-depressive disorders during the elated phase, when a woman may typically seek more sex and become obsessed with sexual thoughts. Increased sexuality rarely occurs without other manifestations of elation. Women become more interested in their bodies and appearance. They may spend unusual amounts of money on new, extravagant clothes and often plan or even decide to have plastic surgery.

Mary Linn's elation from hyperthyroidism went on for a year before she was diagnosed with Graves' disease. She had been married for ten years and had four children. She told me:

My sex life became very different all of a sudden compared to what we had in the past. I became the boss all the time, taking the lead in instigating sex. If my husband wasn't willing, I would get really upset.

The weird part, though, is that I would think of sexual things I had never considered before. I did them on my own without ever being told about them. All my friends are Christians, and we don't go around talking about sexual things, and that was probably the most confusing thing to my husband. He asked, "Where are you getting these ideas?"

Most partners who see such a drastic change in the woman they have known for some time become suspicious and totally confused. Eric, Mary

Linn's husband, thought that his wife's heightened sexual arousal was the result of an affair. She said, "I don't think this will ever make sense to him. He is still very confused. Sometimes we talk about it, and he tries to get me to explain to him, and I try my best, but I don't think I'll ever have an answer or truly understand how Graves' can cause this hyperintensity."

Mary Linn's change in personality fits the description of hypomania. She had never experienced such an obsession with sex, either before the onset of her Graves' disease or after its treatment. In fact, all aspects of Mary Linn's hypomanic behavior were uncharacteristic for her. Certainly the sexual manifestation was unusual, but she was also buying atypical items, she was giving her children a different kind of attention, and she began having a different kind of relationship with her parents. She notes:

> I am still recovering today. Now I think that it's funny. It's funny because it's not like me. It even embarrassed me. Now, everything has really gone back to as close to normal as I can remember it. I have gained back the weight. I have a pile of clothes I can't wear. Even the lingerie—it's too tight. I'm too embarrassed to give it to anyone. My sexual drive came down to what it used to be before Graves' disease.

Sexual Problems in Men

As I said at the start of the chapter, thyroid imbalance is much more common in women than in men, and its effect on women's sexual function is quite often more complex. Yet men suffering from thyroid imbalance may also experience drastic changes in sexual activity. Hypothyroid men often experience a lack of desire and a blunting of fantasies. Even if they are excited or stimulated, erection may not occur. If the hypothyroidism is severe, the erection may be transient, causing an interruption of the sex act. As in women, the tiredness and depression make men disinterested in sex and unable to fulfill their partner's sexual needs.

A hyperthyroid man loses the patience to engage in foreplay to excite his partner. He may become obsessed with the physical act and may not allow his partner to reach an adequate level of excitement before intercourse. One wife of a hyperthyroid man complained:

> It was boom, and it was over with. Before, we would engage in a lot of foreplay, and afterward we'd sit in bed and talk for hours. Then, for several months when John was hyperthyroid, he wanted to have sex almost every day. After maybe one or two minutes of kissing, he would just like to have intercourse. I was not ready. It was frustrating, and I could not refuse. I got angry so quickly.

Hyperthyroid men may also lose the emotional aspect of making love. Sex becomes just a physical activity. Both Richard and his wife noticed a change in his sexuality. Richard said:

At the beginning, sex was something very important—and it wasn't just sex, it was making love, and there is a difference! Then later, sex became just sex. There was a period when we just stopped. Before, we would have sex two or three times a week, and it got to maybe once every three weeks. Later on, the desire just went away. The amazing thing about Graves' disease is that it makes you emotionally bland to everything around you. You have so much energy that you feel you need to be doing something physical all the time.

Other men become sexually interested in the morning, but in the evening, they are physically exhausted and have neither the desire nor the physical strength to perform sexually. As one man said, "In the morning, I would be Superman. By the time I get to bed, I am so tired!"

Hyperthyroid men also lose their normal orgasms. One hyperthyroid man said:

Before, sex lasted a lot longer and maybe even more than one time. Now it is only one time and sometimes not even that. With Graves' disease, you're going at 100 percent of what you should be, and all of a sudden, you're at minus 20 percent. You're so exhausted. Anytime between eight and ten in the evening, you crash. It is like you expended all the energy you had, and then you are left with nothing.

Toward a Better Sex Life

Theoretically, once a woman's thyroid imbalance is corrected, her lack of interest in and avoidance of sex should subside and her fantasies and usual drive should return. Unfortunately, this may not always be the case. Patients may then believe that the change in their sex life is due to reasons other than the thyroid. Some attribute it to age, and others remain perplexed by their loss of sexual interest. As I noted in Chapter 2, a thyroid imbalance is a significant stressful event. Some women may continue to suffer from depression or post–traumatic stress syndrome after the imbalance is corrected. Depression and post–traumatic stress syndrome could in themselves cause a lack of sexual interest. Once distance has come between two partners, they may find it hard to resume their lives as if nothing had happened. The continued lack of interest may also become a challenge to intimacy. Nevertheless, using techniques of gradual excitement and relearning how to enjoy sex can be quite helpful.

You need to practice regular sessions of stimulation and caressing—at first without actually engaging in intercourse. Some of these techniques are described in books like *The Gift of Sex: A Guide to Sexual Fulfillment*.[8] Have your partner rediscover your erogenous zones. You need to train your brain to respond to the stimulation that elicits arousal and excitement.

If sexual problems and symptoms of depression persist after correction of your hypothyroidism, consider changing your thyroxine treatment to a T4/T3 combination (see Chapter 17). This has helped many women with persistent depression and lack of sexual interest. If you are also taking an antidepressant, ask your doctor whether this medication could be the source of the sexual difficulties. Men with sexual difficulties caused by an antidepressant can be helped by taking yohimbine (Yocon®). This medication works on the venous system in the penis to induce and maintain an erection. If you are postmenopausal, discuss with your doctor the use of small amounts of testosterone. This reduces depression, headaches, and loss of energy and restores libido,[9] although it could cause some hair growth as well. Also, look into optimizing your estrogen replacement therapy. Estratest, a hormonal preparation that combines estrogen and small amounts of testosterone, is one of my preferred treatments for menopausal women with persistent sexual difficulties.

Some couples who have experienced distancing and continue to suffer from lingering sexual problems after a thyroid hormone imbalance has been corrected may find it helpful to consult a psychotherapist or sex therapist. To obtain a list of sex therapists, contact:

American Association of Sex Educators, Counselors, and Therapists
P.O. Box 238
Mt. Vernon, IA 52314

The sexual effects of thyroid imbalance described in this chapter are very common. In many couples, they are the main cause of relationship problems. In other couples, they are catalysts for relationship problems that are triggered by changes in the behavior and personality of the thyroid patient. This is one of the many facets of the big question, "Is it my brain, or is it my thyroid?" Thyroid patients and their partners must resolve this issue themselves or seek help from a sex therapist if the problem continues after the thyroid imbalance is corrected.

Important Points to Remember

- Optimal thyroid hormone levels are crucial for having normal libido and normal physical responses that lead to sexual fulfillment.

- An overactive thyroid can cause painful intercourse and a loss of interest in sex, or it can result in raging libido and careless behavior.
- An underactive thyroid often results in blunted sexual appetite, lack of lubrication, and painful sex.
- Sexual problems can continue after correction of a thyroid imbalance. You and your partner need to learn about these effects, discuss them openly, and seek help from a sex therapist if psychological problems and distancing persist.

9

"YOU'VE CHANGED":

When the Thyroid and Relationships Collide

Women and men are fundamentally different in how they communicate and interpret each other's language, behavior, and emotions.[1] Many couples come to recognize their real differences, accept them, and eventually learn to deal with them.

The intrusion of a thyroid imbalance into a couple's relationship very often exacerbates these differences. Subtle changes in how the afflicted person speaks and acts alter the dynamics of the relationship. Thyroid patients, particularly those suffering from an overactive thyroid, often become moody, anxious, angry, and irritable.[2] And many begin to have a distorted perception of their partner's behavior. Unfortunately, their partners may not understand what causes these changes. Inability to cope with changing demands and difficulty in communicating can lead to chaos, with misunderstandings, false expectations, and arguments over trivial matters. For many people, the relationship becomes a burden.

People with a thyroid condition are having terrible trouble understanding themselves and their new, confusing feelings, so they are unlikely to understand their partners. Indeed, thyroid patients are so overwhelmed by their new emotional problems that they cannot cope properly with the stress of the relationship, which becomes a cycle of reactions and counterreactions. Both partners then share the mental stress provoked by the thyroid condition.

Typically, when one of the partners is suffering from thyroid disease, the relationship undergoes two distinct phases, each characterized by its own distinct dynamics and thyroid-related effects. The first phase begins with the intrusion of the thyroid condition and ends when the diagnosis is made. In this phase, relationships frequently deteriorate and may even end because of the lack of understanding of what precipitated or caused the relationship problems. The second phase follows diagnosis.

In phase one, the intrusion is, in most instances, insidious. More often than not, the personality of the afflicted person changes drastically. Although people with thyroid conditions are capable of hiding their suffering to some extent, the disease quickly alters their behavior and language so significantly that other people easily recognize the change. As long as the cause of the change remains undetermined (that is, the thyroid condition has not yet been diagnosed), the couple will be unable to pinpoint the origin of their problems. The relationship suffers proportionately to the length of this period, which could last months or even years.

The paradox in this phase is that people with thyroid ailments do recognize that unusual things are happening within their bodies and minds, but they are unable to understand them, qualify them, or even describe them accurately. At the same time, their distorted perception of themselves and the world around them causes them to regard their partners' behavior as inappropriate. The thyroid sufferers truly believe that their partners are the ones who have changed and are responsible for their own emotional upheaval. In turn, spouses and other loved ones often react by blaming the patient. Hence, thyroid patients may experience guilt feelings resulting from disagreements that worsen their existing anxiety, stress, anger, and depression.

Distancing is inevitable because the patient becomes unable to deal with the stress of arguing. Although both hypothyroidism and hyperthyroidism can lead to similar behavioral changes, certain changes may be more characteristic of one condition than the other. Let's take a look at some of the changes that can ignite fighting, arguing, and distancing.

Ten Ways That Thyroid Conditions May Change Your Personality and Relationships

Many years of working with and observing people with thyroid conditions have allowed me to identify the following ten types of thyroid-related changes that cause trouble for many couples.

Thyroid patients often become impatient and irritable and may display excessive, unreasonable anger. A thyroid imbalance may make you excessively critical and lead you to pick fights with those around you and snap at them. Often anxiety and worries underlie the criticism and anger that people with thyroid imbalances direct toward others. Ironically, though, people with thyroid conditions do not handle criticism well themselves. Take Janice, for example. She had been happily married for four years when she began experiencing tiredness, anxiety, and weight gain. She then suffered for two years before being diagnosed with hypothyroidism at the age of twenty-seven. Janice tended to blame her husband's attitudes for their disturbed relationship. She said:

> For instance, if I did not want to spend money on a certain thing and he wanted to, I would be unreasonably angry, and I would say things that were inappropriate. I told him he was selfish and that he wasn't working toward a common goal. I perceived any decision he made or anything he said or did as inappropriate. It is a miracle we are still together after what we went through in the past two years.

The situation Janice faced is all too real for people with thyroid ailments. They feel compelled to lash out at the very people to whom they need to turn in times of anxiety. In essence, their behavior is controlled by their affliction.

Another hypothyroid woman told me, "There was a lot of yelling and bickering at home. I was frequently very angry. I was disrespectful to my husband and would snap at him when he asked questions because I was upset about the bills or our financial situation. No matter what he did, I would not have been satisfied." Clearly this report goes to the heart of the matter in depicting the incredible conflict within the patient. For the person experiencing the disease, there is no right answer, and anxiety generates discord.

Similarly, Camille, a thirty-two-year-old housewife who suffered from an overactive thyroid due to Graves' disease, told of a family life filled with constant fighting, screaming, and arguing. She said, "Before I was diagnosed, I wasn't getting along well with my parents, which was annoying to me. I had a short temper with them. At home, I have been very crass and sarcastic with my kids. If one of my children left a shoe lying in the middle of the room, I got really annoyed and picked up the shoe and threw it across the room. I couldn't believe I did that. It was not the way I would normally react." This illustrates patients' common tendency to experience a sense of disbelief regarding their unexplained behavior. They know their behavior deviates from what is "normal" for them, but they have no clue as to why.

Another example reveals the common thread of discord that thyroid patients experience in their relationships. Darlene started noticing symptoms of hyperthyroidism three months after her wedding. She and her husband started fighting over trivial matters and ended up seeking help from a counselor. She confessed:

> There are certain things that I should have compromised on. If I had been in a calmer mood, I would have been able to handle that. I did not have patience with

my husband. Before the symptoms of hyperthyroidism, I tended to be less emotional. My husband is Jewish, and I'm Catholic. He didn't want to go home for Christmas. We had a big argument about that. He ended up going home by himself. If I had been more patient, we could have sat down and worked things out.

Darlene worked in a store's customer service department. She experienced the same impatience at work as she had at home and began having problems with her colleagues. She explained the situation like this: "I was lacking patience with the customers all the time. Many times I started crying over trivial matters. I had a big argument with my supervisor. She was irritating me! People say that I would talk really fast. I knew something was wrong, but I had no idea what. I didn't know about hyperthyroidism, where things move quicker."

Darlene's experience is typical of how people with an overactive thyroid are unable to explain their behavioral changes adequately. They feel as if everyone else is to blame, and their behavior is fueled by emotions laced with anger. The fast pace at which hyperthyroid people's brains work may make them regard everybody else as slow and lead them to rationalize the irritability and anger.

People with thyroid conditions may make unrealistic demands of partners, spouses, or family members. They frequently ask others to do things for them, and they also tell others how to do things. A hyperthyroid woman who had serious marital problems as a result of her Graves' disease told me, "I would tell my husband he was never home and that I needed him home. He is a student, and he is not at school full-time, and I would get upset because he was not home to help with chores. But in fact, he was doing the best he could, and still I was not satisfied." This example shows how patients are incapable of viewing their relationships rationally. They cannot see situations clearly and may even provoke their partners with their unrealistic expectations.

Thyroid patients, particularly those with hypothyroidism, want peace and quiet. They feel the need to withdraw from activity and noise. They have a low tolerance for sound. In essence, they wish to insulate themselves in a surrealistic world of tranquillity. One hypothyroid patient told me, "I would want peace and quiet at home. If I didn't get it, I would start shouting at my children and at my husband. Anything that made a lot of noise or movement irritated me. The TV was a nuisance to me. I couldn't watch it. The children's making a lot of noise was a frustration."

Patients may become withdrawn from friends, and they do not want to talk or go out with people. They may lose all interest in doing things with their partners. A good example is Angel, a twenty-five-year-old woman who was suffering from an underactive thyroid. She said:

All I wanted to do was sleep. I couldn't seem to get enough rest. Nothing made me happy. Ted wanted to take me out to eat, and I didn't want to go. He wanted to go to a movie, and I'd say no. If he rented a movie, I'd just fall asleep. I didn't want to be intimate. I didn't want to cook or clean. Then he would get frustrated, and I'd get really emotional and mad. He didn't understand that I'm more tired than he is.

He would try to talk to me, and it was so hard for me to tell him, "Ted, would you just shut up?" He just wanted to tell me about his day and to hear about my day. Questions, questions, questions, talk, talk, talk—and I was so irritable. At first, I think I wanted him to just shut up, then I didn't really want him to shut up.

I just want to feel better and to have more energy. One year ago, I could not have been happier. I felt good, looked good, and we were going out all the time.

Hypothyroid patients want to be left alone. They just want to sleep and withdraw from those around them. In some cases, they realize the people around them are doing the best they can, but they still want to maintain their isolation.

People with thyroid conditions may require more attention from their partners and often feel that they are not getting enough attention. They feel that whatever a partner might do to comfort them is not enough. Ironically, those with thyroid imbalances have mixed feelings about their loved ones. They want their loved ones to be there for them—but only on their terms. In other words, if loved ones do not follow the "rules" laid out for them by the person with the imbalance, he or she will not hesitate to turn on them. Many thyroid patients told me something like this: "I preferred him just to be there, hold my hand, and listen to me, but not to say anything. When he would say things, it would make me irritable and angry."

Mona, suffering from postpartum hypothyroidism, fought with her husband more than she ever had before. She felt she did not get the attention she needed. "The only thoughts I had during this time were that my husband was not helping me with the things that I needed. I had reached a point where I would have hit him in the face in public. I wanted to feel I was cherished. I was feeling very unattractive, like you do after you have a baby. I was extremely overwhelmed and overtired."

People with thyroid ailments may show a lack of commitment to doing things at home or for the family. They may not want to be asked to do things or may become angry if asked. A common source of disagreement is hypothyroid people's declining interest in doing things around the house. Because they are exhausted, they have difficulty handling even minor chores. Just going to the store can be an insurmountable task.

One patient summed this up as follows:

I felt that as long as he didn't ask anything of me, like cooking dinner or going out when I didn't want to, I was comfortable. I wished he would have understood my emotions and feelings and symptoms, but he didn't at first. He kept pushing me. I guess he thought I was being lazy. I felt something was really wrong. I didn't want him to ask me to get out of bed, but he would. He felt it was all in my mind. He wasn't being empathic or sympathetic, so I would get angry with that.

Thyroid patients may exhibit unexplained hatred toward partners, spouses, relatives, and friends or contradictory, rapidly changing feelings. This problem is aptly demonstrated by the case of Jackie, who developed postpartum hypothyroidism. She described the situation like this:

I had a very good relationship with my parents before. When my baby was two months old, I experienced a lot of irritation and anger toward my mother, who used to be my best friend. My mother became angry that I had become so withdrawn from her and so disrespectful. I was very hurtful to her, but I was sick and couldn't deal with her. I didn't feel connected to her at all. I didn't want her to come to my house. I didn't want her to help me in any way.

Jackie's case is typical in that she realized her relationships had changed, but she felt helpless to do anything about it. She knew things were not the way they used to be, but she was unable to see things in proper perspective. To her, feelings of hatred were unavoidable and unchangeable.

Similarly, Sylvia, who was very much in love with her husband and had had what she called a serene, peaceful relationship with him, told me, "My emotions toward my husband were shifting back and forth. Sometimes I liked to be with him and sometimes not." These shifting feelings are quite common among hyperthyroid patients. When coupled with the types of changes in sexual interest described in Chapter 8, they become a serious source of distancing and conflict.

Thyroid sufferers may become overly anxious about how their emotional changes and health are affecting their ability to do their jobs and earn a living. When work-related anxiety is brought home, it often leads to arguing, angry outbursts, and increased irritability. Poor job performance or even job loss due to hypothyroidism or hyperthyroidism's adverse effects on thinking and reasoning further lowers self-esteem. Issues pertaining to financial security and financial responsibilities often arise, burdening the relationship even further. In other cases, people with a thyroid condition become trapped in their work. Many patients, in trying to hold on to their jobs, devote most of their attention and remaining energy to the effort to maintain their job performance. This tremendous burden on the brain will often be expressed in outbursts at home as patients' frustrations and inability to fulfill emotional and physical responsibilities in their private lives affect partners or families.

Amanda, a teacher with a hypothyroid condition, described this conflict to me. "I became irritable with students," she said. "I had to exercise a great deal of self-control so that I wouldn't fly off the handle. This would tire me out so much that, when I got home, I was useless to my husband. I felt guilty, like I wasn't really all there to do the things we wanted to do. We would go dancing, and I couldn't remember to move my foot out for each step. It was very noticeable." When patients focus on doing the best they can at work, their home life inevitably suffers, because they have no energy left for family duties and obligations.

In the same fashion, a hyperthyroid person can become obsessed with work, which may alienate his or her partner. This was true for Kenneth, a thirty-two-year-old salesman who took on another part-time job when he hit the manic period of hyperthyroidism. His wife, frustrated by his behavior, said:

> For the two years that he was doing the part-time job, we grew apart. He was all work. I couldn't even catch him. Then he slept during the weekend. During that time, he had very little to do with us because he had to work. I felt that it was "Kenneth's life," and then it was me and the kids' life.
>
> People would say, "How do you put up with him?" "He is crazy." "How does he work like that?" "You don't have a life." You start examining your life then and asking yourself what you really have. I felt like he didn't love me or care about me. I saw the same distance between him and the kids and his parents. I kept telling him we were growing apart. I told him, "You're going to wake up one day and we are going to be miles apart." Whatever I told him, it didn't register.

Extreme anger and irritability may lead to violence. Whitney, a thirty-one-year-old woman, was living by herself and had been dating a man for a couple of years when she became hyperthyroid. She used to love this man, and they were making wedding plans when things gradually began to change. In her words:

> I had a fairly normal life. As my symptoms progressed, it seemed I was in conflict with everyone. I was disagreeing with everything. People would hurt my feelings easily. The man I was dating at that time refused to understand what I was going through. He was dismissing me and saying it was stress or that I was acting like a baby. He made me feel very small about my problems. He said I was lazy. I was so fatigued from my thyroid condition, but I did not know it. I am not a lazy person!

I remember the intense anger I felt. One day I sat and fantasized about driving my car through his garage. It seemed like a wonderful thing to do. I didn't act upon that. I wouldn't even think of that today. I became more combative. We had lots of arguments that always ended up with me crying and walking out; my emotions would overtake me.

My emotions caused me to have a continuous internal battle. I had no tolerance or patience. When it is your nature to be generous, giving, kind, tolerant, and basically easygoing, and then you're the complete opposite, it is hard to cope. I became mean and nasty, and I didn't know why I was unhappy. I had tantrums and violent spells. I actually could have killed someone.

Violent actions and thoughts plague many thyroid patients. In this way, the patients may become harmful to themselves and others and could end up facing legal problems as well as the problems associated with the disease itself. The thyroid patient's anger may sometimes be expressed as verbal or even physical violence, as was the case with Ryan, a middle-aged engineer.

Jeannine, Ryan's wife, said, "It was not so easy to talk to him. It was like he was on drugs. He was verbally abusive all the time. He is like a volcano: any little thing causes it to erupt."

Ryan related an episode that illustrates how trivial, unimportant matters can trigger bouts of anger and violence:

One day, Jeannine's sister stayed with us. She didn't like me, and she irritated me quite a bit. I sat down and listened to what my wife had to say, and then when I decided to say something, her sister locked herself in the bathroom because she didn't want to hear what I had to say. It totally infuriated me. I went to the bathroom door and started to knock on it. I told her to let me in the door. When she said no, I said, "Let me in the damn door!" When she said no again, the next thing I knew, my arm had just gone through the door. I don't even remember hitting the door, but my arm was through the door, and she was standing up in the shower screaming. I didn't hit her, but I felt like hitting her. She came back in the den, and I told her what I had to say, and I said, "Now if you want to go the bathroom, you can."

Jeannine was a passive and submissive person. She remained in the marriage despite the lack of communication, anger, and distance between her and Ryan.

Hyperthyroidism may make someone act in ways that others may perceive as inconsistent and irrational. Paul and his father were partners in running a gas station. When Paul became hyperthyroid, the business began to do poorly because of his irrational behavior and aggressiveness with customers. As a result, Paul and his father eventually stopped talking to each other.

Friends would ask Paul's wife, "Why is he acting so nervous, and why does he have to speed to go somewhere when he is not in a hurry?" She said, "We would fly out of the driveway like it was an emergency. He acts as if he is crazy. Everything has to be fast."

According to Paul, "My personality really changed drastically. I got to where I really couldn't relax at all, and even at home, I couldn't stand to sit on the couch. I had to be doing something, or I would go into a mood swing where I would get agitated with any little thing." Paul's case is typical with regard to alienation and extreme personality change.

The Partner's Four Most Common Reactions

Not knowing that there is a physical or chemical reason for the personality change, the partner of the person with a thyroid imbalance often becomes confused. The reactions to this new situation vary from person to person. The spouse has been used to living with one person and now must live with a new person who has different perceptions, feelings, and emotions. The differences in perception and language between men and women become a real issue for most spouses because, for some time, they have coped with and adjusted to certain differences—and now those differences have changed. Lack of understanding can generate inappropriate reactions that may contribute to more arguing.

Here are some common reactions of partners:

Partners may pull away from the person with the thyroid imbalance. The distancing, which is the spouse's typical response, initially reflects avoidance of problems. The patient perceives this pulling away as a lack of caring, understanding, and empathy—as a statement that the partner is indifferent. Because of the lower self-esteem generated by thyroid imbalance, the patient tends to feel more anger and may attribute some of his or her problems to the distancing behavior.

This can be seen in the case of Sondra, who was suffering from hypothyroidism and was as confused as her husband about what had happened to their relationship. "We used to get along so well," she said. "I became irritable. I felt he was not really empathic with me for some reason. He does not talk to me very much anymore." Sondra focuses on the distance as a cause more than an effect of her behavior. The lines become blurred for patients when they try to fathom exactly what caused the relationship changes.

Partners may refuse to accept the personality changes associated with thyroid conditions and react with anger and criticism. This typically causes the fighting to escalate. The spouse may go overboard with criticism, which exacerbates the patient's feelings of low self-esteem. The patient may be blamed for deliberately creating arguments. "He took away my motivation and my self-esteem," one hyperthyroid woman said. "He makes me feel awkward about being sick. He asked me if I was doing it for attention. He doesn't have a clue that it is embarrassing. I never felt like he understood what I was going through. We would fight over stupid stuff, like what kind of shampoo to buy." After this couple had seen a counselor for several months with no improvement in their relationship, her underactive thyroid was diagnosed. When the husband learned that his wife's changing emotions were due to her thyroid condition, they stopped going to the psychologist, and he became understanding, flexible, and compassionate.

Partners may be unable to cope and become depressed and anxious themselves. When the wife has a thyroid condition, the husband may become anxious, realize the severity of their problems, and make an effort to understand or talk things over. He may even suggest counseling. During her hyperthyroidism, Ashley experienced a lot of anxiety and mood swings. Her husband, who is somewhat dependent, became anxious, which generated depression. Ashley said, "Initially, I was the one who had a lot of anxiety and anger, but quickly he also became nervous and had bouts of anger. Then we both had higher anxiety."

A few partners may recognize that their loved one has definitely changed and will make an effort to find a medical reason for the changes. Lynette, who had been married for fifteen years, had been very close to her husband since they were children and was supportive of him when he was in law school. They had learned to live with each other and were very close. Initially, when Lynette started having symptoms of hypothyroidism—such as outbursts of anger, irritability, and weight gain—he was quite supportive. He did not know that the problem was physical, however. Although Lynette became angrier and more irritable, they were so close that her husband quickly learned to adapt to the situation, and he concluded that Lynette's behavior stemmed from her weight problem. In a reassuring tone, he repeatedly told her that what was bothering her the most was really the weight. "You have to exercise and try to stay on a diet," he kept telling her. She followed his advice and worked out at the gym, but her condition remained unchanged. After her physicians dismissed Lynette as not having a medical problem, her husband continued to be supportive and started searching self-help books, which led him to suspect that she had a thyroid condition.

A thyroid patient experiencing a change in personality may not necessarily recognize that he or she is the source of the problem, although the person usually does recognize that problems exist. At this stage, however, most people who are close to someone with a thyroid imbalance do not make an effort to understand. Other partners, seeing that the relationship is deteriorating rapidly, often suggest that the couple see a psychologist. Under these circumstances, counseling may or may not be helpful because the source of the problem—the thyroid condition—is not recognized, and the irrational behavior, uncontrollable anger, and irritability continue, which perpetuate the arguing. Often, despite counseling, the couple grows farther apart, and this may lead to a divorce, particularly if the thyroid condition has not been diagnosed and its role in the couple's problems recognized early enough.

At times, even basic communication may become a problem. Gene, the husband of a hyperthyroid woman, said, "What she is thinking comes out of her mouth several times. Either she might tell me something three times before I get angry, or she may think she told me something and she never uttered the words, and then she becomes infuriated."

When couples have preexisting problems, those problems may be exacerbated by the intrusion of the thyroid imbalance, and arguing can mount to unbelievable levels. Without counseling, the relationship will inevitably founder.

Relationships after Diagnosis

Once the condition has been diagnosed, the couple is frequently relieved because they have found an explanation for their problems. The treatment of the thyroid imbalance generally leads to a gradual resolution of the emotional stress, guilt feelings, and mental effects. Still, this often means that these factors may linger for several months or even years, depending on the complexity of the thyroid condition and its treatment.

After being diagnosed with hypothyroidism, Jamie was started on thyroid hormone treatment. She has not fully recovered and feels quite guilty about not being able to keep up with her husband or provide him with the attention he needs. She said:

> I am depressed because I feel like I can't give my husband what I want to give him. I still am not able to be there for him and to do things with him. I want to be intimate like I felt in our first year of marriage. I enjoyed having sex with him, going out, and doing things with friends. Then, after I changed, I didn't want to be intimate with him. That same touch would make me bristle. It was like I had an aversion to him. I felt like telling him, "Just leave me alone." Then I started feeling guilty.

After a few months, though, Jamie's personality returned to normal. Her husband, Andy, knew she had a thyroid imbalance, and Jamie's doctor had explained that it would take a few weeks until the thyroid was regulated. Andy said, "I became used to the change from her being happy to being a person who would snap. She never hollered at me, but she came back quickly with 'Leave me alone!' I knew this was not her." In this type of situation, both partners feel guilty, but the patient experiences the greater guilt because he or she feels responsible for having brought the disease into the relationship.

Monica, a thirty-three-year-old accountant, experienced a similar situation. She had suffered from Graves' disease for more than a year. The intrusion of the thyroid condition into her relationship with her partner, Jack, led to a cascade of arguing, fighting, and distancing. Monica recognized that her behavior was the cause of some of the problems and felt guilty because she realized that she was not easy to live with.

"I have to say I'm probably hot-blooded also," she said. "I am this way about everything—kids, money, work. I'm sure it is hard for Jack. I can imagine that he had a hard time trying to decide what I was going to feel like today or maybe what I would feel like in thirty minutes. I probably was very hard to please."

To cite another example, one day a patient who had been suffering from Graves' disease for three years walked into my office. For the first time, her thyroid seemed to be well regulated, so I was surprised when she told me that she was getting a divorce. She said she had not felt this good for such a long time. Her mood swings, irritability, and anxiety had resolved. She had started working out and had been feeling good about herself. I told her that usually people get divorced before diagnosis, when their thyroid condition is affecting them the most. She said:

> I had been having marital problems for so long! It was an unhealthy relationship for a long time, and in fact, I feel that the stress of the marriage could have caused my Graves' disease. I felt like I had lost so much. I didn't have a job, money, or any control over my life or my health. Even though he was bad for me, I didn't have the courage or the strength to divorce him when I was ill. But now I have regained my self-esteem, and I see more clearly. I am more self-confident. I had to wait to feel this way to have the courage to divorce him.

What Partners Need to Know

Many people with thyroid disease have indicated the importance of receiving support and understanding from their partner or spouse after they are diagnosed and started on treatment. One hypothyroid woman said, "When I did see the doctor and was diagnosed, then my husband started being sympathetic and supportive. He let me sleep, and he would keep my son away from me, but it wasn't until after I was diagnosed. This was so helpful. That helped me recover quicker. Our arguing just stopped."

The partner's support and understanding are crucial for recovery because patients are still not the same as they used to be. They are still unable to control the anxiety, mood swings, anger, and irritability adequately.

Spouses of thyroid patients should also be involved in the management of the thyroid condition. A well-informed spouse will have a significant beneficial impact on the patient's recovery from the emotional effects and suffering due to the thyroid condition. Sometimes the spouse's support may even be as instrumental as the treatment provided by the physician.

Peter, a supportive husband, told me about his wife, who was still being treated for her thyroid condition. "When I see her slipping away," he said, "I know now what that is about, and it is not because she needs another pill. The process of recovery is slow and gradual. I think that thyroid patients need a lot of rest, and I encourage her to get it. Now I don't get upset when all she wants to do is sleep."

Many husbands, not understanding the impact of a thyroid imbalance, may refuse to put up with their spouses. Some may blame women for using hormones as an excuse for bad behavior. It is just as important for male partners to learn how hormones affect mood as it is for women with thyroid imbalances to become informed about their own condition. The imbalance in the brain takes time to normalize. Partners, unaware of these effects, quite often believe that the thyroid sufferer's reactions are psychological.

Some men embrace this challenge. When Loretta got remarried, her husband knew about her thyroid condition. He was an intelligent man and began to educate himself by reading about thyroid disease and its effects. He very quickly realized that he needed to be one of the primary supports for Loretta's recovery and to help her with her suffering. He was very much in love with her and became interested in her condition to the point that he knew perhaps even more about thyroid disease than Loretta did. He came to every office visit and was the one asking questions about therapy, testing, and the effects of thyroid imbalance on the body.

Other spouses, though, prefer to remain ignorant about the disease and its symptoms. When a partner chooses this method of coping with the situation, the patient is left feeling ignored and even guiltier. This will only exacerbate the situation and make the patient's suffering linger indefinitely.

The examples provided in this chapter illustrate how the intrusion of a thyroid condition can easily disturb the harmony of family life. Understanding the emotional aspects of a thyroid imbalance will not only help both patients and family members maintain their relationships; it will also help reduce the stress that can affect the course of the thyroid condition.

10

OVERLAPPING SYMPTOMS
AND SYNDROMES:

Fatigue, Chronic Fatigue, Hypoglycemia, and Fibromyalgia

" I am tired. I am exhausted. I cannot function the way I used to!" I hear these complaints from patients all the time. Many of them come to me because for some time they have been unable to function as before. The tiredness and feeling of exhaustion have robbed them of any sense of joy in everyday life and have interfered with their lives at all levels. Obviously when someone suffering from fatigue sees a specialist in thyroid disease, the tired person often has a notion that a thyroid imbalance may be a contributing factor. Frequently I see in the patient's expression that I am his or her last hope.

Typically, these patients have already seen quite a few doctors for the same complaint and often bring with them copies of records and tests that had been requested by other physicians. The tests and the causes considered inevitably vary from physician to physician. The interpretation of fatigue tends to differ depending on the training, experience, and interest that a physician may have in a particular field of medicine. Most physicians, when faced with the symptom of severe fatigue, are primarily concerned with identifying a major physical condition causing the fatigue. The most common diseases that cross physicians' minds are hepatitis (either alcoholic or viral), an acute or chronic infection such as tuberculosis or HIV, Lyme disease, diabetes or kidney problems, anemia, cancer, multiple sclerosis, or a cardiac condition. In the most general sense, the list of potential causes of fatigue is almost endless.

But when it comes right down to it, major medical conditions are found in only a small percentage of people struggling with fatigue. Each year, doctors record nearly 500 million patient visits to their offices for fatigue.

People say that they're tired so often that it is frequently ignored: feeling tired has become part of the normal way of living. If a person is suffering from several other symptoms, he or she might initially mention only the tiredness and exhaustion because of a perception that all the other symptoms are either part of the tiredness or caused by it. Many people figure, "This is stress. Everything will be fine." Many doctors, too, will often dismiss complaints of tiredness with the recommendation that the patient get more exercise, eat a better diet, or lose weight. Frequently this allows the symptoms of significant unexplained suffering to continue.

Being tired is indeed a common complaint, and only if you insist that you are more than just fatigued are your symptoms likely to be taken seriously by friends, relatives, or physicians. Studies of fatigue have suggested that there is a continuum ranging from "healthy–normal" fatigue to severe and debilitating fatigue. Surveys of European and American communities have shown that fatigue is a common symptom and occurs in 6.9 to 33 percent of men and 10.9 to 42 percent of women.[1] One study conducted in a primary care setting showed that fatigue of a month's duration or more was reported as a major problem among 19 percent of men and 28 percent of women.[2]

In most people, however, fatigue is the result of more than one factor. In order to narrow down the potential causes of fatigue, one has to go through a checklist of symptoms. At times, the process seems to involve detective work (see the list of "Potential Causes of Fatigue" at the end of the chapter).

Doctors consider fatigue to be one of the prime hallmarks of depression. If your endocrine system is working well, expressing the symptom of fatigue often leads to a search for hidden depression. If a physician uses the conventional medical criteria, he or she may ultimately come up with a diagnosis of depression. Quite often when sleep disturbances, decreased interest in pleasure, and appetite changes occur, physicians may think that the full criteria for depression are met. But regardless of whether the tiredness is generated by an infection, a physical condition, poor nutrition, or toxins, it will often lead to frustration and guilty feelings about not being able to accomplish what we need to accomplish. Tiredness causes increased sleep problems; sleep is interrupted by worries and waves of anxiety; when you feel drained, you tend to eat more to boost your energy. The effects of tiredness on sleep, self-esteem, and weight will inevitably induce confusion about what you may be suffering from.

The same level of confusion may exist if the main reason for your fatigue is a depression or anxiety disorder. These disorders can cause physical symptoms such as pain and gastrointestinal symptoms. The occurrence of these physical symptoms may cause your doctor to search for a physical disorder.

The Tripod of Wellness

Our well-being is under the scrutiny of three major systems—the brain, the endocrine system, and the immune system (which I call the tripod of wellness). These three systems, constantly interacting, allow us to appropriately react to and fight anything in the environment that threatens and interferes with our mental and physical health. The interactions among these three systems are so tight that in some cases a disturbance of one system ultimately will alter the functioning of the other two components of the tripod of wellness.

As an endocrinologist, I feel privileged to specialize in a major system of the body that regulates the largest and most significant components of human physiology. The endocrine system affects most facets of our well-being from minute to minute.

Countless patients who have suffered fatigue as the result of a dysfunction of the endocrine system have wandered from physician to physician searching for help, when all it would have taken to uncover the source of their suffering was a blood test.

Although thyroid hormone imbalance is undoubtedly the leading cause of fatigue related to endocrine gland problems, deficiencies of the pituitary gland and the adrenals should be considered as well. In one way or another, most hormones regulate bodily energy levels. They are the chemicals that are dispersed to most vital organs and oversee the basic functions of the cells in your body. A typical example of a malfunctioning endocrine gland that results in extreme tiredness and exhaustion is adrenal insufficiency, or Addison's disease. In nearly 70 percent of cases, this condition is due to an autoimmune attack on the adrenal glands. The attack and the destructive process that takes place in the adrenal glands are reminiscent of Hashimoto's thyroiditis, the leading cause of hypothyroidism, also an autoimmune disease. In fact, patients suffering from autoimmune disorders, including Hashimoto's thyroiditis and Graves' disease, are more prone to becoming afflicted by Addison's disease and vice versa.

Physicians often diagnose Addison's disease only when the disease and the cortisol deficiency have progressed to critical levels. Recently I saw a forty-two-year-old woman who had lost nearly twenty pounds over two years. Her fatigue and exhaustion had become debilitating. Her muscle weakness and loss of appetite were so severe that she had seen ten physicians. Some diagnosed her with depression, others with chronic fatigue syndrome (CFS) or food allergies. Her misery turned out to be due to a deficiency of the adrenal glands, which also made her become depressed. I gave her hydrocortisone treatment, and her fatigue and other symptoms resolved over the next month.

The pituitary gland, the master gland that controls most endocrine glands—including the thyroid, the adrenal glands, and the sexual glands—receives messages from both the brain and the glands that it controls. The pituitary gland, although tiny and hidden in a small socket of the bone at the base of the skull, has tremendous effects on various aspects of bodily functioning. If this gland were to be destroyed by a tumor, for instance, or by an abrupt reduction in blood supply (as might occur during severe hemorrhage), you would begin to suffer from hypopituitarism, a deficiency in the hormones produced by the pituitary gland. Among the wide array of effects that may result from hypopituitarism are an underactive thyroid, an underactive adrenal gland, a deficiency in sexual hormones, and a deficiency in growth hormone. The end result is the occurrence of a wide range of symptoms including fatigue, depression, and low blood pressure.

Although growth hormone promotes growth in children (a deficiency in infancy or childhood will result in dwarfism), growth hormone deficiency in adults was, until recently, thought not to affect their health. However, recent research has shown that a deficiency in growth hormone often results in fatigue, reduced capacity for exercise, muscle weakness, impaired cognition, mild depression, and decreased muscle mass.[3]

Another study concluded that, in some patients, a dysfunctioning pituitary gland causing a deficiency of growth hormone could account for fibromyalgia,[4] a condition that produces debilitating fatigue and a host of other physical and emotional symptoms. These patients have low levels of insulin-like growth factor (IgF1), a chemical normally produced by the liver under the influence of growth hormone that helps to carry out the functions of growth hormone. This research has shown that a growth hormone deficiency could account for as many as one-third of all cases of fibromyalgia.

Once a dysfunction of the endocrine system such as a thyroid imbalance or a growth hormone deficiency occurs, the other two components of the tripod of wellness (the brain and the immune system) are almost inevitably affected. A person with a thyroid imbalance or hypopituitarism, for instance, may become depressed and overwhelmed with stress. The depression causes the immune system to weaken, resulting in infection. Depression and infection result in more tiredness.

This cascade of one system affecting another and thereby worsening the fatigue has a wide range of implications. The first is that it reduces the likelihood that a doctor will consider an endocrine problem as the source of the suffering, because now other systems of the body are involved as well. The second implication is that if a person has more than one condition causing fatigue, symptoms of both conditions may escalate, making it highly likely that one of the conditions will be overlooked. Finally, the escalation of symptoms can become extreme in some patients, who may end up suffering from chronic depression, fibromyalgia, and chronic fatigue syndrome.

Many patients who were diagnosed with fibromyalgia or chronic fatigue syndrome and later found to be hypothyroid ask me whether having the two conditions was just a coincidence or whether the thyroid disorder triggered their fibromyalgia or chronic fatigue syndrome.

The answer is not always straightforward. The relationship among a thyroid imbalance, fibromyalgia, and chronic fatigue syndrome may be comparable to the relationship that exists between a thyroid imbalance and stress or depression. Did the stress or depression generated by a thyroid imbalance weaken the immune system, making the patient vulnerable to fibromyalgia or chronic fatigue syndrome? Or did the overwhelming stress and depression caused by the fatigue and the physical symptoms of fibromyalgia or chronic fatigue syndrome affect the immune system, resulting in a thyroid imbalance? The relationship among stress, depression, and disorders such as fibromyalgia and chronic fatigue syndrome is complex, but reflects interactions among the brain, endocrine system, and immune system. An infection with a virus such as a retrovirus seems to play a major role in the occurrence of CFS. People exposed to high levels of stress may not recover from a viral illness as swiftly as people with lower stress levels (or better stress-coping mechanisms). Now we understand that it is the psychological vulnerability of some people that makes their immune system weaker, and this causes the viral infection to linger for a long time.[5] In essence, psychological factors and stress appear to promote the development of chronic fatigue syndrome. Symptoms of depression have been found in 35 to 70 percent of patients with CFS,[6] and depression often precedes the onset of CFS.

Researchers have uncovered increasing evidence that chronic fatigue syndrome may even represent a particular type of chronic depression. The immune disturbances that occur in depression and CFS are in fact the same. But in some patients the depression may be caused by the fatigue, the chronic nature of the illness, the social stigma associated with the diagnosis, and the fact that no cure has yet been found. Isn't this quite reminiscent of the stress/thyroid escalation? For most people suffering from chronic fatigue syndrome, it is virtually impossible to determine which problem initiated the cascade of events—stress, depression, viral infection, disturbance of the immune system, or disturbance of the endocrine system.[7]

A series of studies have also established that the endocrine system is often disturbed in patients suffering from CFS. Many, for instance, are found to have low cortisol levels, an indication of slowing of the adrenal glands. But again it is not known whether such disturbances are the cause of the disorder or they are the consequence of the depression and the stress associated with the disorder.

A similar relationship exists between changes in brain chemistry and the occurrence of fibromyalgia, another common cause of severe fatigue.[8] Fibromyalgia may begin following an emotional stress, such as an automobile accident or a work-related accident. Some patients are emotionally disturbed and depressed or have suffered from a depression in the past. Stress could conceivably trigger fibromyalgia by making the pituitary gland slow down the manufacture of growth hormone.

Another example of how stress can affect growth hormone is the growth failure seen among abused children. The stress inflicted by the abuse causes the pituitary to produce much less growth hormone.[9]

Thyroid imbalance is also a possible precipitating factor for or even the direct cause of fibromyalgia and chronic fatigue syndrome. It is equally possible that these two conditions could trigger an autoimmune reaction of the thyroid gland. This explains why some patients who are diagnosed with fibromyalgia are found to have an underactive thyroid. Correcting the thyroid imbalance promptly will halt the cycle of symptoms and the worsening of fibromyalgia. In some patients, hypothyroidism can cause a typical case of fibromyalgia that can be cured with thyroid hormone; in other patients, the fibromyalgia will take on a life of its own and may not resolve after treatment of the underactive thyroid.

Fibromyalgia can also be triggered following treatment of an overactive thyroid. Poor correction of an overactive thyroid or repeated rapid swings of thyroid levels during treatment (causing abrupt shifts from hyperthyroidism to severe hypothyroidism) can provoke the onset of fibromyalgia (see Chapter 15). The reason for this is likely to be the tremendous amount of stress and disturbed emotions caused by these abrupt shifts.

Doctors often diagnose fibromyalgia months or even years after a person has been diagnosed with hypothyroidism. Often the patient has complained of fatigue, aches, and pains before therapy, but these symptoms were initially attributed to the hypothyroidism. After the thyroid has been adequately regulated, however, the patient continues to complain of these and a few other symptoms that, taken together, are consistent with fibromyalgia.

Thyroid Imbalance and Fibromyalgia

Fibromyalgia affects 5 percent of the population and accounts for approximately 20 percent of referrals to rheumatologists, specialists in conditions characterized by inflammation or pain in muscles and joints. As with thyroid disorders, this condition predominantly affects women. More than 80 percent of those who suffer from fibromyalgia are women, and the usual age range is twenty to fifty.

As in patients with thyroid imbalances, the physical symptoms, particularly the pains and aches, perpetuate a vicious cycle in which emotional distress, sleep difficulties, pain, and fatigue are mixed and amplified.

For years, the lack of an identifiable basis for fibromyalgia led many physicians to deny that the condition even existed. Many patients might have been tempted to conclude that their symptoms were "in their head." In 1990, however, the American College of Rheumatology issued criteria for the classification and diagnosis of fibromyalgia.[10] These criteria include a history of musculoskeletal pain in several areas of the body for at least three months and pain and tenderness in at least eleven of the eighteen trigger point sites by finger examination. The pains and aches often persist, although they may wax and wane. You may become sensitive to pressure applied to painful spots or even to clothing. You may also suffer from headaches and morning stiffness and tiredness, which can improve through the day and recur in late afternoon and evening. Fibromyalgia will typically make you experience nonrefreshing sleep. Many say that their sleep is light and restless. The easy fatigability with minimal exertion may alter the person's life at work as well as at home. Several other symptoms may also be associated, such as irritable bowel syndrome, urinary frequency, emotional distress, anxiety, and irritability.

Before accepting the diagnosis of fibromyalgia, discuss other disorders with your doctor. Some of the symptoms of fibromyalgia are also symptoms of connective tissue disorders, such as rheumatoid arthritis, Sjögren's syndrome, polymyalgia rheumatica, polymyositis, and lupus. These conditions, too, can cause a generalized pain syndrome, as can parathyroid disease and osteoarthritis. Also, many patients with fibromyalgia suffer simultaneously from a connective tissue disorder such as Raynaud's phenomenon or Sjögren's syndrome.

Doctors refer to fibromyalgia caused by hypothyroidism as "hypothyroid fibromyalgia," as opposed to "euthyroid fibromyalgia" (meaning fibromyalgia not caused by a dysfunctioning gland). Nearly 12 percent of all cases of fibromyalgia are caused by an underactive thyroid.[11] If you have been diagnosed with fibromyalgia, you need to have a TSH test to make sure you are not hypothyroid. If hypothyroidism remains undiagnosed and fibromyalgia lingers, symptoms of fibromyalgia may persist even when the underactive thyroid is finally treated.

Melinda, aged forty-two, was suffering from numerous symptoms quite typical of fibromyalgia with a significant component of depression. When she was diagnosed with hypothyroidism after three years of "physician shopping," she was happy and relieved, thinking that all of her problems were due to her thyroid. Although correction of her thyroid imbalance did result in some improvement, it did not completely resolve her suffering.

During Melinda's first visit to me, before she was started on thyroid medication, her husband said:

Every 60 or 120 days, she will sit down and write a list of how she's feeling in anticipation of seeing a new doctor. These symptoms range from being dizzy, to one cheek going numb, to an uncontrolled spasm in this muscle, to weak knees, to depression, to dry eyes, pains and aches in her joints, stiffness, sleep problems, aches in muscles, and legs and toes tingling. It is rare that these lists get to the doctor's hands because it's easy to type the list, but there is a fear in handing it to the doctor. He or she looks at this long list of symptoms that Melinda says she is experiencing all the time and concludes that either this is one physically and mentally sick puppy and it's beyond me or this can't be happening.

My findings indicated that Melinda was suffering from two separate conditions, fibromyalgia and hypothyroidism. Her hypothyroidism might have caused the fibromyalgia and was exacerbating its symptoms. As noted earlier, after treatment of her thyroid imbalance, many of Melinda's symptoms improved, but many related to the fibromyalgia persisted.

Doctors' frequent dismissal of patients like Melinda and the lack of support, education, and recognition of the syndrome often lead to physician shopping. After having wandered from one physician to another, many people with fibromyalgia find themselves subjected to quackery, seeking help from unreliable healers. Many may accept dangerous treatments that have not been proved effective.

Fibromyalgia, whether caused by or co-occurring with an underactive thyroid, is not necessarily a crippling disease. There are ways to control the symptoms. Small doses of tricyclic antidepressants, such as amitriptyline (Elavil), may be quite helpful to restore the quality of sleep and improve the pain and fatigue. A muscle relaxant taken in the evening may be helpful in improving aches and pains and sleep problems in fibromyalgia patients. Achieving aerobic fitness and avoiding a sedentary lifestyle will gradually improve the symptoms. Excessive exercise, on the other hand, can exacerbate the symptoms. Massage has helped many patients. I have found that avoiding caffeine in the afternoon and evening improves the quality of sleep. Also, patients should avoid too much noise at night. Hypnotherapy seems to be more effective than physical therapy in persistent fibromyalgia. Counseling, acupuncture, and biofeedback have helped many patients, as well. Recent research showed that T3 (Cytomel) administered at high doses (120 micrograms) daily could resolve all symptoms of fibromyalgia and even cure the condition.[12] However, high doses of T3 can produce adverse effects. Lower doses are better tolerated and may help patients relieve some of the symptoms.

In a recent trial, the subcutaneous administration of growth hormone daily was found to be effective in improving the symptoms of fibromyalgia, particularly the aches and pains, fatigue, and reduced capacity for exercise in patients with low IgF1 levels.[13]

Thyroid Imbalance
and Chronic Fatigue Syndrome

The Centers for Disease Control define chronic fatigue syndrome as a new onset of persistent or relapsing debilitating fatigue or easy fatigability that does not resolve with bed rest. Authorities on chronic fatigue have set a standard that the fatigue be severe enough to reduce average daily activity to below 50 percent of the previous "normal" activity level and that it last for a period of at least six months.[14] Other symptoms that may occur in chronic fatigue syndrome are:

- Chills
- Sore throat
- Painful regions
- Generalized muscle weakness
- Muscle pain
- Prolonged fatigue after exercise
- Headaches
- Joint pains
- Neuropsychological symptoms
- Sleep disturbances

Most symptoms develop abruptly. For the diagnosis of chronic fatigue syndrome to be made correctly, the criteria stipulate that you have at least six of the symptoms just mentioned plus at least two of the following: low-grade fever, pharyngitis, and swollen lymph nodes in the neck and armpit regions.[15]

Epidemiologic studies, conducted in several countries, have shown that the frequency of chronic fatigue syndrome is 0.3 to 1 percent.[16]

The psychological impairment can lead to social pressure and isolation. Patients may be described as crazy or lazy. Therefore, as is the case with thyroid patients, people suffering from CFS are often relieved when they finally learn that their symptoms are not "in their head" but are due to a physical condition. Although the neuropsychological symptoms of both depression and chronic fatigue syndrome may be similar and in fact are sometimes indistinguishable, certain physical effects may differentiate the conditions. In depression, the physical effects are often diffuse, and the patient may exhibit a combination of headaches, musculoskeletal pain, and gastrointestinal distress in addition to sleep and sex disturbances, guilt feelings, self-criticism, and pessimism. Some symptoms that are quite characteristic of CFS but not of other conditions causing debilitating fatigue are low-grade fever, enlarged lymph nodes, pharyngitis, and night sweats. Because CFS and hypothyroidism share many of the same symptoms, many patients who suffer from severe fatigue, poor sleep, aches, and pains are erroneously diagnosed with CFS.

Melissa, aged thirty-nine, was diagnosed by her chiropractor as having chronic fatigue syndrome a year ago. She had been struggling with fatigue and many other symptoms, and a friend referred her to me after recognizing that many of Melissa's symptoms were characteristic of hypothyroidism.

When she first came to my office, Melissa said:

> I wish I could feel the same way I used to. I wish I could have the energy I used to have and that the mood swings would go away! I feel like I'm in somebody else's body.
>
> The chiropractor told me I had chronic fatigue syndrome—"Epstein-Barr syndrome," she said. I was told there was no treatment for it. My hair has been falling out.

Because the chiropractor had labeled Melissa's ailment chronic fatigue syndrome, she suffered unnecessarily for an entire year. I concluded that her symptoms were in fact attributable to hypothyroidism and depression rather than chronic fatigue syndrome, and blood tests confirmed the underactive thyroid. An exam did not show enlarged lymph nodes in the neck and armpit regions, nor did Melissa have the low-grade fever or pharyngitis frequently seen in CFS. Appropriate treatment with thyroid hormone resolved all her suffering.

When Melissa came back a few months later and her thyroid levels were normal, she said:

> It seemed like everything changed. All that was left was the pain from my back. Everything else I was complaining about went away. My energy level went up so much. I cannot say I am tired anymore. It felt like this huge lead weight had been taken off my head. Like I had been compressed for years. I started losing weight. The crazy muscle spasms went away. The vision problems got a lot better. I stopped seeing the flashing lights.

Although there is no cure for CFS, a few treatments have been shown to help some patients. These include injection of high doses of immunoglobulin, intramuscular injections of magnesium sulfate, and consumption of high doses of essential fatty acids. The serotonin precursor, 5 hydroxytryptophan, can be helpful in some people.

Hypoglycemia: The Mysteries of Blood Sugar

Hypoglycemia, a below-normal blood sugar level, can cause several nonspecific symptoms such as fatigue, headaches, and rapid heartbeat. Other common symptoms are inability to concentrate, confusion, bizarre behavior, trembling, anxiety, sweating, and hunger. Many of the symptoms occur because the brain is not receiving enough sugar and ordinarily will resolve rather quickly when you eat carbohydrates.

Many of the symptoms of hypoglycemia result from the activation of the autonomic nervous system, the same system that causes some of the physical symptoms of an anxiety disorder. Hypoglycemia, widely publicized in lay magazines and books, is often cited as a common cause of tiredness, poor work and study performance, and sexual dysfunction.[17] As a result, many people suffering symptoms due to depression or anxiety disorder are erroneously diagnosed as hypoglycemic.

The standard test for hypoglycemia is an oral glucose tolerance test, which consists of measuring blood sugar before and several times after the ingestion of glucose. In healthy people not suffering from hypoglycemia, the blood sugar rises after glucose ingestion and then gradually decreases to low levels two to three hours after glucose intake. The levels will typically return to normal. It has been estimated that 20 percent of normal healthy people have a reactive low blood sugar two to three hours after food intake but no symptoms.[18] Doctors will make the diagnosis of true reactive hypoglycemia only if you have experienced symptoms when the blood sugar is low during the glucose test.

I have seen quite a few people who were placed on five to six small meals a day by doctors who diagnosed hypoglycemia. Some of these people were labeled hypoglycemic for quite a long time, yet the source of their symptoms turned out to be depression or an underactive thyroid. Even though the explosive epidemic of mislabeling seemingly everyone as hypoglycemic that occurred in the 1970s and 1980s[19] is slowly receding, this problem has continued to affect a substantial number of people.

Many times people are convinced that they have hypoglycemia because their symptoms improve after they consume carbohydrates. As I've noted, patients suffering from depression, anxiety, or a thyroid imbalance often experience an improvement in mood and anxiety levels when they eat frequently and consume carbohydrates. This is due to biochemical reactions in the brain that, for example, may increase levels of serotonin.

If you were diagnosed as hypoglycemic based only on symptoms, or if your glucose test was not interpreted correctly, you may become debilitated by the diagnosis itself. Many supposed hypoglycemics refuse to eat in restaurants, don't drive a car, or become "dietary cripples" who are deathly afraid of certain food choices.

Consider Tammy, who went to see her general practitioner for nervousness, profuse sweating, irritability, and shakiness—all of which are symptoms of both anxiety and hypoglycemia. Her physician diagnosed her as hypoglycemic and instructed her not to eat fruit or sugar. Because she had seen her father, who had also been diagnosed with hypoglycemia, have similar attacks, Tammy's obsession with hypoglycemia caused her to carry protein foods with her at all times. This went on for an entire year until finally she was diagnosed with Graves' disease.

If true hypoglycemia is not the reason for the symptoms of fatigue and anxiety after a meal, why, then, do some people experience fatigue, sleeplessness, difficulty concentrating, and even rapid heartbeat and sweatiness? If you absorb sugar faster, insulin levels in response to the sugar surge are, in general, higher. This often happens when thyroid levels are high. The result of a rapid rise in blood sugar is a high increase in insulin levels in the bloodstream. This typically causes the blood sugar to drop quickly after the abrupt rise. Even if you do not experience clear-cut low blood sugar, the rapid decline of blood sugar could trigger an exaggerated response of the adrenaline-activated nervous system, which results in symptoms.

In essence, a person can experience symptoms of hypoglycemia without actually having hypoglycemia. Typically, the rapid blood sugar fall and the symptoms it causes occur between one and two hours after a meal. Find out exactly when your symptoms occur in relation to your food intake.

The timing of symptoms is important in differentiating true hypoglycemia from what I call the "rapid blood sugar drop syndrome." With true reactive hypoglycemia, symptoms typically begin three hours after meals. They also coincide with a low blood sugar reading. In the rapid blood sugar drop syndrome, in contrast, the symptoms occur earlier and do not coincide with a low blood sugar reading. They do not occur every day and may depend on your mood and on what you have eaten.

The type of foods consumed determines the magnitude of the rise in blood sugar. Researchers have developed a scale called the glycemic index that scores foods according to the degree of rise in blood sugar that occurs after they are eaten. The higher the glycemic index, the higher the insulin response and the more rapid the subsequent fall in blood sugar. Simple sugars have a higher glycemic index than complex carbohydrates. What determines the glycemic index is not only the type of carbohydrates (simple versus complex) but also the amount of fat, protein, and fiber, as well as the method of food processing and cooking. Thus, to avoid a rapid drop in blood sugar, select foods that have the lowest glycemic index. (See Chapter 18 for a more thorough discussion of the effects of different foods on blood sugar.)

Equally disturbing are vague suggestions that connect hypoglycemia to hypothyroidism[20] and imply that hypoglycemia is a common occurrence in hypothyroidism. These have led some people to conclude that a person suffering from symptoms of hypoglycemia could be treated with thyroid hormone. Thyroid specialists often see patients who were diagnosed as hypoglycemic because of symptoms of fatigue, headaches, and sleep disturbances and who were then placed on thyroid hormone treatment for their condition.

Making the Diagnosis

To determine the likelihood that you are suffering from chronic fatigue syndrome, fibromyalgia, hypothyroidism, or a combination of these conditions, complete the following questionnaires and score yourself for each of the symptoms you are experiencing.

QUESTIONNAIRE A:
SYMPTOMS COMMON TO FIBROMYALGIA,
CHRONIC FATIGUE SYNDROME, AND HYPOTHYROIDISM

Indicate whether you have been experiencing each of the following symptoms. When you answer "No," proceed to the next symptom; when you answer "Yes," score the severity of your symptom (1 = mild, 2 = moderate, 3 = severe) before proceeding to the next one.

Fatigue	Yes	No	_____
Lack of endurance	Yes	No	_____
Dizziness	Yes	No	_____
Joint stiffness	Yes	No	_____
Depression	Yes	No	_____
Anxiety	Yes	No	_____
Difficulty concentrating	Yes	No	_____
Muscle weakness	Yes	No	_____
Headaches	Yes	No	_____
Worsening PMS	Yes	No	_____
Mood swings	Yes	No	_____
Irritability	Yes	No	_____
Word mix-ups	Yes	No	_____
Joint pains and aches	Yes	No	_____
Swollen fingers	Yes	No	_____
Brain fog	Yes	No	_____
Panic attacks	Yes	No	_____
Memory blanks	Yes	No	_____
TOTAL SCORE			_____

Add up your total score. If it is higher than 15, you may be suffering from fibromyalgia, chronic fatigue syndrome, or an underactive thyroid and should proceed to questionnaires B, C, D, and E.

QUESTIONNAIRE B:
CHRONIC FATIGUE SYNDROME/FIBROMYALGIA

Have you suffered, for six months, from fatigue occurring
    even at rest and not relieved by rest that has affected
    your ability to participate in your usual work, social,
    or personal activities? (If you answer yes, give
    yourself 10 points.)   Yes No ____
Do you feel exhausted, dizzy, and about to faint
    after a hot shower? (If you answer yes, give
    yourself 5 points.)   Yes No ____
Do you feel drained and exhausted for more than
    twenty-four hours after exercising? (If you answer
    yes, give yourself 5 points.)   Yes No ____
Did your symptoms begin abruptly? (If you answer
    yes, give yourself 5 points.)   Yes No ____
Have you experienced since the onset of the fatigue,
    but not before, any of the following symptoms
    in a persistent or recurrent fashion? If so, score
    the severity of each symptom as follows: 1 = mild,
    2 = moderate, 3 = severe.

Changing joint pains	Yes	No	____
Bad days, good days	Yes	No	____
Trouble sleeping in the middle of the night	Yes	No	____
Increased thirst	Yes	No	____
Dry eyes, dry mouth	Yes	No	____
Visual blurring	Yes	No	____
Rapid heartbeat	Yes	No	____
Loss of appetite	Yes	No	____
Nausea	Yes	No	____
Severe malaise	Yes	No	____
TOTAL SCORE			____

If your score is 25 or higher, you may be suffering from either
fibromyalgia or chronic fatigue syndrome and should proceed to questionnaire C.

QUESTIONNAIRE C: FIBROMYALGIA

Have you had for at least the past three months pain
  or achiness in many parts of your body, affecting
  both sides of the body (right and left), above and
  below the waist and in the midbody (that is, any
  part of the spine)? (If you answer yes, give
  yourself 5 points.)   Yes No _____

Has your doctor been able to trigger pain by
  pressing on eleven of the eighteen spots on
  your body called trigger points? (If you answer
  yes, give yourself 10 points.)   Yes No _____

Have you experienced any of the following
  symptoms? If so, score the severity of each
  symptom as follows: 1 = mild, 2 = moderate,
  3 = severe.

Muscle spasms   Yes No _____
Numbness and tingling   Yes No _____
Sensitivity of your eyes to light   Yes No _____
Bruising   Yes No _____
Irritable bladder   Yes No _____
Irritable bowel   Yes No _____
Eye pains   Yes No _____
TOTAL SCORE   _____

If your score is 25 or higher, you may be suffering from fibromyalgia.
Regardless of the score, proceed to questionnaires D and E.

QUESTIONNAIRE D: CHRONIC FATIGUE SYNDROME

Do you experience recurrent or persistent fevers?
(If you answer yes, give yourself 10 points.)   Yes No _____
Have you had tender lymph nodes lasting for several
weeks? (If you answer yes, give yourself 10 points.) Yes No _____
Have you experienced any of the following symp-
toms? If so, score the severity of each symptom as
follows: 1 = mild, 2 = moderate, 3 = severe.

Night sweats   Yes No _____
Sore throat   Yes No _____
Increased thirst   Yes No _____
Frequent infections   Yes No _____
TOTAL SCORE   _____

If your score is 25 points or higher in questionnaire D, you may be suffering from chronic fatigue syndrome. Now, regardless of your scores in questionnaires B, C, or D, proceed to questionnaire E.

QUESTIONNAIRE E: HYPOTHYROIDISM

Have you experienced any of the following symptoms for at least one month? When you answer no, proceed to the next symptom; when you answer yes, score the severity of your symptom (1 = mild, 2 = moderate, 3 = severe) before proceeding to the next one.

Hair loss   Yes No _____
Dry skin   Yes No _____
Constipation   Yes No _____
Slow pulse   Yes No _____
Increased appetite   Yes No _____
Weight gain   Yes No _____
Sleep apnea (heavy snoring and brief, intermittent
cessation of breathing during sleep)   Yes No _____
Yellow palms   Yes No _____
Muscle cramps   Yes No _____
Increased sleep   Yes No _____
TOTAL SCORE   _____

If you score higher than 10 in questionnaire E, you may be hypothyroid. If you also scored 25 or more in questionnaire C or D, you may have both hypothyroidism and chronic fatigue syndrome or fibromyalgia.

Potential Causes of Fatigue

DISORDERS OF THE ENDOCRINE SYSTEM
- Hypothyroidism
- Hyperthyroidism
- Addison's disease
- Pituitary deficiency (shortage of growth hormone)
- Multiple deficiencies of pituitary function
- Cushing's disease
- Diabetes

DISORDERS OF THE IMMUNE SYSTEM AND INFECTIONS
- Lupus
- Polymyositis (a rare muscle disease); dermatomyositis (a rare disease causing weak muscles and a skin rash)
- Sjögren's syndrome
- Polymyalgia rheumatica
- Pernicious anemia
- Rheumatoid arthritis
- Epstein-Barr virus infection
- HIV infection; AIDS
- Other viral illnesses
- Tuberculosis
- Lyme disease
- Fungal disease

DISORDERS OF BRAIN CHEMISTRY
- All depressive disorders
- Mood swing disorders

MISCELLANEOUS CONDITIONS
- Fibromyalgia
- Chronic fatigue syndrome
- Anemia
- Cancer
- Alcoholism
- Heavy-metal toxicity
- Medications (beta-blockers; antidepressants)
- Drug abuse
- Liver disease
- Heart failure
- Chronic lung problems

- Sleep apnea
- Parkinson's disease
- Multiple sclerosis
- Lymphoma

Important Points to Remember

- If you are suffering from fatigue, do not assume that your other symptoms are caused by the fatigue. To help your doctor uncover the source(s) of your fatigue, describe *all* your symptoms as precisely as possible.
- To find out what is causing your fatigue, you and your doctor may have to go through a detective-type process of checking the many organ systems that can produce fatigue.
- If no obvious disorders are found to cause your fatigue, disorders of the endocrine system such as deficiencies in the pituitary and adrenal glands should be considered.
- Remember, a person may have more than one disorder causing fatigue. Thyroid imbalance can coexist with other conditions that typically cause fatigue, including fibromyalgia and chronic fatigue syndrome.
- Keep the tripod of wellness (the endocrine system, the immune system, and the brain) in mind while you are trying to find out what is causing your fatigue.
- If you have fibromyalgia, a thyroid imbalance could be the cause.
- Do not easily accept the diagnosis of hypoglycemia unless your symptoms coincide with low blood sugar levels.
- To avoid being misdiagnosed, use symptom questions that help you determine which one of the three overlapping syndromes (fibromyalgia, chronic fatigue syndrome, and thyroid imbalance) is causing your symptom(s).

PART III

WOMEN'S THYROID PROBLEMS:

Your Symptoms Are Not All in Your Head

11

PREMENSTRUAL SYNDROME
AND MENOPAUSE:

Tuning the Cycles

From puberty to menopause, women's bodies and brains are influenced by continuous cycles of hormones. These hormones are crucial not only for reproduction but also for the nature of a woman's feminine identity. Sex hormones—including estrogen, progesterone, testosterone, and DHEA—play an important role in regulating the functioning of various organs (such as the skin) as well as many bodily systems, including the musculoskeletal, circulatory, and immune systems. Sex hormones also play an important role in thinking and memory, and they interact with chemicals in the brain that have been implicated in the regulation of mood, emotions, and sex drive.

The well-defined pattern of women's monthly cycles is tightly regulated by messages from the hypothalamus and pituitary gland. The control of these messages by higher brain centers and the countereffects of hormones on brain functioning are reminiscent of how the thyroid hormone system works. Even though the thyroid system and the sex hormone system are two independent systems governed by the same "master gland," the pituitary, there are important relationships between the two.

First, thyroid hormone levels significantly alter the levels and action of sex hormones. A thyroid hormone imbalance frequently causes either heavy, prolonged menstrual periods (especially in hypothyroidism) or brief, scanty menstrual periods, or even cessation of periods (in hyperthyroidism and also in severe hypothyroidism). Thyroid hormone, which affects sex hormones, is critical for conception and throughout the duration of pregnancy.

Second, sex hormones seem to play a role in the occurrence of thyroid disease. The increased prevalence of thyroid conditions—notably, autoimmune diseases—among females begins to be noted at puberty. As a woman enters her reproductive years, the frequency of both Hashimoto's thyroiditis and Graves' disease increases sharply. At menopause, the frequency of

Hashimoto's thyroiditis and low-grade hypothyroidism also increases, with 13 to 15 percent of postmenopausal women having some thyroid hormone deficit.[1] One study showed that Hashimoto's thyroiditis occurred more frequently in women who had a longer reproductive span (that is, more years between puberty and menopause).[2]

Other facts clearly indicate that sex hormones have a major effect on the activity of the thyroid gland and may even affect the triggering of an autoimmune reaction in the thyroid. For instance, many women with dormant Graves' disease may have a flare-up in the first trimester of pregnancy or after delivery. The important hormonal changes that occur after delivery also seem to account for the high frequency of postpartum thyroid disease. The triggering or worsening of thyroid conditions throughout these periods of hormonal shifts is probably related to effects of the sex hormones on the immune system. For instance, the sex hormone progesterone may affect the immune system and could play a role in the occurrence of autoimmune thyroid disorders.

In addition to these causal or triggering effects, sex hormones have a significant effect on how a thyroid imbalance is expressed. Mental symptoms, such as mood swings and depression, and the way the patient perceives these symptoms, are very much influenced by sex hormone fluctuations. The chemistry of both the brain and the body is influenced in normal and abnormal conditions by the thyroid and sex hormones. A thyroid hormone imbalance will exacerbate the symptoms of hormonal shifts, so a woman who usually has few or no symptoms related to hormonal changes will begin to experience more symptoms when a thyroid imbalance occurs.

These complex ways in which thyroid problems magnify suffering are most apparent during three important periods of the hormonal cycle: the luteal phase of the menstrual cycle (after ovulation, when an egg is released—the time when most women experience premenstrual syndrome, or PMS), the postpartum period, and menopause. This chapter focuses on the relationship between the thyroid, luteal phase syndrome (PMS), and menopause. (Postpartum depression is discussed in Chapter 13.)

PMS: Chemical Imbalance
or Hormonal Shifts?

During the last part of the menstrual cycle (that is, five to seven days prior to the menstrual period), many women suffer mood swings, irritability, anger, loss of energy, difficulty concentrating, appetite changes (particularly food cravings), anxiety, depression, loss of interest in ordinary activities, exhaustion, and sleep pattern changes. This constellation of symptoms, casually called premenstrual syndrome, is reminiscent of a depressive type of cyclic mood disorder. During the course of the reproductive years, this cyclic change in emotions and mood often begins in an insidious fashion. Gradually, women who experience PMS learn to cope with the episodic and recurrent suffering.

Because the symptoms of PMS are similar to those of cyclic depression, it's often thought that the underlying reason is a subtle chemical imbalance responsible for the mood swings. PMS tends to become more noticeable to the woman during the last few days of the menstrual cycle. This is when estrogen levels, after increasing following ovulation, tend to decline. At the same time, the levels of progesterone, which had been produced in great quantities in the second part of the menstrual cycle, tend to decrease as well. These hormonal shifts have been thought to be the basis for premenstrual syndrome. Hormonal shifts also explain the physical discomfort—including bloating, aches and pains, and headaches—that you may experience during PMS.

Premenstrual syndrome is one of the least understood syndromes in medicine. Endocrinologists, reproductive endocrinologists, psychiatrists, and gynecologists have all attempted to understand the basis for the syndrome, yet none has been able to declare authoritatively what causes PMS. For the most part, the various specialists have addressed only the facets of the syndrome that apply to their field. Endocrinologists have found multiple abnormalities that could account for the fluid and salt retention that occurs during the premenstrual period. Reproductive endocrinologists and gynecologists have explained the changes in hormone levels occurring in the last part of the menstrual cycle, which account for some of the physical effects of premenstrual syndrome. Psychiatrists have focused on the emotional aspects of premenstrual syndrome and have provided some criteria for making a correct diagnosis.[3]

Researchers from the various fields have proposed that the cause of premenstrual syndrome could be an increased sensitivity in some women to hormonal shifts or a neuroendocrine abnormality in the chemicals of the brain or a subtle cyclic mood disorder brought on by hormonal shifts. A further possibility is that the hormonal shifts could be just the triggering or aggravating factor leading to the onset and perpetuation of symptoms.

Some women may have an underlying subtle chemical imbalance that predisposes them to suffer PMS. Thyroid hormone, cortisol, and sex hormones (that is, estrogen, progesterone, and androgens) modulate the amount of chemicals in the brain and their effects on the body and mind. These same brain chemicals have been implicated in mood disorders. The interaction of hormones and chemicals could lead to the physical and emotional suffering experienced in premenstrual syndrome.

The Difficulties of Diagnosing PMS

At least half of all women experience some discomfort during the premenstrual period, but the majority of them have mild changes that they perceive as normal and similar to what other women experience. Asked whether they have symptoms of premenstrual syndrome, such women will typically respond, "Oh, yeah, I have those." As with many mental conditions, psychiatrists have proposed rigid criteria for determining whether a woman has PMS. They have defined what they have called the "late luteal phase dysphoric disorder" among women with severe symptoms. Only 5 percent of women actually fulfill these criteria and are diagnosed as having PMS.[4] Many other women who experience the typical, less severe symptoms of premenstrual syndrome do not fulfill these criteria and are not considered to have true PMS.

Severity of premenstrual suffering tends to worsen as a woman gets older. The worsening of the mood swings and the feelings of loss of control intensify with time and reshape the suffering, giving it different dimensions and expressions that become very confusing to the patient as well as to a doctor attempting to diagnose PMS or thyroid imbalance or menopause.

The symptoms of PMS can worsen during the time the woman is about to become menopausal so that the symptoms of PMS and menopause, which are similar, may be intermingled. In some women, the emotional discomfort, mood swings, and irritability are exacerbated in a cyclic fashion on a monthly basis and occur several days each month, even in women entering menopause. At this stage of their reproductive lives, women are often surprised to hear that PMS could be causing their discomfort.

Although premenstrual syndrome is typically described as occurring for five to seven days before the menstrual period, its duration can actually be much longer—up to fifteen to twenty days of the menstrual cycle. Often, as symptoms worsen, they also extend over a longer period of time.

Women who suffer from chronic, undiagnosed mood or anxiety disorders in addition to having PMS can find it particularly difficult to get diagnosed properly. Because both PMS-type symptoms and mood disorders are quite prevalent in the general population, many women who have an underlying subtle to moderately severe mood disorder, often of the depressive type, also experience premenstrual syndrome. In these women, the emotional suffering related to their mood disorder worsens in this vulnerable period of the menstrual cycle. For several days before the menstrual period, these women experience a mixture of discomfort and suffering related to both the PMS and the mood disorder, with the symptoms sometimes becoming severe and disabling. This intensification of symptoms represents a strong argument in favor of a subtle chemical imbalance in the brain's being at the root of PMS.

The following examples of mixed disturbances illustrate the difficulties physicians encounter in accurately diagnosing patients suffering from premenstrual syndrome. The examples also illustrate the importance of brain chemistry being the common denominator for both PMS and other mental disturbances.

In the case of Alyssa, a thirty-five-year-old housewife, a chronic anxiety disorder overlapped with symptoms of PMS and rendered her situation quite confusing. She suffered from cyclothymia, an intermittently depressed mood lasting for periods of a few days, as well as the chronic anxiety. Alyssa's PMS had begun six to seven years earlier and recently her symptoms had been worsening. In midcycle, her mood swings became more severe, and her anxiety symptoms worsened. Although she had visited several physicians, her symptoms had become so confusing that she was given many diagnostic labels but no definite help. She said:

I know when I'm ovulating. I ovulate, and I start walking the path through hormonal hell. My moods get darker, and the depression gets worse. I live most days with some type of discomfort. I get more numbness and tingling in my toes. My periods are extremely painful. The migraines are worse. It's like a knife going through the top of my head.

My mood and emotions are on a roller coaster. I want to get a divorce from my husband about once a month. Once, I asked him to leave. It was shocking. There was nothing he could do that was right.

The closer I get to my period, the harder it is for me to focus or concentrate. I feel like I have lost my mental capacity. Also, the closer I get to my period, the more exaggerated all the other symptoms are. I shake more, my heart palpitates more, I'm colder, my muscles spasm more. I experience an anxiety over what my body is doing. I will get a rage of anxiety just resting.

Every day before I go to sleep, I think I'm going to have a good day tomorrow. It rarely happens. I want to go and crawl in a corner and put my hands over my head and disappear from the face of the earth.

Alyssa noted that her mood swings and depression had gotten worse approximately six months before the doctor told her that she had hypothyroidism. Only after she was successfully treated for hypothyroidism did she notice a significant improvement in her PMS.

Thyroid Hormone Imbalance: The Link to PMS

Endocrinologists have studied various facets of the body's hormonal systems in order to explain some of the symptoms occurring in premenstrual syndrome, such as fluid retention, bloating, and breast tenderness. They have found some abnormalities in many hormonal systems, including the thyroid system. Since thyroid hormone changes levels of brain chemicals known to affect emotions and mood, several researchers have attempted to determine whether PMS could be caused by a thyroid imbalance.

Dr. Peter Schmidt and his coworkers from the National Institutes of Health showed in a study of a large number of women fulfilling the clinical criteria of premenstrual syndrome[5] that 10.5 percent of women with PMS had a thyroid imbalance, frequently low-grade hypothyroidism. Utilizing TRH stimulation testing, the most sensitive test available for detecting a very minor thyroid hormone deficit, they also found that 30 percent of women with PMS who have normal basal TSH levels had a minor thyroid imbalance. The frequency of low-grade hypothyroidism determined by TSH measurement in large samples of women of reproductive age has generally been 3.6 to 7.5 percent, so the rate found in this study was higher than expected.

An open trial conducted by Dr. Nora Brayshaw showed that a high dose of thyroid hormone caused relief of symptoms in women with PMS. Most of the women studied had low-grade hypothyroidism.[6]

These results, although not confirmed by other studies, suggest that thyroid imbalance, including low-grade hypothyroidism, may play a role in the occurrence or exacerbation of PMS in some but not all women. It is possible that a deficit of thyroid hormone in the brain is the basis of premenstrual syndrome in some women. The similarities between the symptoms of hypothyroidism and those of premenstrual syndrome make this hypothesis plausible. Some of the common symptoms include weight gain, poor regulation of temperature, lethargy, irritability, mood swings, and anxiety. The effectiveness of thyroid hormone treatment in some women who suffer from PMS but have normal thyroid glands is reminiscent of the effectiveness noted in women suffering from depression.

Martha, a thirty-two-year-old manager, had never had symptoms of PMS until two years before her gynecologist made the diagnosis of hypothyroidism. She said:

Initially, I was happy most of the time. Then, two years ago, I started getting tired and depressed and having headaches before my period. Little by little, I became very emotional and couldn't get out of bed. I would get up, shower, get dressed, and just sit there.

For several months, my periods would last two weeks, so it was like basically the whole month on PMS. I would be irritable the whole time. When I was diagnosed with hypothyroidism and started thyroid hormone treatment, my symptoms started decreasing. My headaches started decreasing, and then my symptoms went away.

Martha's case is not unique. Another woman who was found to have Hashimoto's thyroiditis had first gone to her doctor complaining of PMS.[7] A thyroid hormone deficit can generate a host of PMS symptoms.

Hyperthyroidism as a Cause of PMS

Mild hyperthyroidism can go unnoticed for years. It can wax and wane, or flare up, especially during periods of stress. Some women notice the effects of mild hyperthyroidism on the body and mind only during the premenstrual period. Many women diagnosed with Graves' disease who have had some experience with PMS state that Graves' disease can be described as PMS multiplied many times. The symptoms of hyperthyroidism and PMS may be so similar that you may attribute symptoms of hyperthyroidism to worsening PMS. The following example illustrates how mild, low-grade hyperthyroidism can manifest itself as PMS.

Courtney, a forty-year-old physician, suffered from low-grade hyperthyroidism for years. She had numerous rounds of thyroid testing over the years, with several of the tests showing normal thyroid function and some showing very mild hyperthyroidism. None of the physicians Courtney had seen felt that she should be given antithyroid medications. Her history was especially noteworthy in that the only time she had symptoms was during the premenstrual period. All the symptoms she described were those of premenstrual syndrome. After treatment of her thyroid condition, she has experienced no significant symptoms of PMS since. According to Courtney:

I noticed even before medical school, when I was younger, nineteen or twenty years old, that I felt uncomfortable when I spent my vacation in the South, especially in the summer, when the temperature is warmer. My hands were a little sweaty. During wintertime, I almost never wore gloves. I didn't feel that I needed them. I also experienced rapid heartbeat. When my son was born, I was twenty-five. That's when my doctor checked my thyroid and told me that it was not severe enough to treat.

My residency was very stressful. I lost weight. My hands often shook, and at night I experienced much anxiety.

The menstrual symptoms began when I was twenty. They became worse over the years. When the menstrual period is over, I feel like I'm all right, not as depressed as before the start of the menstrual period, which are more vulnerable days for me because I cry. I can't control myself. I don't handle reasonably what's going on.

When I had PMS, I got intense, agitated, and irritable. The volume was turned up on my emotions. Sometimes I felt like an eight-track tape that changed channels a lot.

How Thyroid Dysfunction Can
Exacerbate PMS

Many women whose PMS symptoms are worsening are found to have a thyroid dysfunction, the most common being low-grade hypothyroidism. For women suffering from mild premenstrual syndrome, the occurrence of a thyroid imbalance may aggravate PMS symptoms.

Billie was thirty-two when her gynecologist diagnosed a goiter. Thyroid testing showed hypothyroidism. Billie had started having PMS at the age of twenty but coped with the symptoms quite well. Over the preceding three-year period, though, her symptoms had gradually worsened. She saw numerous physicians, who recommended different treatments without results. The worsening of PMS resolved when her hypothyroidism was corrected.

Before treatment, Billie described her symptoms as follows:

I have been suffering from these symptoms for some time. I wanted to break up with my boyfriend, or I didn't like him or something. Then I started noticing that, even when he was gone, I still had that. My symptoms became much worse in the past three years. It was like clockwork. Same feelings, same anxiety. A physician diagnosed PMS and prescribed Prozac. Prozac helped a little, but then I had side effects. I stopped taking it.

I had gotten it down pretty much. Twenty days out of the month I am okay. I know any day I'm waiting for it to come. All of a sudden, it feels like something comes in my body and takes over.

My mind all of a sudden changes. My appetite goes crazy. I never can get satisfied. The imbalance almost drives me crazy. My emotions become overwhelming.

It comes and goes in waves. I would cry and not know why. One minute I would be on top of the world and be doing things with my family, and then five minutes later something would make me mad and I would be yelling at my friends or husband. I'm not the same person. It's like dual personalities.

I went to a PMS specialist. He handed me a brochure and said, "This is what PMS is, and I'm sorry I have nothing to tell you. Take these birth control pills and see if that helps." They made me tired and made me gain weight. Another doctor read my history and told me that I might be suffering from a bipolar disorder. One doctor told me I had cyclothymia.

Billie's PMS became much more severe at the onset of her hypothyroidism. With thyroid hormone treatment, her mind felt clearer all the time and her symptoms improved. She said:

I stayed on more of an even keel. My appetite was more regular. My energy level was more consistent. I didn't do a lot of things at one time. I was more methodical. I usually try to get a lot of things going at the same time—baking, cooking, doing laundry. I don't tire out as I did. I'm calmer. My responses are more thought out. I didn't have any other improvement like this with any other medication.

Hyperthyroidism can also worsen symptoms of PMS. Many women who are familiar with PMS symptoms and have developed Graves' disease have indicated that their PMS symptoms significantly worsened when they became hyperthyroid.

Victoria, a thirty-five-year-old housewife who had suffered from PMS for many years, experienced a worsening of her symptoms when she developed Graves' disease. As in Billie's case, the worsening subsided after correction of the hyperthyroidism. Victoria said:

I had been treated for PMS with medication since my marriage ten years ago. It had subsided between pregnancies and returned and got progressively worse after the second pregnancy. I was teary a lot, and I would cry at things that were not real issues. I would think everything my husband did was wrong, and I hated his guts. I wanted him out the door. That was one of the reasons I went for a medical checkup back when I was first married, because it was something I never noticed until I had to live in the same house with somebody all the time.

At that time, my gynecologist put me on a mild diuretic before my period, and the PMS resolved somewhat. Since my last pregnancy, it was as much the teary, weepy thing as it was the lashing out. Later on, I went back complaining of PMS from ovulation on. I was spending half of my life being completely out of control and feeling high levels of stress. The slightest thing would set me off.

When my cycle is about to come, perhaps one week before the menstrual period, my irritability is worse. I want to eat all the sweets I can find. I want to sleep and will avoid sex. I feel tired and sad. Once my cycle comes and goes, the rest of the month is okay. I focus on whatever I am doing.

My gynecologist had put me on birth control pills. I went back, and she said I might be perimenopausal and I would do well to take progesterone, which would help the symptoms. I'm from a dry part of the country and I was sweating all the time, but I just thought it was this climate. [Such sweating is, of course, a symptom of hyperthyroidism.]

In trying to explain thyroid disease to women who don't have it, I use the analogy that Graves' disease feels like PMS intensified by a factor of about one thousand—the emotional behavior, being crazy, angry, crying, and all that. I felt like that all the time. I couldn't really differentiate between PMS and Graves'. I had PMS before—slight irritability, crying a little more than normal, feeling kind of sluggish and a little breast tenderness, slightly out of control emotionally.

Thyroid hormone excess or deficiency gives a different shape to premenstrual syndrome. It not only amplifies preexisting PMS symptoms but also adds new symptoms to the mix. The additional suffering differs depending on the type and severity of the thyroid imbalance.

Whereas hypothyroidism during PMS introduces more sudden depressed moods, crying spells, feelings of despair and loss of control, sleepiness, guilt feelings, and anger, hyperthyroidism during PMS introduces more anxiety symptoms, restlessness, and altered sleep patterns. Hyperthyroid women experiencing panic attacks may find that those attacks increase in both frequency and severity during the last part of the menstrual cycle. In general, the mood swings, irritability, and anger become mixed with a higher degree of anxiety and agitation during the premenstrual period.

When hypothyroidism and PMS coexist, there is often a lack of sexual desire and impaired sexual arousal in women during the premenstrual period. Hyperthyroid patients also have decreased sex drive during PMS. Some women, however, may experience increased interest in sex and a heightened sexual arousal.

Because the effects of a thyroid imbalance, whether hypothyroidism or hyperthyroidism, contribute to the occurrence or worsening of PMS, we can say that hormonal shifts and a brain chemical imbalance are probably the basis for PMS symptoms. And a change in T3 levels in the brain amplifies the effects.

The Thyroid and Perimenopause

Endocrinologists have noticed that the occurrence of hypothyroidism in the perimenopausal period (the roughly five to ten years leading up to the onset of menopause) often represents a more significant stress than when it occurs at other times. Also, the symptoms of hypothyroidism may intensify as a result of the hormonal shifts that precede menopause. A long-standing, untreated thyroid condition during the perimenopausal period can cause more depression, irritability, and anger and may trigger personal problems and more menopausal symptoms.

Symptoms of menopause and hypothyroidism are astonishingly similar, leading many patients suffering from mild hypothyroidism to be dismissed as menopausal. If a woman is in the perimenopausal or postmenopausal period, the first thing that tends to come to a gynecologist's mind is that symptoms of mood swings or fatigue are due to a hormonal imbalance. A woman may even suggest this possibility to the physician. Should these symptoms persist despite adequate hormone replacement therapy, only an astute and thorough gynecologist might eventually test the thyroid as a possible reason for the symptoms.

The Thyroid's Effect on Menopause

In the next two decades, nearly 40 million American women will face menopause, and a significant number of them will be at risk for having a thyroid imbalance. At menopause, many more women develop Hashimoto's thyroiditis and hypothyroidism. The frequency with which women develop these disorders also increases with aging. The effects of thyroid diseases on menopausal women may prevent them from coping with the various physical and emotional stresses that occur after menopause.

A thyroid imbalance can confuse or exaggerate symptoms of menopause. The passage from regular menstrual periods to cessation of menstruation is not only a marker for the end of the reproductive years but also a critical period during which hormonal and sociocultural influences reshape how a woman perceives herself. She becomes more vulnerable to depression and impaired cognitive function.

Currently, many women live one-third of their lives after menopause. Despite the recognition of the need for comprehensive care for women and of the importance of preventive medicine and education to assure women's good health, health care delivery systems have not emphasized the importance of early detection and adequate treatment of thyroid imbalances. Education about thyroid disease should be part of a woman's health program, particularly at midlife.

Even though *menopause* refers specifically to the cessation of menstruation, during the transition period, estrogen levels gradually decline, and the menstrual periods become more irregular and frequently heavier until they stop altogether. As with PMS, thyroid disease during menopause may have a significant effect on how a woman perceives her menopausal symptoms and even on the nature of those symptoms.

Early research, consisting of poorly designed studies, led to the common assumption that during menopause, most women would inevitably experience hot flashes, night sweats, vaginal dryness, and many other symptoms, including depression, irritability, weight gain, insomnia, and dizziness. Recent studies, however, have suggested that the actual experiences of menopausal syndrome are much less negative than women had been led to expect. Contrary to many published reports, depression and emotional instability are not universal. This lack of reliable information about menopause increases women's anxiety and negative feelings, which perpetuate the symptoms.

Women vary significantly in how they perceive menopause. Women reporting menopausal symptoms are likely to be those who are under high levels of stress and who have particularly negative beliefs about menopause. The horrible descriptions of menopausal symptoms presented by the media and lay magazines may increase fear and anxiety about menopause. According to a study conducted in Great Britain, 44 percent of general practitioners surveyed indicated that the anxiety experienced by their patients about menopause had increased due to the influence of the media.[8] Some women may come to view menopause as inevitably a time of despair and plunge into melancholia. Christiane Northrup, a doctor and women's health specialist, said "expectations of problems in menopause lead to problems."[9]

The physical and emotional symptoms of menopause have been assumed to be due to a decline in estrogen levels, a decline that presumably would be corrected by estrogen replacement therapy. Estrogens certainly have major interactions with brain chemicals that affect cognitive functions and mood. What seems to have a greater effect on the occurrence of such symptoms, however, is the amount of stress experienced prior to menopause. Studies done in Japan and the United States have shown that the expression of the symptoms of menopause and the frequency of these symptoms differ significantly between Japanese and American women.[10] The differences are so striking that they can be explained only by sociocultural factors. For instance, approximately 38 percent of American women experienced a lack of energy, compared to only 6 percent of Japanese women. Some 30 percent of American women experienced irritability, whereas this symptom was reported by only 12 percent of Japanese women. Many other symptoms of menopause, such as depression and trouble sleeping, were on average three times more common in American women than in Japanese women. American women also complained of more hot flashes and night sweats than their Japanese counterparts.

Among Japanese women, the highest rate of depression was found among premenopausal women, whereas among American women, the highest rate of depression occurred among women who were about to become menopausal. Depression during menopause seems to be predicted by a history of previous depression. A woman with a tendency toward depression may feel unable to control the changes that occur during menopause and may then perceive those changes in a more negative way. The depression worsens, and stress is perceived as overwhelming.

For most women, hormonal changes probably do not account for all the changes in well-being or the physical symptoms of menopause. Hormonal changes do seem to play a role in the occurrence of hot flashes and night sweats, however. The frequency of hot flashes appears to be much lower than previously thought, occurring in 50 to 60 percent of women.

One study found that stress from bereavement, divorce, or friends moving away is closely associated with the psychological and physical symptoms of menopause.[11] Other factors, such as low educational and socioeconomic status, are also associated with more symptoms of depression than are generally found among middle-class women. Women with lower monthly incomes were shown to have a higher incidence of nervous complaints at menopause.[12] People with a tendency toward mood swings often feel more helpless when they anticipate and cope with life changes. Further evidence suggesting that menopausal symptoms are linked to brain chemical changes is that a history of premenstrual syndrome is associated with an increased chance of having menopausal symptoms.[13]

Based on the evidence just provided, it becomes easy to understand that a thyroid imbalance occurring prior to menopause is likely to predispose a woman to the occurrence of menopausal symptoms. In a Canadian study, women who experienced health problems, in particular arthritis and thyroid problems, before menopause were more likely to experience depression during menopause.[14] This explains why women with hypothyroidism suffer from more headaches, depression, constipation, and other "menopausal" symptoms, even when they have been adequately treated with thyroid hormone.

Of equal importance is the awareness that the mind-body effects of a thyroid imbalance may be more pronounced in a menopausal woman, even if the imbalance is minimal.

For menopausal women and women about to become menopausal, relaxation techniques, adequate correction of the thyroid imbalance, and lifestyle factors are crucial to prevent or treat the lingering effects of thyroid imbalance (see Chapter 16). The effects of sex hormones, thyroid hormones, and environmental stress influence mind and body. How these effects manifest in mood or physical discomfort varies from woman to woman. So how a physician diagnoses his or her patient's suffering depends on the physician and what appears to be the source of the most prominent symptoms. One physician may blame hormones, another may cite stress, and a third may implicate depression or anxiety. Regardless of the type and severity of suffering due to hormonal effects on women's cycles—whether the premenstrual period, the postpartum period, or menopause—you should be more attuned to have the thyroid component detected and corrected as early as possible.

Important Points to Remember

- If you are a new PMS sufferer, an underactive or overactive thyroid may be the cause of your symptoms.
- If you have suffered from PMS but your symptoms have recently worsened and your menstrual periods have changed, have your doctor consider a thyroid imbalance.
- PMS is essentially a brain chemistry disorder, and changes in hormones

that regulate your brain chemistry appear to be important contributing factors. Keep in mind that thyroid hormone is a major player in brain chemistry.

- If you have experienced a severe thyroid imbalance in your reproductive years, you are likely to experience unpleasant times at menopause. Adequate thyroid treatment and relaxation techniques may be the solution.
- Menopause is a vulnerable time for women. The frequency of thyroid imbalance (Hashimoto's and hypothyroidism) increases sharply during this period.
- The symptoms of menopause and thyroid imbalance are quite similar. If you begin to experience depression, fatigue, and mood swings, do not necessarily attribute your symptoms to menopause. Have your doctor test your thyroid.
- Thyroid imbalance worsens symptoms of menopause and vice versa. Unless all the effects of menopause and thyroid imbalance are addressed, your symptoms may continue and escalate over time.

12

INFERTILITY AND MISCARRIAGE:

Is Your Thyroid a Factor?

Even before the era of sophisticated, precise thyroid testing, doctors were aware of the effects of thyroid imbalance on reproduction. At the turn of the twentieth century, physicians administered thyroid hormone to women to improve their fertility and treat menopause. Today's doctors recognize that adequate thyroid hormone levels are essential to help regulate the production of sex hormones (that is, estrogen and progesterone) and the hormonal cycle responsible for ovulation. Both an excess of thyroid hormone and, more commonly, a deficiency of the hormone alter the harmonious functioning of the reproductive system and sometimes prevent ovulation. Even if ovulation and conception occur, a thyroid imbalance can lead to a deficit in progesterone, which can render the uterus unsuitable for implantation of an embryo. This, in turn, prevents a normal pregnancy.

A number of important advances have occurred in the past decade in the field of infertility medicine. Less publicized have been the findings that link thyroid hormone imbalance with impaired reproduction, infertility, and miscarriage.

Both an underactive thyroid and an overactive thyroid can cause infertility problems and affect the outcome of a pregnancy. Nevertheless, because hypothyroidism is much more common than hyperthyroidism, thyroid-related infertility and miscarriage problems are more frequently caused by an underactive thyroid. For this reason, this chapter focuses on hypothyroidism as a cause of these difficulties.

Infertility is a common condition. Doctors estimate that one of every six couples of childbearing age has a problem with fertility.[1] With modern infertility protocols, which are frequently expensive and time-consuming, approximately two-thirds of all couples can be treated and successfully conceive.

Infertility can be considered a type of chronic illness. The afflicted person lives with a constant but shaky hope that "it" will go away or be cured. An inability to conceive can generate a profound feeling of failure, which can lead to a state that psychologist Erik Erickson described as "stagnation and personal impoverishment."[2] Many infertile couples become obsessed with their childlessness and feel inferior when they see other people with babies. The countless doctor appointments, the expenses, the effects on employment, and the monthly hopes and expectations may eventually overburden the couple and cause them to feel they have no control over their lives, leading to depression and marital problems.

Quite frequently, women being treated for a thyroid imbalance enter infertility programs with no idea that their thyroid condition could be preventing conception and a normal pregnancy. Even more alarming, a significant number of reproductive endocrinologists and gynecologists who treat infertile couples are unaware that a minimal thyroid imbalance can compound or even cause infertility. Nor do many of these doctors realize the importance of detecting subtle thyroid abnormalities.

Although we don't know how frequently minimal hypothyroidism contributes to infertility, recent research has clearly demonstrated that it is an important contributing factor. One study showed that approximately 25 percent of women referred to one infertility clinic had low-grade hypothyroidism.[3]

If you're experiencing problems with fertility, discuss with your gynecologist the possibility of a thyroid imbalance before you spend two years engaging in an infertility protocol. Ask to have your thyroid tested. Often an imbalance will show up only if you have a TRH (thyrotropin-releasing hormone) stimulation test.[4] Among patients found to have low-grade hypothyroidism, the infertility may be reversed with thyroid hormone treatment.

Because thyroid testing is not routinely done when patients enter fertility clinics, many women with minimal hypothyroidism struggle for a long time attempting to conceive. Maria, aged thirty-three, had gone through infertility protocols for almost two years. She was outraged when she learned that she had had symptoms of hypothyroidism for some time but that her gynecologist had not checked her thyroid at the outset of her treatment. She told me, "I had a hard time getting my weight off, and there were some other telltale thyroid signs that I think a doctor who was knowledgeable in this area should have been able to see." Maria became pregnant two months after beginning thyroid hormone treatment.

In the past four years, I have cared for five women with minimal hypothyroidism whose infertility problems were reversed within two to three months after they began thyroid hormone treatment. Prior to the thyroid problem's being identified, all of them had suffered significant emotional and financial burdens as well as altered relationships with their spouses. In four of these cases, the infertile women wondered whether their marriages could survive. Although infertility usually affects both partners, the person suffering from infertility usually has greater feelings of guilt, inadequacy, failure, and low self-esteem. Given our culture's tendency to blame women, however, infertile women take on even more guilt and suffering than men, and their feelings of inadequacy are magnified.

The Burden of Stress and Anxiety

Quite frequently, when a woman is infertile, her husband makes her feel it is her responsibility to become pregnant. One patient described her situation as follows:

> My husband told me it was my "job" to get pregnant. I remember the therapist telling me, "I think part of the reason you feel so bad every month when you're not pregnant is because your husband has told you that is your job, so you're failing at your job."
>
> My husband thought of it as my sole goal. My measure of self-worth became whether the pregnancy test came back positive or negative. So every time the test came back negative, I felt like a complete and total failure. This made me even more depressed. Because I had to suffer in silence, it made it harder to deal with all these emotions. I was filled with sadness.

Generally speaking, infertile couples feel so bad, sad, or ashamed of their problem that they do not tell other people about it. Cut off from friendly support, the infertile person or couple often feels isolated and struggles even more with the emotional upheaval brought on by this problem. It is very important for women to reach out for support during this time. RESOLVE, a national support group for women with infertility issues, has chapters that meet regularly in all major cities around the country. RESOLVE members help each other with medical information and emotional support.

The effects of infertility on a woman suffering from a thyroid dysfunction become exaggerated when she is unaware of the thyroid imbalance. The multiple effects of the thyroid imbalance on the woman's emotions render the suffering quite unbearable and exacerbate the conflicts between spouses. Typically, if she were not hypothyroid, the woman could hide her sadness from friends or relatives, because it would be related to her infertility. When she is hypothyroid, even minimally, the effects of thyroid imbalance may make her depression worse and leave her unable to cope with the stress of infertility. Take steps to prevent this escalation. If you are becoming increasingly depressed over your infertility problem, get a TSH test.

The anxiety that occurs during the months when a woman is taking fertility drugs typically intensifies any anxiety caused by thyroid problems. She worries about whether she will become pregnant this month and how this will change her life. Due to the incredible anxiety she faces, the disappointment of a negative pregnancy test result may be magnified. As a consequence, some women experience worsening PMS and increased anger, mood swings, irritability, and arguing with their husbands.

A hypothyroid woman who is obligated to have intercourse even on days when she may have an aversion to sex often feels even more guilty and inadequate. If her husband is not sympathetic or supportive, or misunderstands her lack of interest in sex, the arguing and distance between them can increase. Roselyn, a thirty-three-year-old secretary, has been married for five years. She had tried to conceive for three years and had gone through infertility protocols with no success. The cause of the infertility was, however, a low-grade hypothyroidism that was uncovered only when they almost gave up the idea of having a baby. Roselyn said:

I could not believe how much stress I felt from trying to get pregnant. Month after month, we spent thousands and thousands of dollars. I had to make the two-hour round-trip to my doctor's office ten to twelve days a month. There was no apparent reason that the fertility protocols I tried were not working for me. It was totally unbelievable. What made it even worse for me was that I didn't feel like I got a lot of support from other people. When I would tell someone we were trying, they would just say, "Oh, all you have to do is relax. My best friend and her husband went on a second honeymoon, and she got pregnant!" I knew that in my case relaxation had nothing to do with whether I got pregnant. Finally, I just stopped talking about it even to my closest friends.

My infertility affected every aspect of my life. My husband is extremely introverted, and he doesn't discuss things with people besides me. So that made it much harder. My PMS has gotten worse, and I often find myself crying and sad. I was experiencing a lot of anxiety and couldn't sleep at night.

When the time of the month came when we had to have sex, I almost dreaded it. I was starting to resent even being touched by my husband. Important aspects of sexuality, like intimacy and spontaneity, are lost when you're going through infertility because the doctors tell you when to have sex, how to do it, who is supposed to do what, where to do it, and for how long. That's not the way it is supposed to be. For me, it just led to a lot more stress.

I couldn't understand what was happening. Nothing made any sense! The fighting and arguing between my husband and me kept escalating over the months. We started going to a therapist, sometimes five or even seven days a week.

I got hysterical. I ranted and raved. The monthly disappointment of not getting pregnant was just unbelievable. I would wait and wait and think, well

I'm going to be pregnant. No, yes, maybe . . . and then, sure enough, I wasn't pregnant. It was totally devastating.

Everything I did had to be planned around when I needed to be at the doctor and when I needed to do this and that. There were many times that I really felt like just giving up. I think my husband got to that point, too.

I kept asking myself, "Is this even worth it?" Without even taking into consideration my time and other inconveniences, I bet we spent over $50,000. That was money out of our pockets.

Because of the repeated failures, Roselyn became quite depressed. As she described it, "I finally quit my job and stayed home. I didn't cook; I didn't do anything. I just sat around the house all day."

Many women like Roselyn become obsessed with their condition and undertake their own determined search for the cause of their infertility. Roselyn eventually became inspired to go to the library and do her own research. She says:

I looked at every infertility book. One book mentioned the thyroid. In this case, my doctor resisted, telling me it would cost $150 to run that test. I thought to myself, I'm already spending $500 every time I come in here, so what's another $150? He agreed to run the test, and to his surprise, it showed I was hypothyroid. At the time, I was angry that this test had not been performed $50,000 and a year earlier.

When I began taking thyroid hormone, there was an improvement in how I was feeling—the cold, the dryness, the hair. I was a little aggravated that it took a couple of months. I thought you could just start me on thyroid hormone on Monday and I could be pregnant on Tuesday. It didn't work that way. Even so, it was the first step in getting me out of what was the worst situation I have ever been in in my entire life.

I also wonder whether anyone would ever have figured out that I had a thyroid problem had I not pursued the fertility research. I even had fertility-related surgeries before I was diagnosed as hypothyroid. Now I think all that was unnecessary.

To avoid the needless suffering that Roselyn went through, ask your reproductive endocrinologist if thyroid testing is part of the infertility work-up. If not, have your doctor request the test.

When Inadequate Hormone Treatment Leads to Infertility

If you have already been diagnosed with an underactive thyroid and are being treated for it, your infertility may be caused by an under- or overcorrected thyroid imbalance. If you are taking thyroid hormone to treat hypothy-roidism, make sure that your treatment is adequate before trying to become pregnant. Insufficient dosage can also cause infertility.

One evening I was giving a talk on the health effects of mild hypothy-roidism to a patient support group made up of laypeople. As I was pointing to a slide illustrating that minimal thyroid hormone deficiency could be responsible for both infertility and miscarriages, I noticed the face of a young lady sitting in the back. She noticeably brightened up, and her expres-sion changed from frustration to what appeared to be relief and hope. Fol-lowing the lecture, she asked me a few questions about how a small deficit in thyroid hormone could affect ovulation and then indicated that she had a thyroid condition and would make an appointment to come and see me. She stated that she had been frustrated and that her stress levels had become high as a result of being unable to conceive. One week later, Felicia was in my office. She told me:

> I was diagnosed hypothyroid at the age of nineteen. I was then placed on thy-roid hormone by my physician. My thyroid has been at the same level for probably the last eight years. I had been going to an internist who once a year had been running TSH tests, and it had been staying pretty stable. He would maybe adjust the dosage once in a while, but it was never anything drastic. I got married four years ago, and we were ready to have children. Initially, we had the attitude that if it happens, it happens. We weren't really on a schedule at any point. It was maybe a year and half after we were married that we started to concentrate on it, and nothing happened. I had been seeing a gynecologist who happened to be an infertility specialist.
>
> I have been going through cycles of drugs to induce a pregnancy, and we have not been successful. I was wondering if my thyroid had anything to do with it.

I asked Felicia whether she had other symptoms. "I did notice that I started to get bad night sweats, and I was suffering from hair loss and very dry and scaly skin. I mean you could run a brush across it and it would flake off, especially on my legs," she said.

Her marital relationship was affected significantly. Her husband con-stantly blamed her and made her feel as if something were wrong with her. She explained:

> It made me feel less of a woman. I began to envy women who don't have to go through all the battles of medications and timing and ovulation testing.
>
> The worst part was the distance that grew between me and my husband. Sex became a chore after a while because you are concentrating on it so much that it isn't spontaneous and fun anymore. Then you come to the end of the

month and you're still not pregnant, and you have to face at least another whole month of this routine that is now old and tiring.

In reviewing the records that Felicia had brought, I noticed that her TSH levels in the past two years, while she had been taking 0.15 milligrams of synthetic L-thyroxine, were 6.0 and 4.5 (normal TSH is 0.4 to 4.5 milli–international units per liter). The fact that her levels were high suggested to me that she was not taking enough thyroid hormone. If that were the case, I thought the resulting mild thyroid hormone deficiency might account for her infertility. I increased her L-thyroxine dose to 0.175 milligrams and asked her to wait a couple of months before resuming the fertility drugs.

Two months later, Felicia got pregnant immediately without fertility drugs. "We thought there is no way that it could have worked like that because of all these other obstacles that we had encountered in the past. It is amazing that we tried with medications for two years and we were not successful, and with a small increase in the dosage, I became pregnant right away."

When she returned to my office six weeks pregnant, Felicia was both happy and angry. She said, "What upsets me the most is that my internist knew I was struggling with infertility. I do feel like we wasted a lot of time and money because no one considered that the thyroid was a problem."

Any woman who has an infertility problem should have her thyroid checked. This simple test may help prevent much of the struggle, mental stress, and financial burden associated with infertility. Even a minute thyroid imbalance can result in correctable infertility. By the same token, any woman who is currently being treated for a thyroid imbalance or has previously been treated for such a condition should be thoroughly tested before attempting to conceive.

Beyond Infertility: When Miscarriage Intervenes

As difficult as infertility is, its hardships can pale compared to the trauma of a miscarriage. Many women, especially those who have had repeated miscarriages, experience tremendous stress and may also suffer from low self-esteem, depression, and marital conflicts.

Although recurrent miscarriages can be due to genetic problems or to a wide range of medical conditions, a high rate of recurrent miscarriages has also been demonstrated among women with thyroid imbalances. The relationship between pregnancy and thyroid problems has been known for some time. Three to four decades ago, gynecologists treated women who had multiple miscarriages with thyroid hormone, which was noted to prevent further pregnancy loss in a significant number of women. Recent research has shown that minimal thyroid imbalance can cause recurrent miscarriages and an inability to carry a normal pregnancy.[5] Even Hashimoto's thyroiditis not severe enough to make the thyroid gland underactive may be associated with miscarriages.[6] Studies have concluded that 2 to 3 percent of pregnant women are hypothyroid.[7] An underactive thyroid can result not only in miscarriages but also in birth defects and other problems that could compromise the health of both the fetus and the pregnant woman.[8]

Emily was happily married and, at the age of thirty-five, had her first child. Two years later, she decided to have a second child and stopped taking birth control pills for five months. Soon afterward, she says:

> I started gaining weight like a bear preparing for winter. The only difference was that I was barely eating and I was exercising daily. The weight problem started taking over my life. I was severely tired and depressed all the time, and all I wanted to do was sleep. When I decided to seek help, I went to a weight-loss clinic.
>
> The physician informed me that I had a goiter and suggested that I see my personal physician before beginning the weight-loss program. When my doctor informed me that I was pregnant, I thought the weight gain and the excessive lethargy were due to the pregnancy. The pregnancy made me excited, and I even ignored the thyroid problem.

Emily was already thinking about a name for the baby, but at the end of the first trimester, she had a miscarriage. She did not understand how this could have happened and felt that she had failed her husband and family. Her guilt and depression were disproportionate to those that a miscarriage usually causes, probably because of her hypothyroidism.

While Emily was telling me her story, I was somewhat amazed that her physician had found a goiter but did not test her thyroid function. In retrospect, it was clear that she had many symptoms of hypothyroidism. The miscarriage was probably related to hypothyroidism because, two months later, tests were performed and showed that her thyroid was indeed underactive.

Emily's thyroid imbalance was diagnosed early on, and she had only one miscarriage. Months later, her thyroid hormone levels returned to normal with treatment, and she had no difficulty carrying a pregnancy to term. Any woman who has had several miscarriages should be tested for a thyroid problem. Even mild thyroid imbalance never suspected by physicians can cause a pregnancy to fail.

Important Points to Remember

- Thyroid imbalance, and low-grade hypothyroidism in particular, may be the overlooked reason for your infertility problems.
- Before you spend two years pursuing an infertility protocol, discuss with your gynecologist the possibility of a thyroid imbalance, and ask to have your thyroid tested. Often the imbalance will show up only if you have a TRH stimulation test.
- Infertility can make you depressed because you may feel as if you have failed at your "job" of becoming pregnant. Thyroid imbalance may worsen your depression, leaving you unable to cope with the stress of infertility. If you are becoming increasingly depressed over your infertility problem, consider the possibility of a thyroid imbalance.
- If you find yourself trapped in the dilemma of lacking sex drive and feeling obligated to have sex, consider the possibility of a thyroid imbalance as the culprit for both the low sex drive and the infertility.
- If you are taking thyroid hormone to treat hypothyroidism, make sure that your treatment is adequate before you try to become pregnant. Insufficient and excessive dosage can also cause infertility.
- Thyroid disease is an often-overlooked cause of recurrent miscarriages as well. Have your thyroid checked if you have repeatedly failed to carry pregnancies to term.

13

POSTPARTUM DEPRESSION:

The Hormonal Link

For most women, bringing a new baby into the world represents happiness, joy, and relief. It also brings increased worries, responsibilities, sleepless nights, and quite often, tremendous stress. Because of these factors as well as hormonal changes that occur in the postpartum period (immediately after birth), a significant number of women experience tension, anxiety, and mood swings. Many also experience anger, difficulty sleeping, and crying spells. For most women, these emotional changes last for two days to a week and then resolve, although some new mothers may continue to suffer mild to moderate mood swings for several weeks.[1] Nearly 15 to 20 percent of women who complete a pregnancy experience longer-lasting postpartum depression that may range from mild to severe. These women suffer low self-esteem, crying spells, increased emotionality, sadness, sleep disturbances, and over- or undereating.

The postpartum period is also a time in which women are vulnerable to thyroid dysfunction. The vulnerability stems from the dramatic hormonal changes of the postpartum weeks and months, and also very likely from the added stress of parenting and life changes. Many women experience postpartum depression as a result of a thyroid imbalance. Thyroid dysfunction in the postpartum period can intensify a woman's perception of stress and increase the difficulties of coping with the demands related to having a new infant. The interactions between the brain and the thyroid in the postpartum period are not limited to the effects of stress on the immune system, which can be a potential triggering factor for autoimmune attacks on the thyroid. This mechanism, although possible, does not account for most postpartum thyroid problems.

Overt postpartum mental disorders have been recognized since antiquity. Descriptions of patterns of mental disorders related to childbirth have been available since a report by the Frenchman Jean Etienne Dominique Esquirol in 1838.[2] Nonetheless, postpartum mental disturbances were seldom talked about until recently, and women afflicted with postpartum depression hid their suffering out of shame. Serious interest by the medical community in postpartum conditions and recognition of both the high frequency of such suffering and its effects on the woman, child, and family began in 1980, when an English physician[3] organized a conference on postpartum psychiatric illness. This led to the founding of an international organization to promote advances in knowledge and treatment of postpartum psychiatric illnesses. Scientific advances in the field of psychiatry, the formation of support groups, and increased public awareness through media coverage have since revealed much of the hidden suffering of postpartum women.

Over the past two decades, thyroid researchers have shown that autoimmune thyroid diseases, including Hashimoto's thyroiditis and Graves' disease, frequently occur during the postpartum period. Various forms of autoimmune-related thyroid imbalances affect as many as 10 percent of postpartum women. Implicating stress as a major triggering factor for the autoimmune attack has been a difficult task, as it has been for autoimmune thyroid diseases occurring at other periods of a woman's life. One recent study, however, showed that women experiencing most of the symptoms of depression have a higher frequency of positive antithyroid antibody, a marker for autoimmune thyroid disease, even though their thyroid function is normal.[4] This finding provides evidence that stress could precipitate not only Graves' disease but also the most common autoimmune thyroid condition, Hashimoto's thyroiditis. It also implies that mind-body medicine; family and spousal support; learning how to cope with stress; and the use of relaxation techniques such as yoga, tai chi, and meditation could help women manage or alleviate the additional stress and depression so often experienced during the postpartum period and potentially minimize autoimmune reactions to the thyroid.

In many postpartum women who develop a thyroid imbalance, an important predisposing factor has been well documented: the presence of an autoimmune thyroid disease. Women who have a positive antithyroid antibody in the last trimester of pregnancy are more prone to postpartum thyroid dysfunction.[5] One study showed that 76 percent of patients with postpartum thyroid dysfunction had a positive antithyroid antibody in the postpartum period.[6] We just don't know yet how much stress will set the stage for thyroid dysfunction in postpartum women.

Fluctuations in the levels of bodily hormones have been held accountable to some extent for the occurrence of postpartum psychiatric conditions. Postpartum symptoms are increasingly thought to be tied to the rapid fall of hormone levels (that is, estrogen and progesterone) from the high levels during pregnancy to the low levels of the prepregnancy state.[7] Doctors have also recognized that hormonal shifts play a role in the triggering of autoimmune thyroid disease. What is perhaps unique to the postpartum period is that the effects of the hormonal shifts, coupled with the suppression of the immune system during pregnancy, could result in an autoimmunity condition after pregnancy.

Although postpartum depression is linked to positive antithryoid antibodies and thyroid dysfunction, before-birth (antenatal) depression, which is also common, does not seem to correlate with thyroid problems.

Because of the high frequency of depression and thyroid imbalance in the postpartum period, doctors should test thyroid function whenever a postpartum woman reports mental and emotional symptoms, including depression. Although it's important to do this so that the doctor and patient can explain and treat the depression, it's also crucial for the woman's future health to correct any thyroid imbalance that has been triggered. The fastest route to healing postpartum depression that coexists with a thyroid imbalance is to treat the thyroid imbalance, which can contribute to, exacerbate, and perpetuate the depression. But that may not be enough. Relaxation techniques and exercise will help you become in control again.

How Common Are Postpartum Depression and Thyroid Imbalance?

More than a century ago, a committee of the Clinical Society of London noted the role of thyroid imbalance in causing postpartum mental changes.[8] This first report not only emphasized the high frequency of psychiatric symptoms due to a thyroid hormone deficit but also pointed out that many of the patients with an underactive thyroid became ill after childbirth. It has since become apparent that a thyroid imbalance contributes significantly to the occurrence of postpartum mood changes.

As noted at the start of the chapter, the estimated frequency of mild postpartum depression in the general population is in the range of 15 to 20 percent of all women. Most women are depressed for a few weeks and then get over it spontaneously, whereas in more severe cases, the depression may last up to a year.

In many cases, both the women themselves and their gynecologists attribute the emotional troubles that occur in the postpartum period to just caring for a new baby. Quite often, women struggle through this depressive state without receiving treatment or support from their spouses or families.

In fact, most husbands of women going through postpartum depression have trouble coping with the changes in their wives' mood and behavior, which tends to isolate the women further and exacerbate their depression. Therefore, postpartum depression is, more often than not, undiagnosed, and its symptoms are frequently attributed to stress. This depressive cycle is often difficult to break in severe cases without psychiatric and medical intervention.

In general, because psychiatric help is sought only in extremely severe cases of depression, when a person becomes suicidal, and because many women suffering from postpartum depression are not diagnosed, we do not have an accurate understanding of the true frequency of postpartum depression.

Clearly, however, thyroid imbalance can cause or exacerbate postpartum depression.

In recent years, several studies in which postpartum women had their thyroid function tested and their antithyroid antibody level measured have shown that 5 to 10 percent of all women have postpartum autoimmune thyroiditis.[9] One-half to two-thirds of these women experience hyperthyroidism, hypothyroidism, or both in the postpartum period. One study done in Wisconsin on women evaluated at six and twelve weeks postpartum showed that 11.3 percent of them had thyroid disease and 6.7 percent had either hypothyroidism or hyperthyroidism in the postpartum period.[10] White women seem more likely to have postpartum autoimmune thyroiditis than African-American women (8.8 percent versus 2.5 percent).

The Many Faces of
Postpartum Thyroid Imbalance

The onset of a thyroid imbalance may occur as early as one to two months after delivery, and the imbalance may exhibit different patterns. The most typical pattern is three distinct phases: a transient or temporary hyperthyroidism lasting two to three months, followed by a period of hypothyroidism, and then spontaneous return of thyroid levels to normal. In a significant number of women, the function of the thyroid gland returns to normal by seven to eight months into the postpartum period. In essence many cases of thyroid imbalances occurring in the postpartum period are temporary but do cause symptoms. Some women, however, may have a persistent imbalance.

The reason for this pattern is related to a rapid autoimmune attack on thyroid cells, similar to the condition silent thyroiditis (see Chapter 4), which tends to occur in persons with Hashimoto's thyroiditis. During the first phase, the destruction of thyroid cells results in leakage of thyroid hormone into the bloodstream, causing an excess of thyroid hormone and thus hyperthyroidism. As the destruction subsides, thyroid hormone levels decrease. This frequently results in hypothyroidism because the cells that were healthy and previously making adequate amounts of thyroid hormone are no longer present to maintain normal thyroid levels. Once the patient becomes hypothyroid, thyroid cells begin to regenerate. It takes a few weeks before the thyroid completes its recovery and thyroid hormone levels return to normal.

In general, hyperthyroidism tends to occur earlier than the first two to three months after delivery, whereas hypothyroidism usually occurs at a later point, at around four months after delivery. Cases of hypothyroidism occasionally occur as late as eight months after delivery of a baby.

In some women, the destruction of the thyroid cells and the resulting hyperthyroidism are not severe enough to precipitate a phase of hypothyroidism. In such women, hyperthyroidism is present for several weeks, followed by resumption of normal thyroid function. Many of these women are not diagnosed unless systematically tested.

Another common pattern is that of transient hypothyroidism lasting two to three months. This may be followed either by the recovery of normal thyroid function or by the development of permanent hypothyroidism, which thereafter requires lifelong thyroid hormone treatment. Women who progress into permanent hypothyroidism may have a more severely destructive Hashimoto's thyroiditis than women who recover from hypothyroidism. In some women, dormant Graves' disease may flare up in the immediately postpartum period and cause postpartum Graves' disease.

If you have experienced a postpartum thyroid dysfunction once, you need to know that you are at a higher risk for experiencing postpartum thyroid dysfunction after future pregnancies as well. Also, many women who develop postpartum thyroid dysfunction will have some type of thyroid abnormality later. For instance, one study showed that 23 percent of women who experienced a postpartum thyroid dysfunction were found to be hypothyroid twenty-four to forty-eight months later. The striking finding was that half the women who experienced just hypothyroidism in the postpartum period had continued to suffer from an underactive thyroid.[11] This implies that, once the autoimmune attack has occurred or worsened in the postpartum period, the likelihood of having further thyroid problems increases. The risk for having permanent hypothyroidism later increases when the postpartum thyroid dysfunction has occurred in the last period of a woman's reproductive years. Also, for reasons that are unclear, women who have had multiple pregnancies and previous miscarriages are at a higher risk for having permanent hypothyroidism.

Effects of Postpartum
Thyroid Imbalance on Mind and Mood

In the postpartum period, the effects of a thyroid imbalance on mental health cannot be ignored. Dr. Clifford C. Hayslip and his coworkers from Walter Reed Army Medical Center[12] have shown that women who suffered from postpartum hypothyroidism were depressed and had impaired concentration and memory as well as other complaints more frequently than did women who did not have postpartum thyroid dysfunction. Approximately 70 percent of women who are hypothyroid in the postpartum period become careless and make more mistakes than women whose thyroid function is normal. These women also tend to complain of fatigue, weight gain, cold intolerance, and nervousness. Nearly half the women with postpartum hypothyroidism have nightmares, compared to 5.5 percent of women with normal thyroid function.

Women with postpartum depression feel a lot of guilt about their inability to provide the care that their infants require. They become depressed for a variety of reasons, which differ from one woman to another. Certainly, stress, the unconscious fear of mothering, marital conflicts, and real or perceived lack of support from the husband and family contribute to postpartum depression.

Postpartum depression and anxiety, like other kinds of depression, can range from minimal to quite severe. The rarest psychiatric condition that can occur in the period following birth is postpartum psychosis, characterized by hallucinations, delirium, and agitation. After the psychosis passes or is medically resolved, depression may follow. Although most cases of postpartum psychosis are not caused by a thyroid imbalance, such an imbalance has been implicated in rare cases.[13]

Because the effects of thyroid imbalance on mood and emotions in the postpartum period are little publicized, many new mothers are at risk for suffering significantly at just the time in their lives when they—and their families—would expect to feel the most joy. Typically, the depression due to postpartum thyroid disease is indistinguishable from that of postpartum depression, although, in many instances, the onset of depression due to postpartum thyroid disease occurs later. And many women who have postpartum depression experience a worsening of their depression as a result of postpartum thyroid disease. Yet many patients who have a typical postpartum thyroid dysfunction have no symptoms of depression whatsoever!

Kathy, aged twenty-six, had several symptoms of postpartum thyroid dysfunction. She was diagnosed only after her thyroid function was on its way back to normal. Her symptoms were indicative of hyperthyroidism, which lasted two months, followed by three months of hypothyroidism. But she and her husband, an anesthesiologist in a teaching hospital, had attributed all of her symptoms to the stress associated with having a baby and moving to a different city. Kathy described her symptoms as follows:

> I felt hyperactive after I had my baby. I was running around so much after she was born to the point that I had uterine bleeding again. I was breast-feeding, but I would run around and try to do all these things.
>
> When my daughter was four months old, I lost twenty-six pounds. I felt hot, shaky, and sweaty. I remember sitting in the closet and crying and being very upset. I had rapid heartbeats. We thought it was just stress.
>
> Two months later, I felt depressed and all of a sudden tired and exhausted. I regained the lost weight plus another fifteen pounds. My skin was dry. I was so sleepy that when my little girl napped, I would nap, too. I went to see my doctor, and he said my thyroid was big.

What Kathy described was a period of hyperactivity and hypomania caused by hyperthyroidism, followed by a period of depression, caused by hypothyroidism.

In contrast, Jasmine, a schoolteacher, began having crying spells, mood swings, and periods of anger one week after the delivery of her second child. Gradually, her personality continued to change, and her symptoms worsened. She was twenty-nine years old, had previously been healthy, and had never suffered from depression in the past. Here's how she described what had been happening since the birth of her child as a result of an underactive thyroid that began in the postpartum period:

> I loved my baby so much, but I hated everybody else around me. They couldn't do anything right. I was exhausted. All I wanted to do was take care of the baby and watch TV. I was losing a tremendous amount of weight and was not eating. I didn't make enough milk. I was severely ill, and not having that validated was tough.
>
> I love my husband very much, but at the time, I couldn't stand the sight of him. Then I would think, "Why did he marry me? Look at the basket case that I am." I was trying to take care of the new baby, work, and keep the house clean, and I didn't have the energy to do any of it. As laundry would pile up and things would get dusty around the house, I would get more depressed and have less energy. I didn't think there was any way out.

Jasmine had a clear-cut case of postpartum depression, which was affecting her marriage. TSH testing showed she was hypothyroid. With thyroid hormone treatment, her depression resolved and she became her old self again. Even though her depression responded to the thyroid hormone treatment, it is not clear to this day whether her depression was entirely due to thyroid dysfunction or whether the underactive thyroid made a postpartum depression worse.

Another young woman whom I saw recently was depressed and anxious. She suffered from postpartum thyroid dysfunction, but her doctor had dismissed her anxiety as due to the stress of caring for the baby. She described some of her symptoms as follows:

> I was afraid to hold my baby. My husband took care of him for a long time. I cried. I had nightmares that I tried to hurt my baby. I had a lot of trouble sleeping. I would sleep a couple of hours and wake up in the middle of the night and toss and turn for a few hours and fall asleep.
>
> First, I went to my general practitioner. He put me on antidepressants. I would get shortness of breath. My heart would palpitate a little bit. I get up from the bed and walk around and lie on the sofa. There's not anything in my life to cause depression. I have a wonderful husband and a wonderful little boy.

After postpartum thyroiditis was diagnosed and treated, she became symptom-free when her thyroid condition resolved.

Grace, twenty-nine years old, described her suffering from major depression due to postpartum hypothyroidism after the birth of her daughter. She was feeling alone because her husband was out of town quite often and her mother had just been admitted to the hospital for cancer treatment. She said:

> For about four weeks, I would get up in the mornings and somehow function in a normal manner. Six weeks after I had my baby, I had a complete nervous breakdown. I would still be in my gown and have no recollection of the day at all. One night I went to the store and bought formula and a bottle, and I wrote down all the instructions on how to make formula, and I sat down and could not move. I wanted to cease to exist for a period of time. I wanted to raise my child, but with everything that was happening, or that I perceived was happening, I couldn't deal with it at that time. I couldn't seem to articulate it, or nobody was listening to the type of help I needed. I needed to rest. They had me diagnosed with major postpartum depression. A few days later, they told me I had severe hypothyroidism.

Grace was treated with thyroid hormone and an antidepressant. A few months later, she was doing well, and the antidepressant was stopped. The depression never came back. This underscores again the importance of testing for a thyroid condition whenever a patient feels depressed—and especially when a postpartum mother is depressed.

When a postpartum thyroid imbalance occurs in a patient with a history of depression, frequently the thyroid imbalance triggers depression. Hillary had had trouble with recurrent depression for years and took medication intermittently. Her worst episode of depression occurred after she had her second baby. Her psychiatrist considered postpartum hypothyroidism only after Hillary made two suicide attempts.

Some women with postpartum depression and thyroid imbalance may require antidepressants and psychiatric therapy. Support from her husband, counseling, and medical treatment of the thyroid imbalance will improve the woman's and the family's ability to cope with her depression. Overlooking the thyroid imbalance will result in difficulty controlling the symptoms of depression.

Diana had suffered from depression in the postpartum period due to hypothyroidism. She was diagnosed as having postpartum depression, but she was not tested for thyroid imbalance. She was treated with antidepressants, which did not improve her condition. She said:

> I can't recall having had any problems up until after the birth of my little boy. Seven or eight months afterward, I was real depressed. One doctor I saw said it was impossible to have postpartum depression that long after giving birth. I basically felt worthless. I didn't want to do anything. Another doctor put me on Prozac and then Zoloft. I didn't notice either helping me. No one checked my thyroid until my gynecologist did a blood test, which showed I was hypothyroid.

When postpartum depression and postpartum thyroid dysfunction occur at the same time, one cannot with certainty implicate the thyroid disease as being the only reason for the depression. A thyroid imbalance could be just a contributing factor. Although studies have shown an association between postpartum depression and postpartum thyroid dysfunction, no one can be certain whether the depression would have occurred if the thyroid disease had not been present. Most physicians do not take postpartum symptoms seriously because culturally, it is expected that women will go through some mood changes and emotional instability in the postpartum period. Our society unfairly expects these new mothers to "tough it out" and push their way through the sometimes overwhelming emotional and physical effects of postpartum depression. Doctors, spouses, and families often tell new mothers to ignore their own symptoms and "think of the baby" and the joy they "should" feel. Despite the frequency of postpartum depression and postpartum thyroid dysfunction, physicians often ignore both problems and neglect thyroid testing of depressed women in the postpartum period. This tendency *must* change to prevent serious consequences for both the mothers and the infants.

Important Points to Remember

- In some women, a thyroid imbalance makes postpartum depression worse. Have your thyroid checked if you become overwhelmed by sadness, crying spells, distancing from your spouse, or an inability to care for your baby.
- Thyroid imbalance in the postpartum period often exhibits a pattern of transient hyperthyroidism followed by hypothyroidism, then recovery of normal thyroid function.
- Some women, however, experience only transient hyperthyroidism or transient hypothyroidism. Others develop a permanently overactive thyroid due to Graves' disease or a permanently underactive thyroid due to Hashimoto's thyroiditis.
- Once you have had thyroid trouble after delivering a baby, your risk of having thyroid problems after subsequent pregnancies is increased. Also, you become at risk for having permanent hypothyroidism down the road.
- The postpartum period is a vulnerable one for women, many of whom experience the onset of their thyroid imbalance after delivering a baby.

PART IV

DIAGNOSING AND TREATING COMMON THYROID DISORDERS:

The Journey to Wellness

14

WHAT YOU NEED TO KNOW
ABOUT THYROID TESTS

For years, the public has received conflicting information on how to diagnose a thyroid imbalance properly. Some holistic doctors and alternative practitioners may diagnose you as hypothyroid if you suffer from tiredness and other symptoms of low metabolism. They will use your basal (resting) temperature as an index of low thyroid and will monitor the treatment by having you check your basal temperature three to four times a day (see Chapter 6). Some doctors will treat your allergies, asthma, hair loss, dry skin, and gastrointestinal upset with thyroid hormone, believing that you have an underactive thyroid even if your blood tests are normal. They may tell you that thyroid hormone is not working well in your body and you need thyroid hormone treatment because you are hypothyroid. Many conventional doctors, in contrast, go strictly by blood tests and believe that you have a thyroid imbalance only if your blood tests are clearly out of the normal range.

Because of these differences of opinion, some people have remained undiagnosed even though they sought medical help, whereas others have been subjected to inappropriate and overzealous treatments that were damaging to their overall emotional and physical health. To avoid these pitfalls, you need to know about the most reliable tests for evaluating your thyroid and how to interpret them in light of your symptoms. That way, you won't fall through the cracks and fail to receive the help that you need from your doctor.

Before it was possible to measure blood levels of thyroid hormones, the common practice was to go by indirect clues, such as:

- Basal temperature (an indirect way of measuring a person's metabolism), which is low in patients who are hypothyroid
- Cholesterol levels, which are high in people with hypothyroidism and low in those with hyperthyroidism

- Iodine in the blood, which is low in hypothyroidism and high in hyperthyroidism
- Achilles reflex time (how long it takes the Achilles tendon to relax after contraction), which is slow in hypothyroidism and faster in hyperthyroidism

For the past three decades, doctors have been able to measure the levels of the hormones T4 and T3 in the bloodstream as well as thyroid-stimulating hormone (TSH), the pituitary hormone that tightly controls the functioning of the thyroid gland and the manufacture of thyroid hormone. The pituitary is like a finely tuned sensor that detects even a subtle deficit or excess of thyroid hormone. A deficit of thyroid hormone in the blood will cause TSH to rise, and an excess of thyroid hormone will make it fall.

TSH is now recognized as the most sensitive measurement for alerting doctors to a thyroid imbalance.[1] When the levels of thyroid hormone change slightly, they will often remain within the normal range even though the TSH has already become abnormal. In fact, the majority of those who suffer from low-grade hypothyroidism or low-grade hyperthyroidism have T4 and T3 levels within the normal laboratory range. The normal range for thyroid hormone levels is very wide and is established by averaging the levels obtained from large numbers of people. Because what is a "normal" level of thyroid hormone differs from one person to the next, the normal range used in laboratories needs to be wide enough to include many people. For instance, in many laboratories, the normal levels for T4 range from 5 to 12 micrograms per deciliter of serum, and those for T3 range from 90 to 220 nanograms per deciliter.

Technological advances now allow doctors to measure TSH levels in a very sensitive way, both far below the lower limit and far above the upper limit of the normal range. In general, a normal TSH is between 0.4 and 5.0 milli–international units per liter. The greater the excess of thyroid hormone, the lower the TSH below the normal range; the greater the deficit, the higher the TSH above the normal range. Now doctors can detect any minute excess or deficit of thyroid hormone resulting from an over- or underactive thyroid or from taking too much or too little thyroid hormone medication. So-called second- and third-generation TSH assays developed in recent years can read as low as 0.10 and 0.01 milli–international units per liter, respectively.

This sounds very straightforward. If your TSH level falls within the normal laboratory range, then your thyroid gland is working properly. If it is high, your doctor will diagnose you with an underactive thyroid; if it is low, your doctor will suspect an overactive thyroid and will measure your thyroid hormone levels, which will be expected to be high. But it is not as straightforward as it sounds. TSH is not the only (nor in some cases the most revealing) test. Increasingly, more and more physicians believe that you can be suffering from hypothyroidism even though your blood tests, including TSH, are normal.

The Controversy over Hypothyroidism
with Normal Blood Tests

Nothing is more irritating for persons suffering from tiredness, low mood, and inability to control their weight than to be told that their TSH is normal, only to be told some years later, upon being retested, that they are hypothyroid. During the intervening period, they have continued to suffer needlessly, and their thyroid gland, which was already slightly deficient, has been further damaged, resulting in an even greater thyroid deficit.

How could that be? A person might ask, "My TSH was 3 two years ago, and now it has gone up to 12. Was I hypothyroid then?" Yes, indeed, that might have been the case. The principal reason for the difficulty in detecting a low-grade underactive thyroid when doctors use this most sophisticated and sensitive thyroid test is that, as with T4 and T3, a normal laboratory reading for TSH is established based on levels measured in a large number of people. What is normal for your TSH level may differ dramatically from what is normal for mine.

Here's an example. Let's suppose that your normal TSH level is 0.6 milli–international units per liter when your thyroid is working well. But as a result of a minimal deficit due to Hashimoto's thyroiditis, your TSH went up to 3 or 4. Your body and your pituitary gland had sensed the deficit, and the pituitary had reacted to it, raising the TSH to almost six times its original level. But a doctor may interpret a TSH level of 3 or 4 as normal and assure you that you have no thyroid problems.

In short, many people may be suffering from minute imbalances that have not yet resulted in abnormal blood tests. If we included people with low-grade hypothyroidism whose blood tests are normal, the frequency of hypothyroidism would no doubt exceed 10 percent of the population. What is of special concern, though, is that many people whose test results are dismissed as normal could continue to have symptoms of an underactive thyroid. Their moods, emotions, and overall well-being are affected by this imbalance, yet they are not receiving the care they need to get to the root of their problems.

You don't need to be a thyroid expert to realize from what I have said so far that if your TSH is close to the upper limit of the normal range set by laboratories, you have a higher risk of being low-grade hypothyroid. In fact, researchers are beginning to recognize the upper segment of the normal range as suspicious for hypothyroidism. Nearly a third of patients who are receiving thyroid hormone replacement for hypothyroidism or have a goiter and whose TSH level is in the suspicious range turn out to be hypothyroid when they are evaluated by TRH stimulation testing (a procedure that measures TSH after injection of thyrotropin-releasing hormone into the bloodstream). Recently, one study showed that more than 50 percent of women who have a positive antithyroid antibody marker for Hashimoto's thyroiditis and a TSH level ranging between 2 and 4.5 (considered normal) became clearly hypothyroid (showed a definite elevation of TSH) within ten years.[2] Even when this marker was absent, 30 percent of women with a TSH level in this high–normal range became hypothyroid.

Another study also showed that LDL cholesterol, which is increased in hypothyroidism, can be lowered with fairly small doses of thyroid hormone in persons whose TSH level ranges between 2 and 4.5 milli–international units per liter.[3] In short, many people who have a TSH level in the upper segment of the normal range may be suffering from low-grade hypothyroidism, particularly if they have the destructive disorder of Hashimoto's thyroiditis. It is not uncommon to see TSH levels fluctuate, going from high–normal to levels slightly above the normal range. It is as if the pituitary were trying to adjust normal function from one day to the next. These fluctuations often confuse doctors and make them suspect laboratory errors. "How could a person be hypothyroid one day and normal the next?" is a lament I've heard a number of times from other doctors. In fact, when the deficit in thyroid hormone is minimal, the TSH level rises slightly and could be vacillating up and down across the line marking the upper limit of the laboratory normal range, leading to confusion and misdiagnosis.

Even if the TSH level is in the lower segment of the normal range, a person may still be suffering from low-grade hypothyroidism. If you have symptoms of an underactive thyroid and a goiter, an underactive thyroid may be uncovered by a TRH test.[4]

The wide range of normal levels for TSH is not the only reason someone could be hypothyroid despite normal blood tests. Another possible reason (not scientifically established yet) is that, even though a person may have a healthy thyroid gland that produces adequate amounts of thyroid hormones, the hormones may not work efficiently in the body. Once the thyroid hormone T4 has reached cells, it is converted to T3, the most active form of thyroid hormone. Here it interacts with genes and becomes involved in a wide range of regulations of metabolism and a myriad of biological effects.

It turns out that, locally in bodily organs, the amount of the active form of thyroid hormone is finely regulated as well. This regulation is the most ancient from an evolutionary perspective, having developed much earlier than the appearance of the pituitary gland. In primitive vertebrates such as lampreys, the main mechanism for regulating thyroid balance is found within organs:[5] the central mechanism of hypothalamic/pituitary control is nonexistent. As animals evolved to rely more on the thyroid gland to manufacture thyroid hormone, the hypothalamic/pituitary mechanism became the major system of regulation. Local regulation in organs gradually became a secondary mechanism that controls the availability of the right amount of active thyroid hormone and its effects in target tissue.

It is conceivable that some people may have an abnormality in the process of regulation in the organs that is designed to deliver the right amount of thyroid hormone to the metabolic machinery of the cells. People with this type of regulation dysfunction may suffer from many symptoms of low metabolism and low thyroid. For example, one patient, Judith, came to see me because of tiredness, dry skin, and difficulty losing weight despite dieting and exercise. Her TSH and TRH tests, however, were normal. I explained to her that her symptoms had nothing to do with her thyroid. She replied, "It does no good for me if my pituitary gland is well and is producing normal amounts of TSH and I am not happy." She vehemently told me that if I did not put her on thyroid hormone, she would go see another doctor who would. "All the symptoms that I have are those of a low thyroid," she kept saying. Because I suspected that she would have the misfortune to be placed on a high dose of thyroid hormone by another doctor, I prescribed a low dose of L-thyroxine and insisted that this was only a three-month trial. To my surprise, most of her symptoms went away, and she has continued to do fine. Two weeks later, a forty-two-year-old woman and her two daughters came to see me with similar complaints. Their blood tests were also normal. Perhaps some genetic factor might have been causing them to suffer from an inefficiency of thyroid hormone in their bodies. Their symptoms also improved with thyroid hormone.

Dr. Gordon R. B. Skinner advocated recently in the *British Medical Journal* a trial of thyroid hormone treatment for about three months in persons suffering from symptoms of hypothyroidism.[6] He believes that many people may be hypothyroid despite having normal blood tests. Quite possibly this proposal has merit. However, further research is needed to make sure that the treatment works for reasons that go beyond the placebo effect. (A placebo effect might have been responsible for the thyroid hormone treatment's having worked on the patients I just described.)

The emerging evidence that one can be hypothyroid despite normal blood tests explains the common frustration among people who do not get help despite suffering from tiredness, low mood, and difficulty concentrating. It is one of the reasons why many patients turn to naturopathic doctors or other alternative practitioners after having tried to get relief from conventional physicians. A large number of naturopathic doctors prescribe thyroid hormone for symptoms of underactive thyroid in people having normal blood tests. They believe that some of these people have inefficiency of thyroid hormone in their organs. If this assumption is correct, it may explain why some (but not all) patients report a beneficial effect from the treatment. At this time, however, there is no scientific basis for recommending thyroid hormone treatment to patients with normal blood tests. If your doctor prescribes this treatment, you need to understand that it should be taken on a trial basis and you need to pay attention to the doses prescribed. Make sure that your thyroid levels and TSH remain normal and are monitored regularly during the treatment.

Problems with Thyroid Testing

The most sensitive test for diagnosing hypothyroidism due to damage to the thyroid gland is an elevation in the TSH level. The more severe the hypothyroidism, the higher the TSH and the lower the T4 and T3 levels. Some physicians, however, continue to order T4 and T3 levels without obtaining a TSH measurement in people suspected of having an underactive thyroid.[7] If your doctor relies only on the T4 and T3 measurements and fails to order the appropriate test (TSH), you may not be correctly diagnosed for hypothyroidism.

Prior to an obvious rise in the TSH level, TSH may fluctuate, so that a consistent elevation in the TSH level may not be documented. As I indicated earlier, your doctor may consider a TSH of 4.5 (near the upper limit of the normal range) as normal. This level should be viewed with suspicion, however, because it may indicate that you do indeed have low-grade hypothyroidism.

Conversely, when a person has thyroid hormone excess, the first abnormality to occur is a decrease in the TSH level. Using sensitive TSH testing, physicians should also be able to detect minimal thyroid hormone excess. With low-grade hyperthyroidism, T4 and T3 levels may be normal but TSH may be low. It appears that many primary care physicians easily dismiss this abnormality as a normal finding.

Note that a number of common drugs can affect TSH scores, including the following medications that tend to increase TSH:

- Amiodarone
- Haloperidol
- Metoclopramide
- Lithium

- Morphine
- Aminoglutethimide

The following drugs tend to decrease TSH:

- Cortisone and other glucocorticoids
- Dopamine
- Anabolic steroids
- Heparin
- Somatostatin analogues

If you are suffering from depression or an anxiety disorder, you may have a low TSH reading even though you do not have a thyroid disorder. Research has shown that up to 30 percent of patients suffering from major depression not due to a thyroid condition have a slightly low TSH level.[8] This is presumably caused by the activation of the thyroid system in response to depression. Often the TSH reading becomes normal when your depression or anxiety disorder is treated. To avoid being misdiagnosed as having an overactive thyroid, make sure that your doctor orders a very sensitive (third-generation) TSH test.

Researchers have recently devised a one-step, quick TSH test that is said to provide a reliable reading in ten minutes. This one-step test may soon become widely available in doctors' offices, drugstores, and even as a home test for the purpose of screening for hypothyroidism and monitoring thyroid hormone treatment. This test does not give a specific reading for TSH, however. Rather, it can tell you whether your TSH is lower than 5 or higher than 5. That's all. In effect, you will test positive for hypothyroidism if your TSH is higher than 5. A major limitation of this test is that you might be lulled into thinking that you are not hypothyroid even though your actual TSH reading may fall in the suspicious upper segment of the normal range. Also, this test cannot detect an overactive thyroid. For these reasons, it is not the best test to monitor whether you are taking too little or too much thyroid hormone. Knowing these limitations, you could use this test as a way to detect hypothyroidism. In a sense, the one-step TSH test is like a urine pregnancy test: it has value only if it is positive.

Beyond TSH

Once the TSH test shows evidence of a thyroid imbalance, the next step is to determine the severity of the imbalance. For an underactive thyroid, TSH is very reliable at providing your doctor with a precise measure of the severity of the deficit. The higher the TSH, the more severe the hypothyroidism. In contrast, for an overactive thyroid, TSH has little value for determining the severity of the excess of thyroid hormone in your system.

Another series of tests can be especially helpful in assessing the severity of a thyroid hormone deficit or excess. These include measurements of T4 and T3 resin uptake and free T4 and T3 levels. To understand these tests, let's take a look at how thyroid hormone gets around inside the body.

Thyroid hormone in the bloodstream is bound to proteins that carry it to the organs. This bloodstream hormone represents a form of reserve. One of the main carrying proteins is thyroid-binding globulin (TBG), which is produced in the liver and can be affected by illnesses, liver disease, and medications such as estrogens. The carrying proteins have bound to them more than 99 percent of the thyroid hormone found in the bloodstream. Therefore, total T4 and T3 levels can be high or low if the amount of these proteins is high or low. For example, a woman who is pregnant or takes estrogen will have high T4 levels (sometimes far above the upper limit of normal) while her thyroid system is working properly. High and low total T4 and T3 are quite common and do not necessarily reflect an imbalance. The system is set so that the levels of free thyroid hormone in the bloodstream and organs remain normal.

For this reason, your doctor will often order another test, called a T3 resin uptake (often confused with T3 level). T3 resin uptake gives an estimate of the amount of TBG. When interpreted in conjunction with total T4 or T3, it will provide a more accurate estimate of the level of true biologically active thyroid hormone in your system. For instance, a pregnant woman or a woman taking estrogens will have, in addition to a high T4 level, a low T3 resin uptake. This indicates that the high T4 is due to high levels of TBG. Actually, if you multiply T4 by T3 resin uptake, you get the free thyrexene index (FTI), a better test for assessing thyroid hormone level than T4. The free form of thyroid hormone (called simply free T4 and free T3) can also be measured in the laboratory. Free T4 often provides a more accurate picture of whether there is a deficiency or an excess of thyroid hormone in the body. A free T3 level is requested when the gland is minimally overactive and in some cases of thyroid overactivity during pregnancy.

Doctors use the free T4 and the T4 and T3 resin uptake tests when they need more information on the severity of a thyroid hormone deficit. They also use T4, T3, free T4, and free T3 levels to determine how much excess thyroid hormone is circulating in the body. The higher these hormone levels, the more severe the excess. Doctors also measure these levels when they suspect a thyroid imbalance due to a disorder of the pituitary gland, even when TSH levels are normal.

Getting the Right Diagnosis

If you have decided to be screened for a thyroid imbalance, or your physician has ordered a thyroid test to determine whether you have a thyroid imbalance, make sure that the test ordered is a TSH. As the accompanying table shows, the test will immediately tell you whether you have hypothyroidism (if the TSH level is higher than 4.5 milli–international units per liter) or you should be further evaluated by measuring the thyroid hormones T4 and T3 if you are suspected of having an overactive thyroid (TSH is lower than 0.4 milli–international units per liter). If you have symptoms of hypothyroidism and your TSH is normal, I recommend that you speak with your doctor about having a TRH test to see whether you have an underactive thyroid, particularly if your TSH level is greater than 2 and you have a family history of thyroid disease.

HOW TO DETERMINE THYROID IMBALANCES BASED ON TSH LEVELS

Range of TSH Level (milli–international units/liter	Diagnosis
>20	Moderate to severe hypothyroidism
4.5–20	Low-grade hypothyroidism
2.1–4.4	Normal. Also suspicious for hypothyroidism (if there are symptoms or a goiter)
0.4–2.0	Normal
0.1–0.39	Gray zone for too much thyroid hormone
<0.1	Hyperthyroidism or pituitary problem

The TRH stimulation test brings out any minimal excess or deficiency of thyroid hormone that has not thrown the TSH out of its normal laboratory range. In a person with a healthy thyroid and pituitary, the injection of TRH (200 to 500 milligrams) into the bloodstream will result in a rise in TSH ranging from 3 to 15 milli–international units per liter within thirty to forty-five minutes after the injection. The difference between the highest TSH level and the baseline level defines what is normal and what is abnormal. Blood is drawn fifteen, thirty, and forty-five minutes after injection of TRH.

In low-grade hypothyroidism, the difference between the highest level and baseline level exceeds 15 milli–international units per liter. The reason for this exaggerated response of the pituitary is that when the thyroid gland is minimally failing, the pituitary gland is in a state of alert. It contains greater amounts of TSH, and upon administering TRH (hormone designed to stimulate the pituitary), the pituitary releases high amounts of TSH. When there is thyroid hormone excess, the pituitary has backed off and contains little TSH. The increase in TSH is therefore tiny, and the difference is less than 3 milli–international units per liter. However, this range of normal TSH response may vary somewhat from one laboratory to another.

Even when sensitive TSH assays are used (third-generation assays being the most sensitive), the TRH test may help to establish whether there is minimal thyroid hormone excess. In such situations, thyroid hormone levels are normal and TSH is low. The TRH test is useful only when the TSH falls in a gray zone ranging between 0.1 and 0.4 milli–international units per liter.

No further testing is needed if the TSH is normal and you have no symptoms. If the TSH is high or low, however, your doctor will typically measure thyroid hormone levels. T4 often remains in the normal range until the TSH level exceeds 20 milli–international units per liter. Beyond that level, T4 will tend to fall below normal. But this is not engraved in stone. T4 may still be normal even when TSH has reached 25 or 30.

By the same token, thyroid hormone levels will be normal in low-grade hyperthyroidism. When the gland becomes clearly overactive, both T4 and T3 will exceed the upper limit of the normal range. Many people with an overactive thyroid have a normal T4 level, with their T3 being the only thyroid hormone that has risen above normal as a result of thyroid activity.

It is important to make sure that your doctor has measured your T3 level (not T3 resin uptake) if you are hyperthyroid. Your doctor might overlook severe hyperthyroidism if he or she orders only a T4 test.

The Thyroid Neck Check

In January 1997, during the third annual Thyroid Awareness Month, the American Association of Clinical Endocrinologists introduced the "thyroid neck check."[9] This association recommends that the public learn how to do this simple self-examination for the early detection of thyroid disease.

As I've mentioned, whether a thyroid imbalance results in hypothyroidism or hyperthyroidism, it is often generated by an autoimmune disorder such as Hashimoto's thyroiditis or Graves' disease. Both of these disorders are typically associated with an enlarged thyroid, or goiter. Lumps in the thyroid that can induce hyperthyroidism and lumps that could contain cancer may also become visible. You need to pay attention to the lower part of the neck, where the thyroid gland is located. This is especially important if you have a family history of thyroid disease or symptoms of thyroid imbalance.

You can detect a bulginess or a goiter by extending your neck in front of a mirror and gently turning your head slightly to the right and then to the left. If you see that the surface of your neck area just above the sternum (which is the middle bone of the chest) is uneven or protruding even slightly, you might have a lump (nodule) or a goiter. A goiter could mean having Hashimoto's thyroiditis or Graves' disease.

Another physical sign that physicians check and you can learn to use as well to watch for an underactive or overactive thyroid is the pulse rate. The heart is exquisitely sensitive to changes in the levels of thyroid hormone. Excess thyroid hormone will make your heart beat faster, and low thyroid levels will cause the heart to slow down. If you know your resting heart rate and have developed symptoms of thyroid imbalance, checking your resting heart rate can alert you that your levels have become abnormal. For instance, taking your pulse is one way to tell whether your anxiety symptoms have anything to do with your thyroid. A rapid heartbeat at rest often suggests that you have an overactive thyroid. Make sure, however, that you do not have a fever or an infection, are not dehydrated, and have not consumed caffeine— all of which can raise your resting pulse rate. Also, your pulse rate should be checked while lying down, preferably in the morning. The pulse rate is not sensitive enough to detect low-grade imbalances, however, and it is less reliable if you are older than sixty, since, with aging, thyroid hormone excess loses its ability to accelerate the heartbeat.

Having a Goiter: What Does It Mean?

In the United States, the most common type of goiter after those resulting from Hashimoto's thyroiditis and Graves' disease is a nontoxic goiter, a diffuse enlargement that rarely causes symptoms. It is due to a wide range of growth factors. As with the toxic goiters, a nontoxic goiter may initially be diffuse but over time can become multinodular (containing several lumps). Studies have shown that multinodular nontoxic goiters can eventually become toxic nodular goiters that lead to an overactive thyroid (see Chapter 4).

There are no drugs that can effectively shrink a nontoxic nodule. If, after becoming multinodular, the goiter causes symptoms such as hoarseness or difficulty swallowing or breathing, however, physicians often recommend surgical removal. Several studies have shown that destruction of the goiter with high-dose radioactive iodine is safe and effective. This may be an alternative to surgery.

Although rare, it is possible for a goiter to form because the thyroid gland lacks certain enzymes that it needs to manufacture thyroid hormone. In adults, a mild deficit in these enzymes can result in a goiter even though thyroid hormone levels in the blood are normal. The goiter is the result of the pituitary hormone TSH being stimulated by a minimally defective thyroid. If several members of your family have goiters without an imbalance, it might be worthwhile to have your physician look into it. Iodine deficiency is another cause of goiter, because iodine is one of the main ingredients used by the thyroid to manufacture thyroid hormone. In the United States, goiter is rarely due to iodine deficiency. In many parts of the world, however, iodine deficiency is a common cause of goiter (see Chapter 18).

To determine the cause of your goiter, your physician may order one or several of the following tests:

- *TSH:* This test can help to determine whether the thyroid's activity is normal.
- *Antithyroid antibodies:* If TSH is normal or high and your gland is diffusely enlarged (no lumps), this test can aid diagnosis. It is used to determine whether you have Hashimoto's thyroiditis.
- *Radioactive iodine scan and uptake:* Doctors use this test if you are suspected of having Hashimoto's thyroiditis or an enzymatic defect. They also use it to differentiate Graves' disease (high uptake) from silent thyroiditis (low uptake) and if you are suspected of having a multinodular nontoxic or toxic goiter.
- *Thyroid ultrasound:* This test can rule out the presence of a lump or confirm the presence of one or multiple nodules (multinodular goiter).

Let me add a few words about thyroid tenderness. Most physicians interpret tenderness in the thyroid as a symptom of subacute thyroiditis. But Hashimoto's thyroiditis can also cause tenderness and discomfort. Even Graves' disease can cause tenderness and pain, although this is not as common. This happens when a component of Hashimoto's disease is also present in the gland. If you have Graves' disease and are suffering from a painful and tender thyroid, it may mean that Hashimoto's thyroiditis could take over and you could become hypothyroid in the near future.

When to Measure Antithyroid Antibodies

Antithyroid antibodies are markers in the bloodstream that are released by the immune system when there is an immune attack on the thyroid gland. Although many people with no thyroid disease could have very low concentrations of these antibodies in the bloodstream, high concentrations typically indicate an autoimmune thyroid disease. The antibodies that can be readily measured by commercial laboratories for the diagnosis of Hashimoto's thyroiditis are:

- Antithyroglobulin antibody
- Antimicrosomal antibody
- Antithyroperoxidase (anti-TPO) antibody

Of the three tests, anti-TPO antibody is the most sensitive. These antibody tests, however, are not foolproof. Nearly 10 to 20 percent of people with Hashimoto's thyroiditis do not have high antibodies. (If Hashimoto's is suspected, another diagnostic test may be helpful—thyroid ultrasound. It often shows diffuse inflammation and disturbance of the architecture of the gland resulting from the autoimmune attack. Ultrasound also may help in determining whether a bulge in the thyroid represents an area of intense inflammation due to Hashimoto's thyroiditis or a distinct lump, which could raise some concern about malignancy.)

Once antithyroid antibodies have been found to be elevated and the diagnosis of Hashimoto's thyroiditis is confirmed, do not expect your physician to monitor the levels of the antibody over time. Although my patients sometimes request such monitoring, it serves no purpose and does not affect decisions about treatment. Many people have the immune reaction in their thyroid and high levels of antithyroid antibodies for twenty years or more without problems of underactive or overactive thyroid. They may maintain normal function throughout their lives or could become thyroid-imbalanced in the future. You should also know that one or several of these antibodies may be high in Graves' disease, as well.

The antibody more often released by the immune system in people with Graves' disease is thyroid-stimulating antibody (TSAb), which can be measured in the laboratory. As is the case with the other antibodies, TSAb levels may not be high in some patients with Graves' disease. Although it is sometimes useful to measure this antibody in people suspected of having Graves' disease, monitoring the levels of this antibody serves no purpose. By and large, repeating the measurement will have no effect on the treatment of the condition.

People with autoimmune thyroid disease may have high concentrations of antibodies that are used by doctors as markers for other autoimmune diseases, such as lupus and rheumatoid arthritis. Some of these antibodies are ANA, anti–smooth muscle antibody, and anti-SS DNA. Such patients, however, may not have an autoimmune disease.[10] The high concentrations of antibodies may merely reflect a disturbed immune system mistakenly producing some of these antibodies. Also, if you are suffering from an autoimmune disorder, you are likely to have high levels of antithyroid antibodies. This may or may not be an indication that you have a thyroid imbalance. For instance, as many as 38 percent of children with insulin-dependent diabetes have antithyroid antibodies.[11]

Know Your Risk

A family history of thyroid disease may increase your risk of having an autoimmune thyroid disease such as Hashimoto's thyroiditis or Graves' disease. This increased risk is related to a genetic predisposition.[12] If you or members of your family suffer from an autoimmune condition such as insulin-dependent diabetes, lupus, or rheumatoid arthritis, you also have a much higher lifetime risk for developing an autoimmune thyroid disorder such as Hashimoto's thyroiditis or Graves' disease. Because the genes that predetermine whether you will have a thyroid condition often overlap or are linked to genes that predispose you to other unrelated conditions, it is important to know that the risk for having a thyroid imbalance becomes greater if you or a family member has been diagnosed with such conditions. For example, former president John F. Kennedy had Addison's disease. His son, John F. Kennedy Jr., also suffers from Addison's disease as well as Graves' disease.[13] Some patients have two or more autoimmune disorders and are considered as having a polyglandular failure syndrome. A characteristic association is an autoimmune thyroid disease, Addison's disease, and insulin-dependent diabetes.

Another example is the definite increase in the frequency of vitiligo among people suffering from Graves' disease or Hashimoto's thyroiditis. Vitiligo is the presence of blanched areas on the skin due to the loss of normal pigmentation in these areas. The loss of pigment results from an immune system attack on the skin cells, called melanocytes, that maintain normal pigmentation. The loss of pigmentation may be limited to a small area or affect many areas of the skin. One of the most overlooked autoimmune conditions that could coexist with an autoimmune thyroid disease is Sjögren's syndrome (also called Sicca syndrome). Nearly half of patients with Hashimoto's thyroiditis have subtle features of Sjögren's syndrome, which can progress to cause dry mouth, dry eyes, and vaginal dryness.

Consult the accompanying table to learn about which conditions have been shown to increase the predisposition to autoimmune thyroid disease. This table will also help alert you to other conditions to which you may be predisposed if you have been diagnosed with an autoimmune thyroid disorder and have been or are being treated for it.

AUTOIMMUNE CONDITIONS TO WATCH FOR

Condition	Cause	Symptoms
Pernicious anemia	Deficiency of vitamin B$_{12}$ due to lack of a stomach factor essential for vitamin B$_{12}$ absorption	Numbness, tingling in hands and feet, loss of balance, leg weakness
Rheumatoid arthritis	Autoimmune inflammation of joints	Stiffness in the morning, joint pain (knuckles, wrists, elbows, and so on)
Insulin-dependent diabetes	Autoimmune attack on cells in the pancreas that produce insulin	Increased frequency of urination, thirst, weight loss, blurred vision, ketoacidosis
Addison's disease	Autoimmune reaction to adrenal glands (which normally produce cortisol and mineralocorticoid hormones)	Weight loss, fatigue, epigastric pain, nausea, diarrhea, vomiting, low blood pressure, fainting, dehydration, hypoglycemia, increased pigmentation of the skin
Crohn's disease	Autoimmune inflammation of small bowel	Abdominal pain, diarrhea, bloody diarrhea, fever
Lupus	Autoimmune attack on skin and other connective tissue in various organs including the kidney, heart, and joints	Joint pain, fever, rash over the face or other skin areas, kidney damage, heart and lung problems
Myasthenia gravis	Autoimmune attack on a receptor in muscle cells that is essential for contraction of muscles (acetylcholine receptors)	Muscle weakness, double vision, difficulty swallowing
Sjögren's syndrome	Autoimmune reaction to salivary glands, tear glands, and mucus glands of vagina	Eye irritation, dry mouth, vaginal dryness
Scleroderma	Immune reaction causing inflammation and scarring of skin and connective tissue of many organs	Stiffness and pain of fingers, Raynaud's syndrome (blanching and pain of fingers upon exposure to cold)

AUTOIMMUNE CONDITIONS TO WATCH FOR

Condition	Cause	Symptoms
Primary biliary cirrhosis	Autoimmune reaction to bile ducts causing obstruction of the ducts	Jaundice, abnormal liver function, itching
Oophoritis	Autoimmune reaction to ovaries resulting in scarring	Early menopause, loss of menstrual periods

Your risk of becoming hypothyroid is very high if you have received external radiation for the treatment of head and neck tumors, lymphomas, or acne. One study of eighty-one patients who were treated with external radiation for Hodgkin's disease found that up to 58 percent of them were hypothyroid when tested ten to eighteen years after the radiation treatment.[14] External radiation can also cause nodules and cancer in the thyroid gland. The same risk of underactive thyroid and thyroid nodules applies to people who have been exposed to radiation from nuclear fallout.

Radiation from nuclear fallout and nuclear reactor accidents may cause Hashimoto's thyroiditis, thyroid nodules, and cancer as well as hypothyroidism. Researchers noted that, as a consequence of the 1986 Chernobyl accident near Kiev in the USSR (now Ukraine), which caused the release of radioactive material, including radioactive iodine, hypothyroidism rates increased in nearby areas. Even horses and cattle that were not evacuated from an area near Chernobyl became hypothyroid. People in parts of the western United States who were exposed to fallout from nuclear tests done in the 1950s and 1960s may be at a higher risk for having hypothyroidism as well as thyroid nodules.

In addition to autoimmune diseases and radiation, certain other conditions, discussed in the following paragraphs, might provide a clue that you or family members may be at higher risk for having a thyroid imbalance.

For reasons that are unclear, the reading disability dyslexia may alert you to an increased risk for developing a thyroid imbalance. Dyslexia is characterized by a difficulty in distinguishing written symbols, and dyslexics often transpose letters and confuse right and left. Although their overall intelligence may be high, dyslexic children may perform poorly in school because of difficulties with reading and spelling. Typically, dyslexia affects males in the family. Former president George Bush indicated to me that his son Neil suffered from dyslexia when he was in his very early school years. His trouble had resolved since. Neil, however, has not had thyroid disease himself. On the other hand, President Bush's son Marvin had colitis, also genetically linked to autoimmune thyroid disorders. Marvin also has not had a thyroid problem.

Premature graying of the hair before the age of thirty may indicate that you have genes that predispose you to a thyroid disorder. Barbara Bush had premature graying of the hair, a clue that she was at risk for autoimmune thyroid disease. One small survey among patients with autoimmune thyroid disease suggested that left-handed or ambidextrous men might be at higher risk for having Graves' disease or Hashimoto's thyroiditis.

Dermatitis herpetiformis, a rare condition, may be associated with an autoimmune thyroid disease. People with this condition have fluid-filled blisters with itching and hives over their back and lower extremities. If you or a family member has been diagnosed with this condition, have your thyroid tested.

Celiac disease, a disorder of the small bowel, can also occur in patients with autoimmune thyroid diseases. This condition is the result of a sensitivity to gliadin (found in wheat gluten) and can cause diarrhea and malabsorption. The symptoms resolve when the patients eats a gluten-free diet.

As we have seen, a thyroid imbalance can affect any organ in the body (see Chapters 3 and 4). Nevertheless, there are many symptoms that doctors often fail to associate with thyroid disease. If you are experiencing any of these symptoms, discuss the possibility of thyroid disease with your doctor and have him or her test your thyroid. For instance, the red, itchy patches of hives, also known as urticaria, can occur with either hypo- or hyperthyroidism. In many patients, hives are a manifestation of an autoimmune thyroid disease. Patients with hives have a higher frequency of Hashimoto's thyroiditis.[15] In some instances, thyroid hormone treatment resolves the condition, even when thyroid hormone levels are normal. If your levels are high or low and you have hives, you may get relief from taking antihistamimic medications and from correcting the imbalance.

Easy bruising can be a sign of a thyroid imbalance. It may have something to do with a low count of blood platelets (cells that are essential in regulating clotting) or a malfunction of the platelets. Sometimes several members of the same family have a low platelet count simultaneously with Graves' disease and could experience tiny punctate bleeding spots in the skin (petechiae).[16] An often-overlooked cause of easy bruising in thyroid patients is also the use of nonsteroidal anti-inflammatory drugs (NSAIDs), which doctors frequently prescribe for the aches and pains of arthritis that these patients may experience.

Hair loss has been one of the most common complaints among my thyroid patients. Hair loss occurs during both hypo- and hyperthyroidism and may persist for months even after normal blood levels of thyroid hormone have been reestablished. This symptom can be very distressing and alarming for both men and women who may also be suffering from weight problems, depression, and low self-esteem. The effect of a thyroid imbalance on the health of hair follicles can be so drastic that you may notice clumps of hair on your pillow or hairbrush. Your hair may be coming out on the brush and blocking the drain after a shower. Although you need to report this symptom to your physician, do not be alarmed. Most of the time, your hair will come back. If you continue to have hair loss for months after your blood tests become normal, it's because the hair follicles have not fully recovered from the effects of the thyroid imbalance. Although it may take six months to a year for the new, strong hair to replace the old, weak hair that resulted from an imbalance, your hair follicles will become healthy with good thyroid balance, healthy nutrition, and stress management.

If you or a family member ever suffered from the patchy hair loss of alopecia areata, you may be at higher risk for having a thyroid disorder. This condition results in bald areas in any part of the body where hair normally grows, including the scalp, beard, and pubic area. Although this condition often causes concern and worry, in most instances it will resolve spontaneously over several months. In a few people, the hair loss is unfortunately permanent.

Muscle weakness is a symptom of both hyper- and hypothyroidism, but if you experience periods of paralysis after hard exercise or eating lots of sugar, it may be an indication that you are suffering from "hypokalemic periodic paralysis." The paralysis is caused by low potassium levels and co-occurs with Graves' disease. It tends to afflict Asian people. Often, after you achieve a proper thyroid balance, the decline of potassium levels in your blood will no longer occur, and you will stop having the episodes of paralysis.

The following list summarizes the various conditions that should alert you to the possibility of a thyroid imbalance.

CONDITIONS THAT INCREASE THE RISK OF THYROID IMBALANCE
- Autoimmune disorder (see earlier table, page 235, listing autoimmune conditions that occur with a higher frequency in patients with auto-immune thyroid diseases)
- Dyslexia
- Premature graying of hair
- History of depression
- Manic-depression
- Dermatitis herpetiformis
- Down's syndrome, Turner's syndrome
- Family history of Alzheimer's disease
- History of breast cancer

- Alopecia areata
- Chronic urticaria (diffuse itching) in women
- Polymyalgia rheumatica
- Celiac disease

As I've mentioned throughout, older people, postmenopausal women, and women who are suffering from depression or have a history of depression, anxiety, PMS, infertility, recent miscarriage, postpartum depression, or heavy menstrual bleeding should consider thyroid imbalance as a possible reason for the thyroid-related symptoms.

Determining your thyroid status will, of course, alert you to whether your suffering has been caused by a thyroid imbalance. Knowing your risk can also make you pay more serious attention to this tiny gland that so intimately affects all aspects of your well-being, from mood to relationships. When you know your risk of thyroid imbalance and have become familiar with its symptoms, you will be more likely to have your physician consider thyroid imbalance early on, before the imbalance has robbed you of your overall health.

Diagnosing a thyroid imbalance early will also prevent many of the hidden effects that do not cause symptoms right away but could eventually come to haunt you many years later. The accompanying table lists some of the hidden physical effects of hypo- and hyperthyroidism.

HIDDEN EFFECTS OF THYROID IMBALANCE

Hypothyroidism	Hyperthyroidism
High total and LDL cholesterol	Cardiac rhythm problems
Coronary artery disease	Cardiomyopathy and congestive heart failure
Damage to brain structures	Damage to brain structures
High blood pressure	High blood pressure
Glucose intolerance and diabetes	Glucose intolerance and diabetes
	Bone loss and osteoporosis
Acceleration of aging	Acceleration of aging

When the Pituitary Is the Problem

Pituitary deficiency accounts for a very small percentage of the cases of underactive thyroid: as few as 5 in 100,000 people with an underactive thyroid have a pituitary or hypothalamic problem.[17] Many conditions can cause the pituitary gland to become deficient. The most common are tumors in the pituitary or hypothalamus and destruction of the pituitary as a result of poor blood supply or an infection. Destruction of the pituitary related to poor blood supply, such as can occur after delivery of a baby, can cause the person to have severe headaches and visual problems. An underactive thyroid due to an isolated deficiency of TSH is extremely rare.[18]

In hypothyroidism due to a hypothalamic or pituitary disease, the TSH level may be normal or low. The diagnosis cannot be confirmed unless the thyroid hormone level (particularly T4) is measured. In hypothyroidism due to a pituitary problem, the T4 level will be low. You need to know that you could fall through the cracks if you have a pituitary problem causing hypothyroidism but your physician has requested only a TSH test.

Important Points to Remember

- If you are suspected of having a thyroid imbalance, the first and most important thyroid test is TSH.
- You may be suffering from a "minimal thyroid deficiency" even though your TSH is normal. To uncover the imbalance, you may need TRH testing, especially if your TSH level is near the high end of the normal range.
- If you discover you have a goiter (an enlarged thyroid gland), make sure that you receive appropriate testing. If your thyroid levels are normal or if you have hypothyroidism, an antithyroid antibody test will help determine whether you have Hashimoto's thyroiditis.
- If you have not been diagnosed with a thyroid disorder, learn about the conditions that may predispose you to developing a thyroid imbalance and the symptoms that should alert you that you may have a thyroid disorder. These include several autoimmune conditions, premature graying of hair before age thirty, dyslexia, left-handedness in men, and familial patterns of thyroid disease.

15

TREATING THE IMBALANCE

Being diagnosed with a thyroid imbalance can be a relief for people who have long suffered from its symptoms, because they expect that all their problems will disappear very quickly with treatment. They cannot wait to get on with their lives, feel good again, and function normally. Their doctors will often assure them that their thyroid tests will become completely normal over the next few weeks and they will start feeling good again. Typically, when patients begin the treatment, they will perceive a gradual improvement. For weeks or months, however, they may continue not to feel at their best. Many find it hard to admit to other people, either at work or at home, that they are still not feeling good.

In fact, some symptoms may resolve only after a period of "thyroid stability." Often, after correction of a thyroid condition, emotional effects may persist as a result of what I call the "shake-up" of the brain by the thyroid imbalance. In order to shorten this period of recovery and avoid the persistence of symptoms, you need to work with your doctor to reach and maintain normal thyroid hormone levels as soon as possible. You also need to avoid wide fluctuations in your thyroid levels, which are likely to occur if your doctor has little expertise in treating thyroid disorders.

This chapter teaches you how to reach and maintain a proper balance. It also addresses many of the problems that commonly occur during the treatment of thyroid conditions. It highlights cases of undue suffering resulting from stereotypical treatment approaches and limited awareness of the effects of thyroid imbalance during treatment. It also shows you how to avoid these pitfalls and speed up your recovery.

Finding the Right Doctor

In the initial phase of treatment, many patients struggle with their emotions. On the one hand, you want to express your suffering to your physician. On the other hand, you may be quite inhibited about disclosing your anguish. Many patients become overwhelmed by their symptoms and need compassion and understanding from their physicians. If you are receiving treatment for an underactive thyroid by your primary care physician, make sure that your doctor has a good knowledge of adjusting medication. If difficulties arise, insist on being referred to a specialist.

The emotional effects of hyperthyroidism may make you feel alone and helpless. The physician's attitude will have a significant effect on the way you will feel. You have the right to expect your doctor to explain the nature and effects of thyroid imbalance. Some doctors are not prepared to deal with the emotional and mental effects of thyroid imbalance during treatment, however, and will instead focus almost exclusively on normalizing your blood tests. This can be very frustrating to patients whose emotional and mental changes haven't been explained adequately. Some patients, who haven't been told about the effects of thyroid imbalance, may find themselves wondering whether they are not sick but "crazy." You should expect more from your doctor than just analyzing blood tests and adjusting thyroid medication. Your endocrinologist should explain the dynamics of the disease and lay out what is likely to happen as a result of it.

While treating Cassandra's overactive thyroid with medication, the endocrinologist's primary concern was to adjust the dose of medication and try to achieve normal blood tests. Meanwhile, Cassandra was experiencing unexplained emotional problems. She described her encounters with her physician:

> We would have a very brief discussion and do an exam. Sometimes she would chastise me for not working. I felt she couldn't understand how truly ill I was. I was reporting all the anxiety and depression, and she was very dismissive of that. I went every two weeks for a period of months.
>
> I didn't think enough aggressive measures were being taken to subdue my symptoms. I was so angry with the endocrinologist. I was thinking maybe I wasn't being a good patient. But I was a very compliant patient. I wanted to feel better. It was like I was in a big black hole trying to climb out, and nobody could reach in to get me. I felt helpless. It was very depressing. I felt trapped. My self-esteem was terrible.
>
> One day, the nurse announced I was in the exam room, and I heard the doctor say "Again?" She often didn't communicate with me outside of the office. Her office staff would call, or I would get messages in the mail to adjust my dosage.

I expected her to have a greater understanding of what I was going through symptomatically and emotionally.

Cassandra had great willpower. She wanted to feel normal; she wanted to understand. She wanted to communicate with her physician. She attempted to describe her emotional, debilitating suffering, but her doctor seemed unconcerned. Unlike Cassandra, many people may not feel at ease talking about their suffering. Many have severe anxiety or panic attacks and do not express the symptoms to their physicians for fear of being taken for fools. Yet it is important to express these symptoms, both to ensure better understanding and to obtain optimal treatment. To avoid undue suffering generated by lack of communication between you and your doctor, choose a thyroid specialist who can deal with your emotions.

Nuclear medicine doctors are often involved in the treatment of Graves' disease because they are the ones who calculate the dose of radioactive iodine and administer the treatment to the thyroid gland. Unfortunately, many nuclear medicine doctors feel that they are capable of taking over the care of Graves' disease patients. They seldom have adequate knowledge, however, to assess the response to therapy. They also have very limited knowledge of the clinical and emotional aspects of hyperthyroidism during treatment. Some patients with an overactive thyroid, either on their own or based on recommendations from friends, seek their care from nuclear medicine doctors. This may result in inadequate control of the thyroid imbalance, thus lengthening the period of suffering and adding more frustrations and adverse emotional effects. Many nuclear medicine physicians feel they are astute and experienced enough to determine the exact dose of radioactive iodine that will partially destroy the thyroid gland while leaving exactly enough of the gland to produce adequate amounts of natural hormone. This is often unrealistic.

Treating the Underactive Thyroid

As I've explained, hypothyroidism due to a damaged thyroid gland causes high TSH levels. The higher the TSH, the more severe the hypothyroidism. Your doctor's treatment goal is to give you the amount of thyroid hormone needed to reduce TSH to normal levels. In general, the higher the TSH, the higher the thyroid hormone dose needs to be for you to reach and maintain normal thyroid balance.[1] Therefore, the TSH levels obtained at diagnosis may allow your doctor to predict from the outset the dosage range needed to achieve close-to-normal thyroid levels. Thus, it is not uncommon for doctors to increase the dose gradually over the first few weeks of treatment without monitoring TSH until the estimated dose has been reached and stabilized for a few weeks.[2]

Although synthetic levothyroxine, currently the most widely used form of thyroid hormone to treat hypothyroidism, became available in the 1950s, its use became widespread only in the early 1970s, when researchers discovered that animal-derived thyroid extracts were causing unstable and inconsistent blood levels of thyroid hormones. Desiccated thyroid contains T4 and T3 in variable amounts, depending on the preparation process used by the manufacturer and the iodine content in the diet of the animals from which the thyroid glands were taken. Also, around the same time, scientists discovered that, when people take synthetic thyroxine (T4), some of it is converted to T3 in bodily organs, thus providing stable levels of both T4 and T3. The stability of thyroid hormone levels and TSH levels achieved by using synthetic levothyroxine is also due to the fact that T4 has a very long life in the body. When taken on a daily basis, the thyroxine pill allows for a steady and continuous production of T3 in bodily organs.

Pharmaceutical companies manufacture levothyroxine tablets in different strengths, ranging from 25 micrograms (or .025 milligrams) up to 300 micrograms (0.3 milligrams). The three most commonly used brands of levothyroxine are Synthroid®, Levoxyl®, and Levothroid®. The availability of these different strengths facilitates the fine adjustment of the dose of thyroid hormone so that blood levels can be maintained in the normal "laboratory range" as long as you continue taking the medication. When you fill your prescription, make sure you are not given a generic preparation, since generics may not contain the exact amount of thyroid hormone prescribed.[3]

If your doctor doesn't do the dose adjustments properly, you are likely to continue to experience symptoms for a long time.

For Tracy, whom I recently saw for a second opinion, it took a year and a half to reach normal thyroid levels after her initial diagnosis. She said, "My doctor was having so much trouble getting me regulated to a normal TSH level. Every four months, I'd be going back in and complaining I wasn't feeling well, and sure enough, the blood test would show that I was correct. The adjustments made by my doctor were never enough to make me normal again."

To avoid such problems, I have developed a graduated dosage method that yields excellent results for most people. In the accompanying table, you can identify the dose that you need to reach during this first phase of treatment by looking at your initial TSH level.

GRADUATED DOSAGE METHOD FOR LEVOTHYROXINE

Initial TSH Level (milli–international units per liter)	Dose to Be Achieved at End of First Phase (micrograms of levothyroxine)
< 15	25.0
15–25	37.5
25–30	50.0
30–40	75.0
> 40	100.0

In persons with severe hypothyroidism, the initial dose of thyroid hormone should be small and increased gradually to the dose required. Abrupt and rapid administration of high doses of thyroid hormone to severely hypothyroid patients may cause health problems, especially in older people. For example, while a person is hypothyroid, his or her heart works slowly and has adapted to the low metabolism. Rapid correction of hypothyroidism in someone with a preexisting heart condition, which may be unknown to the patient and physician, could quickly accelerate the heart function and induce a heart attack. Most doctors like to start you at 25 micrograms a day and increase the dose weekly by 25 micrograms until the estimated dose is reached. For patients under forty-five years of age who are otherwise healthy, the dosage may be stepped up faster. In older patients and those with heart disease or anxiety symptoms, the dosage should be stepped up every two weeks.

Severe mood disorders that can be quite alarming may also occur when doctors prescribe high doses of thyroid hormone at the beginning of treatment. Often such patients have a history of high anxiety or emotional problems. These symptoms may occur four to seven days after they begin taking the high dose of thyroid hormone. If you experience mental effects, you need to have your doctor reduce the dose of thyroid hormone immediately. Doctors have had to hospitalize patients because of mania or other reactions to excessive thyroid hormone. Patients may become severely agitated, their thoughts may race, and they may exhibit inappropriate behavior. Some may even experience hallucinations and delusions.[4]

A high amount of thyroid hormone commonly worsens an existing anxiety disorder, which may be a source of confusion for you and your physician. Myra, aged forty-nine, had had a great deal of stress in her life and had been suffering from a generalized anxiety disorder for quite a few years. She was intermittently prescribed Valium and other medications, which helped control her anxiety, and she had learned through the years to manage her symptoms. When she was diagnosed as hypothyroid, her doctor prescribed a high dose of thyroid hormone from the beginning instead of starting her at a low dose and stepping it up gradually. After a few days on the medication, Myra began to experience severe panic attacks and increased anxiety symptoms. She woke up in the middle of the night with a rapid heartbeat, a hot and sweaty feeling, and a choking sensation "as if somebody was pressing on my neck."

She took the thyroid pill for a couple of weeks, but her symptoms kept getting worse. She reached the point of experiencing ten to fifteen panic attacks a day. Finally, she concluded that this might be caused by the thyroid medication and stopped taking it on her own, which caused the anxiety symptoms and panic attacks to diminish. Later, even small doses triggered panic attacks. It became a vicious cycle in which Myra associated the thyroid hormone treatment with a worsening of her symptoms. After I counseled her about the nature and cause of her symptoms, she finally agreed to try the graduated dosage method. The dose was eventually increased, her thyroid levels became normal, and the exaggerated anxiety symptoms were resolved. In fact, Myra now suffers from less anxiety than she did before the doctors diagnosed her thyroid condition. Myra's anxiety disorder was probably caused in part by the underactive thyroid, but when too much thyroid hormone entered her system at once, the anxiety became worse.

Approximately six weeks after you reach the estimated dose that is expected to bring your thyroid levels close to normal, your doctor will typically order a TSH test so the dose can be adjusted. The size of the adjustment needed should be determined based on the result of the new TSH test. How fast this adjustment is made also depends on your age and on whether you suffer from a heart condition.

The dose of thyroid hormone may need to be adjusted once or twice before you reach a normal TSH level. Do not have your TSH tested more often than every six to eight weeks at the beginning. The criterion for successful therapy is to finally get TSH within a normal range and keep it there.

PROBLEMS DURING THE MAINTENANCE PHASE
OF TREATMENT OF HYPOTHYROIDISM

Once your thyroid test levels have stabilized, you need to make sure that your doctor does not prescribe too much or too little thyroid hormone. In one study, 14 percent of hypothyroid patients taking thyroid hormone were overreplaced, and 18 percent were underreplaced.[5]

People taking too much thyroid hormone will have a low TSH reading and may develop cardiac problems.[6] Postmenopausal women will have accelerated bone loss, which predisposes them to osteoporosis.[7] Even minimal thyroid hormone excess may make you irritable and cause you to suffer from undue nervousness, anxiety, or hypomanic behavior.[8]

Consider the case of Catherine, a thirty-four-year-old sales manager who was diagnosed with hypothyroidism by her internist. The dose of thyroid hormone she was receiving exceeded her needs. She began suffering from shakiness, insomnia, and palpitations; she also noted that her eyes seemed to be locked in a stare. She described symptoms of hypomania. "I couldn't sit still for any length of time," she said. "I became too energetic and obsessive-compulsive about cleaning my house and working long hours. I would get up in the middle of the night to clean up."

Catherine felt she was possessed and had lost control of her body. Deep inside, she noted that the person she had become was not her usual self. She experienced rage for no apparent reason and felt compelled to ride a bicycle in a remote area, pedaling as hard and fast as she could until she felt the rage subside.

These changes had occurred so quickly that Catherine didn't understand what was happening to her. She thought she was losing her mind. Her heart was beating at such a fast pace that she was afraid to go to sleep for fear she would have a heart attack in her sleep. "I wanted so badly to be my old self—the me that I knew and loved. I was afraid of this new person, and I wanted to feel healthy again." Catherine did indeed feel healthy again once her dose of thyroid hormone was reduced to a more appropriate level.

Do not increase the dose on your own or insist that your physician increase the dose because you have not felt an improvement and believe that a higher dose would make you feel better. Increasing the dose may cause new problems. Do not decrease or stop the thyroid medication on your own or skip taking it once or twice a week either. Some patients phone their doctors and try to convince them to alter their prescription without testing and/or follow-up. This can lead to a cumulative deficit or excess in thyroid hormone, which can cause a great deal of suffering.

Sophia had been receiving 150 micrograms of levothyroxine daily for three years. One day, she called her physician and mentioned that she had heart palpitations. These were in fact due to anxiety over another family member's health problems. Sophia's physician decreased the dose from 150 micrograms to 75 micrograms and told her to come to his office for repeat thyroid testing three months later. Because of her personal problems, Sophia did not take the time to have a follow-up test until a full year later. During that year, she had a wide range of symptoms that she attributed to stress.

When Sophia finally did return to her physician for follow-up, her tests showed hypothyroidism because she was taking only half the dose required to maintain normal thyroid levels. After the dose was readjusted, her symptoms gradually disappeared. In fact, she became better able to cope with her family problems.

Another unfortunate problem that still happens to some hypothyroid patients taking thyroid hormone occurs when general practitioners instruct them to stop taking their medication. Crystal, who was hypothyroid, was taken off thyroid hormone by her general practitioner when he saw that her thyroid test results were normal while she was taking thyroid hormone. What this physician probably overlooked is that the test results were normal because of the treatment. Three or four months after she stopped taking the medication, Crystal suffered from serious depression and had many symptoms of hypothyroidism. She went back to her doctor, and he said her symptoms were caused by stress. When I tested Crystal and found her hypothyroid, I placed her back on thyroid hormone treatment, and she has done well ever since.

The likelihood that you are under- or overcorrected is extremely high if your physician does not monitor TSH when you are taking thyroid hormone. Many physicians unfortunately continue to run T3 and T4 tests and often try to make treatment decisions based on these tests instead of TSH. T4 and T3 test results are also easily misinterpreted when the levels of the proteins carrying thyroid hormone in the blood are abnormal (see Chapter 14). In addition, several medications can alter thyroid hormone levels. For instance, Dilantin and aspirin may lower the total T4 reading, even though thyroid function is normal.

To achieve a good balance, you need to have your TSH maintained between 0.5 and 2.0 milli–international units per liter while receiving thyroid hormone treatment. A TSH ranging between 2.0 and 4.5 may mean some thyroid hormone deficiency (see Chapter 14). Often all it takes to restore normal thyroid status is a small increase in the dose, which might have significant effects on the way you feel. If, despite having a normal TSH for at least three to four months, you continue to suffer from depression or symptoms of underactive thyroid such as tiredness, dry skin, and pains and aches, you may experience an improvement by combining T4 and T3 in your treatment program (see Chapter 17). Your system may still be lacking some T3 even though your blood test results are normal.

OPTIMIZING YOUR USE OF THYROID HORMONE PILLS

Many foods, nutrients, and drugs can interfere with thyroid hormone absorption. For example, if you take iron (ferrous sulfate) at the same time as thyroid hormone, it will bind with some of the thyroid hormone and block its absorption. Fiber and calcium carbonate, if taken simultaneously with thyroid hormone, may interfere with absorption of the hormone.

Several medications, when taken together with thyroid hormone, can also decrease the availability of the hormone by interfering with its absorption in the gastrointestinal tract. For instance, antacids containing aluminum (Maalox), drugs used to lower cholesterol (cholestyramine, Questran, colestid), and sucralfate (an aluminum-containing ulcer drug) cause decreased absorption from the gastrointestinal tract.

To avoid this interference effect, take your thyroid hormone at least three to four hours before or after you take these medications. I recommend that you take your thyroid pill at the same time every day, preferably before breakfast on an empty stomach with two or three cups of water. Take your nutritional supplements and drugs at lunch and suppertime.

Some medications increase the rate at which your body clears thyroid hormone. If you are taking a stable dose of thyroid hormone and were recently prescribed the drugs Dilantin (phenytoin), Tegretol (carbamazepine), or phenobarbital, you may need a change in your dosage. Do not forget to mention these new medications to the physician treating your hypothyroidism so that he or she can retest your thyroid.

Generally speaking, it is quite safe for women with a thyroid imbalance to use oral contraceptives, even while taking appropriate thyroid medication. Very rarely, oral contraceptives containing estrogen cause a slight increase in the need for thyroid hormone replacement, presumably because estrogens cause an increase in thyroid hormone–binding proteins in your bloodstream. If you have been receiving a stable dose of thyroid hormone and have begun taking an oral contraceptive or hormone replacement therapy, it is wise to have your physician order a TSH test three months after you start the estrogens. By that time, your blood levels should have stabilized so that the TSH test result will be reliable for the purpose of a dose adjustment. If you have taken Tamoxifen, an antiestrogen used for the treatment of breast cancer, for more than one year, you may require more thyroid hormone.[9]

HOW OFTEN SHOULD YOU BE RETESTED?

Some doctors recommend that thyroid tests be done once a year when a patient's thyroid function has returned to normal with a specific dose of thyroid hormone replacement. You may have an unstable thyroid condition, however. Patients with Hashimoto's thyroiditis may have a concomitant Graves' disease that may be more active at some times than at others. If you have hypothyroidism due to Hashimoto's thyroiditis and are taking a stable dose of thyroid hormone, a flare-up of Graves' disease and production of the antibodies that stimulate the thyroid gland may make you require less thyroid hormone.[10] Rarely, it can even cause the rapid onset of hyperthyroidism and require stopping thyroid hormone treatment.[11] Several of my patients with underactive thyroids suffer from frequent fluctuations in the activity of the gland. You need to be aware that the residual activity of the gland affected by Hashimoto's thyroiditis does change and can fluctuate over time.[12] As a result, patients with an underactive thyroid may require frequent adjustments in the dose of thyroid hormone. In fact, in a very few patients who had very unstable thyroid activity causing shifts from overactivity to underactivity, I had to recommend surgical removal of the thyroid in order to maintain normal thyroid levels.

Retesting patients once a year will ignore possibly significant changes in their thyroid activity. Some patients may suffer from the effects of thyroid hormone excess or deficiency and not know it. Because changes in thyroid levels in patients receiving stable doses of thyroid hormone are common, a better recommendation is that thyroid tests be done regularly every six months and that the test results be closely scrutinized in conjunction with a careful assessment of symptoms.[13] If you are hypothyroid as a result of the treatment of Graves' disease, you may need more frequent testing (every three to four months), at least initially.

Three years previously, doctors in her managed care health program had diagnosed Wanda with an underactive thyroid. The thyroid hormone she was taking made her symptoms subside. She was retested once and was told to continue the same dose of medication. A few months later, she began experiencing tremendous stress at home. She complained of many symptoms that her primary care physician never attributed to possible hypothyroidism. She had understood from her physician that her thyroid problem was taken care of as long as she took the medication.

Wanda said, "I was absolutely zonked out. I would walk in and lie down and go to sleep at 6:30. I was very depressed. When I told my primary care physician I was having dizziness, he put me on motion sickness medicine, which I took one time and it made me feel bad."

When Wanda was finally tested again two years later, she was quite hypothyroid. Adjustment of her thyroid medication resolved her tiredness and other symptoms. After that experience, Wanda decided to change her health insurance coverage and her doctor.

Many patients believe that having an underactive thyroid means that the gland has quit working and all they have to do is take the same pill for their entire lives. Therefore, they try to get refills for their medication over the phone, believing that there is no need to be examined or tested. This may result in unhappy surprises.

Correcting the
Overactive Thyroid and Side Effects

If you've been diagnosed with an overactive thyroid due to Graves' disease, understanding the available treatments will allow you to work with your doctor in selecting the best option.

TREATMENT OPTIONS

The three major methods currently used to treat Graves' disease—administering antithyroid drugs, destroying a significant portion of the thyroid gland with radioactive iodine, and surgically removing a significant portion of the gland—address the consequences rather than the cause of the condition.[14]

ANTITHYROID DRUGS

Doctors may prescribe antithyroid drugs such as methimazole or PTU for six months to two years (the average is one year) to maintain normal thyroid levels and hopefully achieve a remission. (You have achieved a remission if, after several months of treatment, you no longer require medication to maintain normal levels of thyroid hormone and TSH.) Antithyroid medications are picked up by the thyroid gland, where they inhibit the production of thyroid hormone. They also have an effect on the immune system, diminishing the autoimmune attack on the thyroid. In general, 30 to 50 percent of patients achieve a remission[15] when they take one of these medications for at least six months to a year. Women in their reproductive years with mild hyperthyroidism and small goiters respond well to this form of treatment.

Methimazole lasts longer in the body and you can take it as a single daily dose if you require 30 milligrams or less, whereas PTU should be taken three to four times a day. With either medication, experienced physicians can often maintain thyroid function in the normal range for as long as the treatment is continued.

Several common minor side effects may occur during treatment and often resolve spontaneously or after the patient switches to another medication. In some instances, the persistence of such symptoms requires stopping the medication. These side effects include:

- Itching
- Skin rash
- Hives
- Joint pains
- Fever
- Upset stomach
- Metallic taste

One of the adverse effects of antithyroid medications that often worries patients is agranulocytosis, a reaction in the bone marrow, which suddenly stops manufacturing white blood cells. This frightening complication, which occurs more frequently in the first three months of treatment, should not cause you undue anxiety because it is quite rare. One study showed that this complication occurs in only 3 out of 10,000 people treated with medication each year.[16] Although physicians usually do not monitor your white blood cell count, it is safer if this is done each time you have your thyroid tested while being treated. If a sore throat, a sore mouth, or an infection occurs, you should report to your doctor and have your white blood-cell count measured. If the white cell count drops significantly, you need to stop the medication immediately. The low white blood-cell count can result in a blood infection. Your doctor will often recommend isolation in a hospital room, antibiotics, and treatment with medications that raise your white blood-cell count to appropriate levels.

Liver damage, another unusual complication of antithyroid medications, is rather serious and often occurs in the first few months of treatment as well. For this reason, your doctor will typically test your liver on a regular basis. If liver tests become abnormal, the medication should be stopped immediately.

Other serious, albeit rare, side effects from using antithyroid drugs include:

- Suppressed production of red blood cells in bone marrow (aplastic anemia)
- Low platelet count
- Inflammation of blood vessels (vasculitis), causing symptoms similar to lupus

If you have tolerated the medication well, you need to stay on it for at least eight to twelve months to give it a chance to produce the remission for which you are hoping. During treatment, you need to be retested (by checking not only TSH but also free thyroxine index and T3) every two months and have your dose adjusted. Typically, the dose is gradually reduced as your requirement for the medication decreases and the activity of the disease slows down. At the end of the treatment period, most doctors tend to stop the medication abruptly to see whether you stay normal without it. With methimazole, I usually decrease the dose first by 5 milligrams daily until the patient has reached a dose of 5 milligrams per day; then the dose is dropped to 5 milligrams every other day, then to 5 milligrams twice a week (on Sunday and Wednesday) before stopping the medication. Only if the TSH remains normal while you are taking 5 milligrams twice a week for at least two months should you stop taking the medication. If the TSH is not normal, you may become hyperthyroid again, and the vicious cycle will resume. If the TSH level becomes low even though thyroid hormone levels are normal, that means your gland still requires medication. In this case, the dose of medication will need to be increased to achieve normal levels again. At this point, you may want to proceed with an alternative treatment or continue the medication for another six-month period before you try stopping it again.

DESTROYING A SIGNIFICANT PORTION OF THE
THYROID WITH RADIOACTIVE IODINE

Another treatment method is to destroy a significant portion of the thyroid gland with radioactive iodine (radioiodine). This method is simple. You are given a small amount of radioactive iodine to drink. The amount is either fixed (10–20 millicuries) or based on the size of your thyroid gland and its level of activity after you have had a radioactive iodine uptake test (see Chapter 14). This method is the preferred form of treatment for toxic nodules and multinodular toxic goiters. Doctors also find this method effective for treating nontoxic goiters that have caused pressure in the neck, including difficulty swallowing.[17] For patients with Graves' disease, this method should be chosen if you are unlikely to achieve a remission with medications or if you have experienced side effects from the medications. Doctors frequently recommend this method for men and people older than forty-five.

Also, your doctor will often prescribe radioactive iodine to treat your Graves' disease if, after a year or two of medication, your thyroid gland continues to be overactive. In general, this method is used if, after you have achieved a remission with medication, your thyroid becomes overactive again months or years after you completed the course of medication.

Even when radioactive iodine is chosen from the outset, some doctors prescribe an antithyroid medication for two months prior to the radioiodine treatment, to bring your thyroid levels down to normal first. I often elect this last approach so that the patient improves—emotionally and physically—and has time to learn more about the condition and the treatment options. Using medications initially will also help determine whether your gland is quite responsive to medication. It will often prevent you from rapidly swinging from hyperthyroidism to severe hypothyroidism. You will be asked to stop the antithyroid medication two to five days before the radioactive iodine treatment and to restart the medication at smaller doses three to five days after the treatment. If the medication you have been taking is PTU, make sure that you are switched to Tapazole® three to four weeks prior to the radioiodine treatment. Recent research has concluded that PTU treatment causes the gland to become more resistant to radioiodine treatment.[18]

The purpose of radioiodine treatment is to destroy enough of the thyroid gland so that the remaining part does not produce excess thyroid hormone. The destruction begins within days after the treatment and may continue over a period of several years. Many patients are led to believe that radioactive iodine rapidly destroys the entire gland, whereas, most of the time, it actually destroys only a portion. In fact, the amount of the thyroid gland destroyed with treatment varies from person to person because glands have different levels of sensitivity to the damaging effect of radioiodine.

Many doctors in the United States prefer this method because it is in general safe and effective. In many European countries and in Japan, doctors favor trying medications first. One treatment with radioiodine may not suffice. Nearly 30 percent of patients treated with radioactive iodine need to be retreated one or more times, and the overwhelming majority of people treated with this method become hypothyroid over weeks, months, or years. Several years after the treatment, as many as 70 percent of people treated with radioactive iodine will become permanently hypothyroid. Very rarely do people become hyperthyroid again many years after treatment with radioactive iodine.[19]

This method should not be used if you are pregnant. If you are a woman of childbearing age, your doctor will typically order a pregnancy test prior to the treatment. This treatment should also be avoided in people having moderate to severe eye disease until the eye condition has become stable. It can cause or worsen eye disease in 15 percent of patients. For this reason, some doctors prescribe prednisone (a corticosteroid medication that slows down the inflammation in the eyes) for several weeks after radioactive iodine treatment, which may reduce the occurrence of eye disease. A recent study conducted in England and Wales showed that patients with Graves' disease treated with radioactive iodine had a mortality rate much higher than the rest of the population.[20] It appears that the increased mortality is probably not related to the treatment, however, but rather to how the hyperthyroid condition compounds the adverse effects of other ailments such as osteoporosis and heart disease.

Many people, when told about the option of radioactive iodine treatment, become concerned that it will cause long-term adverse health effects. There is no scientific evidence so far that the treatment causes thyroid cancer or leukemia. There is debate, however, about the increased risk of cancer of the stomach, hypopharynx, and esophagus. One recent study, for instance, concluded that the occurrence of stomach cancer may increase years after the treatment, particularly in younger people.[21] Because these concerns are not quite settled yet, it is perhaps safer to treat children and adolescents with medications first and consider radioiodine treatment for young people as a last resort.

Children born to women previously treated with radioactive iodine do not experience a significantly increased risk of genetic defects. Nevertheless, if you are treated with radioiodine, you should avoid becoming pregnant within six months after the treatment. It is not known, moreover, whether radioactive iodine received during the reproductive years will have any genetic or carcinogenic effects on future generations.

SURGICAL REMOVAL OF A SIGNIFICANT PORTION OF THE THYROID

Surgical removal of a significant portion of the thyroid gland (subtotal thyroidectomy) is not frequently used in the United States unless special circumstances exist. For example, for patients who choose not to take radioiodine and who have experienced reactions to medications, or have very enlarged thyroid glands and are concerned about eye disease, surgical removal of a part of the gland may be an option. Complete removal of the gland may relieve some of the symptoms in some persons suffering from thyroid eye disease. Another advantage of surgery is the rapid control of symptoms. The patient must be treated with medications (iodine and a beta-blocker) before the operation, however, to avoid complications such as thyroid storm that could develop as a result of surgery.[22]

I tend to recommend surgery for children and adolescents who have not responded to the medication or could not tolerate it. Surgery often cures the condition and prevents fluctuation of thyroid levels and its detrimental effects on mood and behavior. A pregnant woman treated with medication who experiences significant side effects can be treated with surgery during pregnancy.

If you decide to have an operation, choose a surgeon who has continued and proven experience with thyroid surgery. This is crucial because surgical removal of the thyroid can result in impairment of the voice and problems with low calcium due to damage to the parathyroid glands (four small glands right behind the thyroid that control calcium metabolism). To ensure the best outcome, choose a surgeon who has done at least ten to fifteen thyroid surgeries a year for the past two to three years. Ask about his or her track record. The procedure for Graves' disease is subtotal thyroidectomy, although some surgeons may recommend a total thyroidectomy for people with eye disease to help the eye problem. A total thyroidectomy, however, is more likely to cause complications such as low calcium and nerve damage. You also need to remember that, in nearly 30 percent of people who have a subtotal thyroidectomy, the thyroid gland will become overactive again in the future. If that happens, radioiodine treatment will be the best option. If you are planning to become pregnant right away, surgery may be the best alternative.

Many persons with thyroid hormone resistance (high thyroid hormone levels, normal/high TSH) are misdiagnosed as having an overactive thyroid due to Graves' disease and may unnecessarily undergo a partial removal of the thyroid gland.[23] Such surgery is harmful, however, and is likely to impair the patient's future health.

MAKING THE RIGHT DECISION

If you have just been diagnosed with an overactive thyroid due to Graves' disease, you should discuss the three treatment options with your doctor and get advice on which method to choose. Some patients are more comfortable than others with taking the responsibility for contributing to this decision. If you have significant eye disease, you should not rush into radioactive iodine treatment because that may worsen your eye problems. Also, make sure that your doctor has looked for lumps in your thyroid if you have Graves' disease. Research is showing that patients with Graves' disease may be at a slightly higher risk for thyroid cancer, although this is not quite settled. If you do have a lump, a fine-needle aspiration biopsy (see Chapter 20) should be done *before* you receive the radioactive iodine treatment, since this treatment will affect the results of any biopsy performed afterward. If a cancer is present, then the treatment for both the overactive thyroid and the lump should be surgery.

Some endocrinologists recommend the same treatment for all their patients suffering from an overactive thyroid due to Graves' disease. This explains why a patient seen by two or three endocrinologists may be given different opinions with respect to treatment. The method chosen should in fact depend on several factors, including your age, whether you are a woman in your reproductive years, whether your overactive thyroid is severe, and how long you have suffered from hyperthyroidism before the diagnosis was made. The size of your thyroid gland and whether you have significant eye problems are, as I explained, other factors that ought to be taken into account in making the decision.

Claire, like many Graves' disease patients having no knowledge of the condition, became confused during her first visit with the endocrinologist. She said:

I went to see this one doctor, but my first visit was not a good visit. He came in with this one little lab report and said, "Okay, you have Graves' disease. We need to start you on these pills, and you're going to take them every day." He then went on to say, "But it's not going to do any good, so we might as well forget that, and we'll go ahead and give you the radioactive iodine. Let me just go ahead and schedule that, and we'll get it done in two weeks." I didn't like that. I still didn't know what anything was. I went back to my husband's doctor and asked for another referral.

Claire had mild hyperthyroidism and a small goiter. She was treated with Tapazole for one year by another endocrinologist and achieved a remission. She has been off medication for almost two years, and her thyroid function has remained normal. If she had gone ahead with the radioactive iodine treatment, she could have become immediately hypothyroid. To avoid receiving the wrong form of treatment, ask your endocrinologist for specific reasons why one option is recommended over another.

Adriana, a thirty-three-year-old accountant, had suffered unnecessarily for more than a year because she did not receive the right form of treatment. By the time she was seen by an endocrinologist, she had a big goiter and had been severely hyperthyroid for about two years. She described her first encounter with the physician. "We talked about what forms of treatment were available. My understanding was that I had to start with medication to control the hyperthyroidism, and if that didn't work within a few years, I would be given radioactive iodine to destroy the gland, and if that did not work, we could resort to surgery." She left the endocrinologist's office with a prescription for PTU.

Adriana took the antithyroid medication for a year and a half but did not achieve a remission. Many patients like Adriana who have large goiters and severe hyperthyroidism at the outset do not achieve a permanent remission with medications and should be considered for more radical treatment, such as radioactive iodine, from the beginning. Adriana had had to take five to six PTU pills three to four times a day and her thyroid levels rarely reached normalcy, whereas she could have been offered radioiodine treatment much sooner.

"My dosage went up and down all the time," she said. "I was adjusted so often it was like riding a roller coaster. I just felt like the physician did not understand me or how truly ill I was. There was a little improvement, but many of my symptoms persisted. It was like trying to put out a forest fire with a fire extinguisher."

If medications are chosen to treat your condition, you need to commit to taking them daily as prescribed. Otherwise, you will prolong your suffering and be more likely to experience lingering effects down the road. Agoraphobia in particular can make a person unwilling to take medications.[24] Agoraphobia is a form of anxiety disorder that may be triggered by hyperthyroidism, in which the sufferer becomes easily frightened and reluctant to leave home and face new people. If you have become agoraphobic or are experiencing other symptoms of an anxiety disorder, you are likely to do better with radioactive iodine treatment.

Many patients suffering from an overactive thyroid improve rather quickly when they are prescribed, from the outset, a beta-blocker such as propranolol (Inderal). I often prescribe propranolol at a dose of 40 to 60 milligrams four times a day for the first three weeks, then ask the patient to reduce the dose by half for another week or two while thyroid hormone levels are being brought down with antithyroid treatment. If you are treated with a long course of antithyroid medication, you may do better if you also take a tranquilizer such as alprazolam (Xanax). In Chapter 2, I explained how stress generated by thyroid imbalance can become self-perpetuating and how stress can affect the activity of Graves' disease. Reducing the stress and anxiety using mind-body relaxation techniques is certainly effective. But you may also need to use medication for several weeks to alleviate your anxiety symptoms. This will increase your chances of reaching a remission.

In one report from Italy, women who took the benzodiazepine bromazepam (Lexotan) for seven or more months had a much higher remission rate than women who took the tranquilizer for only the first two months.[25] The difference is striking because only 25 percent of patients who took the tranquilizer for seven months or more had a relapse, whereas 75 percent of those who took bromazepam for only two months had a relapse. The author of the report recommended 3 milligrams twice a day during the first month and 1.5 milligrams twice a day thereafter.

You need to know that whatever method is chosen, you could be disappointed. For instance, you may take medications for more than a year and find that you are not responding and have to try another method, or you may be treated with radioactive iodine and find six months or a year later that you need another radioactive iodine treatment. You must be prepared for such disappointments. Sometimes the initially chosen treatment simply does not work, and alternatives must be considered.

WORKING WITH YOUR DOCTOR TO AVOID WILD SWINGS
Whether you are being treated with medication or have received radioactive iodine treatment, fluctuations in thyroid levels can be expected. You need to work with your doctor, however, to minimize the occurrence of major, rapid swings. Major fluctuations can cause you to lose control and experience significant emotional and physical suffering, including anxiety, variations in energy level, anger, and mood swings. Emotional instability may alter your brain chemistry and make you more vulnerable to mental anguish even after your thyroid is regulated. If these fluctuations in thyroid function occur while you are being treated with medication because the dose has not been adjusted smoothly, you will typically experience frustration and despair and your symptoms will persist. Your initial hope of ending your suffering dissipates and is replaced by anger at the physician and feelings of being condemned to suffer.

Katie is an example of a Graves' disease patient whose thyroid condition was inadequately controlled as a result of poor adjustment of the dose of medication. Three months after Katie started the medication, her doctor told Katie she was hypothyroid. "I became tired and lethargic, but the anxiety was still there. Then he stopped the medication and told me to return in two months. Two months later, all my original symptoms had come back. He put me on a lower dose of PTU, but two months later, I was hyperthyroid. I could not stand these fluctuations any longer. I had to find another doctor."

To avoid Katie's misfortune, make sure that you are retested six weeks after starting the medication. Then you need to be retested every two months. Each time when the levels are normal during the course of treatment, I typically decrease the dosage to avoid the occurrence of hypothyroidism. This is the best way to avoid major swings in thyroid levels.

Some early studies showed that combining methimazole at a steady dose to block the thyroid gland with thyroxine to replace the deficit caused by the methimazole (called a block-replace regimen) increased the remission rate. You are given a high dose of methimazole (30 to 40 milligrams daily) in conjunction with thyroxine. The thyroxine dose will be adjusted to maintain normal thyroid test results. More recent studies, however, have not confirmed that the block-replace regimen leads to higher rates of remission. Although the block-replace regimen allows the maintenance of stable thyroid hormone levels throughout the course of treatment,[26] it is likely to cause more side effects from the high dose of antithyroid medication.

People treated with radioactive iodine may also suffer wild fluctuations, which can be minimized or prevented. Although many patients assume that they take the radioiodine cocktail and their gland is destroyed and that's the end of the story, it does not happen that way. Radioactive iodine has an initial "blasting" effect on the gland, which lasts a few months, and an ongoing destructive effect, which begins at the time of treatment and could go on for years—often many years. But what complicates the matter further is that the sensitivity and vulnerability to the radioactive iodine differ from one person to another. This explains why, after treatment with radioactive iodine, the thyroid hormone levels may remain high over the following several months or may plunge to very low levels within a few weeks. Even if you become hypothyroid very quickly after the treatment, the gland may recover, and you can become hyperthyroid again, or you may stay hypothyroid. Research has shown that nearly 15 to 20 percent of people treated with radioactive iodine experience, within the first six months, a temporary hypothyroidism, which lasts several weeks.[27] Under these conditions, if your doctor starts you on high doses of thyroid hormone thinking that you have become permanently hypothyroid, you may easily become hyperthyroid a few weeks later when your gland has recovered some of its function.

This instability of thyroid levels for a few months after the treatment can take a toll on your physical and emotional health. I have even seen a few patients who experienced clear-cut cases of fibromyalgia following the brutal swings of their thyroid levels resulting from their treatment.

While your thyroid gland is being destroyed by radioiodine, you need to receive treatment for as long as is necessary to maintain normal or near-normal thyroid hormone levels. Hyperthyroidism could worsen for a few days after the treatment as a result of stopping the antithyroid medication. One woman who received radioactive iodine treatment said, "It was not explained that I would be more hyper- before becoming hypo-. I woke up in the middle of the night with terrible anxiety. If the doctor had just explained to me what would happen after treatment with radioactive iodine, maybe I would have felt less anxiety and emotion. I would have known why things happened."

Avoid taking high doses of antithyroid medications after radioiodine treatment. A small amount may help bring down thyroid levels while the radioiodine is working, but high amounts can add to the radioiodine's effect and make you plunge rapidly into a severely hypothyroid state. After you receive the radioactive iodine treatment, you need to be retested four weeks later so that your doctor can adjust your medication.

To avoid rapid hypothyroidism and major swings in thyroid levels, discuss with your physician the use of a combination methimazole/thyroxine therapy for the first six months after the radioiodine treatment. I have used this protocol with many patients, and the results are excellent. One week after the radioactive iodine treatment, I prescribe 30 milligrams of methimazole to be taken as a single daily dose. This will bring the levels close to normal. One week after starting the methimazole, I add thyroid hormone replacement at a dose of 0.075 milligrams of thyroxine. The dose of thyroxine may need to be adjusted every two months for the next six months. These adjustments are generally minor. After six months, the methimazole is stopped, and the dose of thyroxine is adjusted according to thyroid tests. The dose of thyroxine is decreased by half if thyroid tests are normal. If the patient is mildly hypothyroid, I continue the same dose of thyroxine. If the patient is slightly hyperthyroid, I have him or her stop taking the thyroid hormone. Two months after the patient has stopped the methimazole and adjusted the dose of thyroxine, the thyroid hormone dose will be adjusted again or stopped to maintain a normal or close-to-normal thyroid function. It is better to have one easily corrected swing of thyroid levels after six months of stability than to have many difficult-to-control swings due to the prominent effects of radioiodine during the first six months after treatment. While following this treatment protocol, my patients have their white blood-cell count and liver function tested each time their thyroid is tested.

Treating Thyroid Imbalances
during Pregnancy

When a woman is pregnant, the demands on the thyroid gland increase significantly. In moderately iodine-deficient areas, the thyroid glands of pregnant women often become enlarged. This has been known since antiquity: ancient Egyptian hieroglyphics depict it clearly. The mother's gland has to provide extra thyroid hormone for herself and perhaps for the developing fetus. In iodine-deficient areas, the frequency of goiter during pregnancy increases because the gland attempts to overcome the deficiency of supplied iodine. But even when the iodine supply is adequate, the size of the thyroid gland may increase during pregnancy.

An underactive thyroid is quite common among women of childbearing age. It is estimated that 2 to 3 percent of pregnant women are hypothyroid when tested during the first trimester.[28] Pregnant women taking thyroid hormone for hypothyroidism often experience a significant increase in their thyroid hormone requirement, and researchers estimate that 80 percent of these women require an increase in the dose. This reflects both the increased need for thyroid hormone and the higher levels of the proteins that carry thyroid hormone in the bloodstream. Without proper thyroid balance, the pregnant hypothyroid woman has a higher chance of miscarrying or giving birth to a baby with congenital malformations.[29] Another possibility is that mental development of the fetus may be hindered, adversely affecting the baby's later intellectual growth.

When a pregnant woman is taking thyroid hormone for an underactive thyroid, she cannot rely on symptoms to signal whether her thyroid is well regulated. For this reason, periodic thyroid testing (every two months) is needed to ensure adequate thyroid levels throughout the pregnancy. Finding out that your levels are off while pregnant does not mean that they cannot be regulated quickly.

If you are pregnant and have an overactive thyroid caused by Graves' disease, you should be treated with antithyroid medications. If you were taking methimazole (Tapazole) before becoming pregnant, your doctor might switch you to propylthiouracil (abbreviated "PTU") because of the possibility of a rare congenital abnormality of the scalp called aplasia cutis.[30] There is considerable doubt about this complication occurring as a result of Tapazole, but many doctors feel it is safer to use PTU during pregnancy. As the pregnancy progresses, the activity of Graves' disease slows down, and the dose of antithyroid medication must be gradually reduced so that thyroid hormone levels remain on the high side throughout the pregnancy. PTU crosses the placenta and can cause hypothyroidism in the fetus if the dose is too high. Toward the end of pregnancy, you may not need to take the medication any longer because the immune attack on the thyroid will have slowed down significantly. But frequent monitoring is the key. I recommend that, if you are pregnant and suffer from an overactive thyroid, you should be tested every month until delivery so that your thyroid levels are maintained at high–normal with the lowest dose of medication.

After delivery, however, the activity of the disease often increases. The medication frequently must be restarted or the dose increased to avoid high thyroid hormone levels after delivery.

Antithyroid medications are excreted in the milk, with PTU apparently present in lower amounts than methimazole. Nevertheless, research has shown that methimazole at a dose of 20 milligrams or less a day is safe for newborns.

Important Points to Remember

- Choose a doctor who is knowledgeable in treating thyroid disorders and who can also deal with your emotions.
- If you are diagnosed as hypothyroid, the dose of thyroid medication that you need to take initially will depend on how high your initial TSH level is.
- Optimize your thyroid hormone treatment by taking your pill before breakfast, and avoid taking it with medication that will affect its absorption.
- If you are treated for an underactive thyroid, once your thyroid tests have become normal, you need to be retested approximately every six months.
- If you have an overactive thyroid, learn about the treatment options and discuss them with your doctor before making the decision. Learn about side effects, too. No treatment is perfect. But choose a doctor who has expertise in treating Graves' disease.
- Work with your doctor to avoid major swings in thyroid hormone levels during treatment. These swings may be a bad experience for you and may cause you to suffer lingering symptoms after the imbalance is corrected.

16

CURING THE LINGERING EFFECTS
OF THYROID IMBALANCE

If you have suffered a thyroid imbalance, your symptoms will typically resolve with adequate treatment. Sometimes, however, even after the physical and mental symptoms of hypothyroidism or hyperthyroidism have disappeared, you may still not feel like your old self. If your imbalance was severe or of long duration, moreover, you may continue to have emotional problems, anxiety, depressive symptoms, and even some residual cognitive deficits. As a result, you may not feel normal even though, technically and medically, you no longer have a thyroid imbalance.

Hyperthyroidism and hypothyroidism shake up your brain. Although you may recover completely if the imbalance is minimal and of short duration, a significant, long-term imbalance could affect your mind for a long time even after you've been properly treated. Thyroid imbalances can affect your brain chemistry in the same way as long-term abuse of alcohol or drugs! Yet your physician may not know about these lingering effects because they have not been widely publicized, discussed, or taught.

In this respect, conventional medicine has been unfair to thyroid patients with persistent symptoms. Because your doctor assesses whether you have been adequately treated for your thyroid condition by measuring blood hormone levels, he or she will look at the lab results and say, "Your thyroid test is normal; your symptoms are not due to your thyroid." Yet you may feel deep inside that your persistent suffering does have something to do with your thyroid. And you would be correct.

Imagine that your water bill has doubled in the past month and you suspect a leak in your house. You call the plumber, who inspects the pipes, sinks, and toilets. Finding no leak, the plumber says, "I can't do anything for you." But the outside pipe that runs from the meter to the house does have a leak. The plumber you called not only didn't see it but may even have believed it wasn't his or her job to deal with it. This situation is analogous to the aftereffects of thyroid disease. Often the symptoms are dismissed by the doctor treating the thyroid condition or the patient is referred to a psychiatrist because of the nature of the symptoms. Even though these symptoms are chronic, they may not fulfill the rigid criteria of mood disorders, so some patients are left further frustrated and misguided.

One of the most widely read endocrinology textbooks states, "Once thyroid hormone therapy is commenced, the recovery from the mental disturbances of hypothyroidism often lags behind the restoration of normal metabolism."[1] Typically, however, doctors fail to mention that the time lag may be quite long. This reality is haunting to the patient, family, and friends and confusing to many physicians.

From Depression to
Lingering Anxiety and Stress

In hypothyroid patients, the most common residual suffering is the persistence of depression that was initially triggered by thyroid hormone deficit.[2] This kind of depression can take on a life of its own, unabated and untouched even after blood levels have returned to normal. A survey conducted in my outpatient clinic tells me that 25 percent of patients whose blood tests have become normal with thyroxine treatment have had persistent symptoms of depression. Many continue to be tired or exhausted and report that they have not returned to their "normal" selves. Hypothyroidism of long duration may also generate a situation similar to post–traumatic stress syndrome, in which the depression triggered directly or indirectly by the patient's thyroid condition affects his or her job or personal life in stressful ways that can become self-perpetuating and even overwhelming.

In some cases, the lingering depression and anxiety may remain unnoticed except for when it emerges every once in a while in response to new stresses. One patient, Rhonda, said, "After I got on a stable dose of thyroid hormone, the depression was better, but as soon as any stressors would enter into the picture, whether finances or trouble at my job, it would come back. As long as I wasn't stressed, and as long as my thyroid level was stable, I was fine."

Many patients with Graves' disease who have suffered from thyroid imbalance for quite some time without treatment become less emotionally tolerant and resilient after their overactive thyroid has been corrected than before the onset of Graves' disease. They may still feel angry and impatient, as well as depressed and anxious. Results of a recent survey published in the *Journal of Neuropsychiatry and Clinical Neurosciences* showed a significant persistent impairment in memory, attention, planning, and productivity in patients with Graves' disease long after their thyroid levels had become normal.[3]

Even two and a half years after their last hyperthyroid episode,[4] patients whose thyroid function had been restored to normal and who were in remission were found to experience anxiety, depression, hypochondriasis, social introversion, and impaired cognitive functions more frequently than normal and more frequently than before they got sick. With maintenance of normal thyroid function, however, these residual effects may eventually subside over time.

Why these symptoms persist is not clear. It is possible that hyperthyroidism, being a form of severe mental stress, can cause residual abnormalities in brain function, as has been shown in concentration camp survivors.[5]

Tiffany, who suffered from Graves' disease for two years prior to being diagnosed, had had stable thyroid tests for at least one year since receiving adequate thyroid hormone treatment. In a follow-up visit, she complained that she was no longer the same as she had been before her illness and was trying to find a reason for the way she was feeling:

> I got in the habit of being that way but not as bad as when I was hyperthyroid. I am more tolerant now, but I still have waves of anger. I feel like I live alone. It is quite possible that I am depressed.
>
> I have two nephews, and if I see them once a month, that's okay, and they only live six miles away from me. I never have been a big eater, but now I crave food, especially in the afternoon when I feel tense and tired. I'm generally a giving person, and now it's like I am not going to give anyone anything. Graves' disease has changed me.

Tiffany's stamina and energy levels are no longer the same as before her illness. Her case and others like hers raise many questions: Is she feeling different and low because she is missing a little T3 that her thyroid gland would normally have produced now that she is relying on T4 pills to maintain normal blood levels? Is a persistent chemical imbalance affecting her tolerance level, mood, and anger? If so, was this a residual, subtle chemical imbalance due to the flooding of brain cells by thyroid hormone when she was hyperthyroid? Or did the overwhelming effect of stress from the hyperthyroidism leave her with some form of post–traumatic stress syndrome?

Whatever the exact cause of the depression and emotional instability that continue to haunt you, you will benefit from engaging in mind-body techniques such as relaxation, yoga, and exercise at least three times a week. (Some people may require daily sessions; for more on mind-body techniques, see Chapter 18.) By doing so, you will help yourself get over these changes, and you will help the tiredness, low coping ability, and concentration and memory impairments to subside. Tiffany's experience was typical. After a few months of relaxation sessions and regular exercise, her temper and tolerance level improved dramatically while her thyroid levels stayed normal.

If your symptoms are severe, you are likely to be helped by antidepressants, such as selective serotonin reuptake inhibitors (SSRIs). In the next chapter, you will learn how combining T4 and T3 may be the solution for your lingering symptoms. (See Chapter 17.)

Using Mind-Body Techniques to Avoid Lingering Effects

Techniques such as music therapy, dance or movement therapy, yoga, or tai chi enhance the strength of your mind and its ability to master your body's functioning. These practices will have a tremendous positive effect on your body image and self-esteem as well. They will also help your depression and may even help you with your communication skills. Choose the technique best suited to your lifestyle. For instance, because of time constraints, you may wish to combine an aerobic exercise program with music therapy. Tai chi combines an aerobic type of exercise and relaxation and has done wonders for many of my patients. If you suffer from lingering anxiety and panic attacks, meditation and biofeedback might be the solution. During biofeedback, sensors are applied to some areas of your body and connected to a device that detects and monitors body functions that are considered to be involuntary but that you can learn to control through practice. Biofeedback is also popular for treating symptoms of depression and anxiety. But even if you choose biofeedback or meditation, do not forget your aerobic exercise.

For some people with other health problems that prevent them from exercising, guided imagery and art therapy can be helpful. In guided imagery, you focus on images or sensations that help you relax. Many practitioners believe that it can also enhance the strength of the immune system. It certainly helps relieve anxiety.

Self-help groups are an important mind-body resource that helps persistent sufferers cope better with their symptoms and speed up their recovery. Meeting as a group, expressing personal thoughts, and exchanging experiences with others have helped many people suffering from conditions ranging from obesity to alcoholism in which the mind, attitude, and behavior play an important role in the recovery process. These groups help you feel and see that you are not alone. Through my involvement as the medical director of the American Foundation of Thyroid Patients, I have repeatedly seen the beneficial effects of group sessions in which thyroid patients meet and discuss their symptoms and problems. You may also want to start practicing a mind-body technique with other patients from the group. To find out about local patient support groups, call one of the main thyroid patient organizations (see the "Resources" list at the end of the book).

Counseling and Psychotherapy

Many thyroid patients need counseling. Counseling and psychotherapy are an important part of mind-body programs. Sessions can be designed to help you overcome your lingering suffering once thyroid tests have become normal. Counseling may also help you resolve many of the personal and relationship issues generated by the thyroid imbalance. The inability to function as before and the relationship problems generate a feeling of loss similar to grief. You may feel that you have lost control of your life and are unable to regain the happiness that you enjoyed before the thyroid disorder. Counseling will help you come to terms with your loss and feel hopeful and optimistic about your life and your future.

Yet many doctors do not counsel their patients. Even in a primary care setting, only a third of patients suffering from depression who need counseling receive a maximum of "three minutes of counseling." Lack of counseling is even worse in prepaid health care plans.[6] Many patients have already gone through a great deal of stress by the time they're diagnosed, and many will continue to deal with personal or job-related problems generated by the imbalance. These psychological issues need to be addressed, and a therapist can help you deal with them.

Supportive psychotherapy is needed most by patients with lingering symptoms of depression and anxiety. There are other practical methods of psychotherapy that can help. In behavioral psychotherapy, the therapist may focus on identifying what in your life is likely to trigger your symptoms. The aim is to help you understand and change the way you react to situations. In cognitive therapy, the therapist looks for patterns of thinking that are likely to cause symptoms. These methods do not address your unconscious conflicts, but they are aimed at correcting your symptoms. The therapy will help you to regain your emotional balance, cope better with the stress, and strengthen your defense mechanisms so that you regain control. Behavioral/cognitive psychotherapy has been shown to be as effective as medication in the treatment of mild depression and anxiety disorder.[7]

You may also need marital or couples therapy. Ask for a referral from your primary care physician or endocrinologist, who will probably know of a few competent therapists who have developed a great deal of experience dealing with marital issues. The couples therapist may be a psychiatrist, a psychologist, or a psychiatric social worker. Get two or three recommendations and meet with the therapists to discuss their training, experience, and degrees before deciding on one and beginning the sessions.

Finally, psychodynamic psychotherapy, which focuses on addressing unconscious conflicts and resolving the root of psychological conflicts, may be necessary for patients whose thyroid imbalance unmasks deep-rooted psychological issues or who have psychological issues independent of the thyroid imbalance. Psychodynamic psychotherapy can be an expensive and protracted type of treatment, but it is the only way to address deeply rooted psychological problems.

Selecting the Right Antidepressant

If your emotional symptoms become overwhelming and you have not been able to break the vicious cycle of depression and stress, you may benefit from taking an antidepressant, which will also help your anxiety symptoms.

When you use an antidepressant, you need to educate yourself about its most common side effects and how often they occur. You also need to know that it takes time for an antidepressant to begin working. Many need at least six to eight weeks to elevate mood. Often, even after eight weeks, increasing the dose can make a big difference. The accompanying table lists the most commonly prescribed antidepressants.

COMMONLY USED ANTIDEPRESSANTS AND THEIR SIDE EFFECTS

Drug	Trade Name	Common Side Effects
SELECTIVE SEROTONIN REUPTAKE INHIBITORS (SSRIS)		
Fluoxetine	Prozac®	Nausea, headaches, nervousness,
Sertraline	Zoloft®	insomnia, fatigue, and sexual
Paroxetine	Paxil®	problems
Fluvoxamine	Luvox®	
Citalopram	Celexa®	
TRICYCLIC ANTIDEPRESSANTS		
Amitriptyline	Elavil®	Urinary retention, constipation, dry mouth, blurry vision, weight
Nortriptyline	Pamelor®	gain, sexual dysfunction, and sun sensitivity; dizziness when
Imipramine	Tofranil®	standing up or sitting down; sedation, heart rhythm problems

Drug	Trade Name	Common Side Effects
TRICYCLIC ANTIDEPRESSANTS		
Desipramine	Norpramine®	
Doxepin	Sinequan®	
ATYPICAL ANTIDEPRESSANTS		
Mirtazapine	Remeron®	Sedation, weight gain, dizziness, dry mouth, constipation
Venlafaxine	Effexor®	Increase in diastolic blood pressure and SSRI side effects
Bupropion	Wellbutrin®	Agitation, anxiety, insomnia, headache, seizures (rarely)
Trazodone	Desyrel®	Sedation, nausea
Nefazodone	Serzone®	Sedation, nervousness, sleep disturbance
MAO (MONOAMINE OXIDASE) INHIBITORS		
Phenelzine	Nardil®	Sleep problems, high blood pressure, sexual problems, weight gain, and—most dangerous—life-threatening interactions with other drugs and some foods
Tranylcypromine	Parnate®	
Selegiline	Eldepryl®	

The efficacy of all the antidepressant medications is similar. Doctors choose an antidepressant based on their experiences with the medication and also take into consideration its potential adverse effects. The SSRIs have become the first choice for many forms of depression because their potential side effects are less common and less serious than those of the other types of antidepressants. Although there are some differences among the various SSRIs, these differences tend to be minimal.

The most commonly used SSRIs include fluoxetine (Prozac), sertraline (Zoloft), and paroxetine (Paxil). These medications not only treat depression but can also be effective in obsessive-compulsive disorders. Zoloft is quite effective if you continue to suffer from panic attacks. Generally speaking, the two most common side effects, which often subside within two weeks, are nausea and headaches. Nausea can be avoided by taking the medication with food. Other adverse effects are insomnia, jitteriness, fatigue, sexual dysfunction, sedation, and agitation. Sertraline tends to cause diarrhea more frequently than the other medications. These side effects also often subside with time.

Do not take a monoamine oxidase inhibitor in combination with one of these medications. Taking the two together may cause "serotonin syndrome," characterized by agitation, diarrhea, involuntary muscle movements, trembling, high temperature, high blood pressure, and even seizures. Taking L-tryptophan or a tryptophan substitute in conjunction with an SSRI may lead to the same complication.

Scientific studies have not yet compared the efficacy of the various antidepressants after blood levels of thyroid hormones have been normalized with treatment. However, I typically use an SSRI first because side effects are less common with this clan of antidepressants.

In case the SSRIs do not work or you have had an adverse reaction to them, the next course of action would be a tricyclic antidepressant such as amitriptyline or nortriptyline or an atypical antidepressant. Tricyclics are effective in treating depression and controlling panic attacks. If you are suffering from agitation and loss of appetite, doxepin will help. If you are sleeping too much, desipramine will have a stimulating effect. The most common side effects of tricyclics are weight gain, sedation, dry mouth, sexual problems, constipation, sensitivity to the sun, urinary retention, blurry vision, rapid heartbeat and heartbeat problems, and dizziness when you stand up or sit down.

Nowadays tricyclic antidepressants have largely fallen by the wayside because they may cause so many side effects. Nevertheless, if your depression has not responded to an SSRI, taking a tricyclic may be the solution. I have found that tricyclic antidepressants are most useful for the patient who has problems sleeping at night (often a patient with Graves' disease) and lingering depression with significant anxiety symptoms.

The atypical antidepressants are a growing group of drugs that affect different combinations of neurotransmitters. In general, doctors turn to them if SSRIs are not effective. I have found no use for mirtazapine in thyroid patients. It has potent appetite-promoting effects and often causes weight gain. Other side effects of mirtazapine are sedation, dizziness, dry mouth, and constipation. Trazodone and nefazodone, however, are useful if the patient is suffering from insomnia. Typically, the insomnia can be effectively treated with doses smaller than the dose that would be needed to treat depression. A small dose of one of these two medications makes an SSRI work better. Bupropion has recently received much media attention for its usefulness in helping people to stop smoking. This antidepressant has an energizing effect on most patients. Its side effects are agitation, anxiety, insomnia, headaches, and, rarely, seizures. Venlafaxine is often thought of as a "souped-up" SSRI. It is a new selective reuptake inhibitor of both serotonin and noradrenaline. It seems to cause fewer side effects and may work if one of the SSRIs has failed to give you the response expected. It might also work faster than the other antidepressants. Some of the side effects that you need to be aware of are an increase in diastolic blood pressure, headaches, nausea, and nervousness.

Doctors now generally view MAO (monoamine oxidase) inhibitors as the last drugs to be considered for treating depression, although they can be helpful in atypical depression. Even though MAO inhibitors are quite potent at alleviating depression, they are troublesome to work with, sometimes causing side effects such as sleep problems, high blood pressure, sexual problems, and weight gain. If you are taking an MAO inhibitor, you need to watch your diet and avoid eating many common foods, such as cheese and chocolate, that contain the chemical tyramine. The combination can trigger severe high blood pressure and other serious health problems. MAO inhibitors can also cause these problems when taken with certain medications.

Lithium carbonate is a potent antidepressant used more commonly in bipolar disorders, especially manic-depression. With patients who do not respond to an SSRI or a tricyclic, some doctors add lithium to enhance the efficacy of the antidepressant. Studies have shown that adding T3 instead of lithium is as effective. For full effect, the dose of lithium must often be increased to 900 to 1,500 milligrams per day. Doctors need to check your blood levels, however, to avoid lithium's toxic effects, including thyroid problems, diabetes insipidus (which causes increased urination), high calcium levels, and kidney problems.

The most commonly used antianxiety medications are Valium, Librium, Xanax, and Ativan (all of which are benzodiazepines) and Buspar (a non-benzodiazepine). Their adverse effects are sedation, confusion (only rarely), and lack of coordination. Avoid taking benzodiazepines for a long time because you are likely to become addicted. This is one of the main problems people encounter when taking a prolonged course of benzodiazepines.

In general, once you are started on an antidepressant, the treatment is continued for at least six months and, if necessary, extended for up to one to two years. Depression can come back even if you are taking an antidepressant medication, including all of the ones I've discussed here. If you have an underactive thyroid and are taking thyroid hormone, using a combination of T4 and T3 rather than T4 alone will help prevent the depression from returning (for details on T4/T3 combination treatment, refer to Chapter 17). Using this combination protocol will help you control the depression better while taking lower doses of conventional antidepressants, which will reduce your likelihood of experiencing side effects from them.

The Persistent Cognitive
Effects of Thyroid Imbalance

"I feel as if my brain aged by ten years," Cheryl told me during her first visit to my office. Cheryl, aged forty-seven, suffered an overactive thyroid that was undiagnosed for almost two years. After receiving radioactive iodine treatment, she became hypothyroid and was prescribed an adequate amount of thyroxine by her former endocrinologist. Although she maintained normal blood test results, she had continued to struggle with some impairment of her intellectual and cognitive abilities.

"My most significant problem," she went on to say, "is that I am unable to concentrate, even on trivial matters. It seems like I cannot process information and act on it as I used to. I forget words, or they elude me in a conversation. I would go into a room and not remember why I went in there. It would take me a few minutes, then I would sometimes remember."

A severe thyroid imbalance may cause a significant impairment in cognitive function, particularly memory and the ability to concentrate and to register and process incoming information. After the thyroid imbalance is corrected, these impairments often subside and treatment halts their progression. Some patients who experience a thyroid imbalance, however, continue to have a deficit in cognitive function after the thyroid condition is treated and corrected. The impairment of these functions may be more profound when the patient is afflicted at a young age.

In some patients, the cognitive deficit associated with prolonged and severe hypothyroidism may be more permanent with regard to memory and temporary with regard to general intelligence and concentration. Treatment also typically stops the progression of memory impairment, but if the thyroid hormone deficit remains untreated, cognitive impairment may worsen with time. Research has suggested that hypothyroidism could cause a direct and perhaps irreversible effect on brain structures, causing the memory impairment,[8] while other brain functions that rely on adequate amounts of neurotransmitters may be restored to normal.

Occasionally, patients previously treated for an overactive thyroid experience significant residual intellectual difficulty that impairs their ability to work. Dr. Hans Perrild, studying neuropsychological function in patients with a previous history of hyperthyroidism, found among his patients four who were granted disability because of a significant reduction in their ability to perform any work.[9] This suggests that people who are afflicted with hyperthyroidism that has lingered for some time may not be the same even ten years after correction of the imbalance.

Impairment in cognitive abilities due to hypothyroidism may range from minimal (detected only by standardized neuropsychological testing) to quite significant (noticeable to the person and close family or friends). In extreme cases, when brain structures are significantly affected by the thyroid hormone deficit, the impairment can even progress to dementia, particularly in older people.

How Thyroid Imbalance Causes Damage
to the Brain: The Link with Aging

In a sense, Cheryl was correct to compare her suffering with an accelerated aging of her brain. As you get older, you become apt to suffer impaired cognition. You may have difficulty remembering names, keeping several things in mind at the same time, and processing information. You may have difficulty finding words, or you may slowly lose the ability to grasp details of what is going on around you.

Why do many people like Cheryl, after a severe thyroid imbalance, experience a deterioration of their cognitive abilities similar to what older people might experience over an extended period of time? Can untreated hypothyroidism lead to irreversible dementia? And does normal aging worsen the deterioration of your cognitive abilities if you experienced a long and significant thyroid imbalance? Recent advances in medical research in this field are revealing the answers to these questions. Research is also suggesting what we should do to improve intellectual faculties and prevent further age-related deterioration of the brain.

Thyroid imbalance of some duration can damage the brain in the same way aging does. With increasing age, the brain becomes more subjected to the adverse effects of free radicals, the toxic oxygenated compounds released during metabolism. These radicals gradually damage major components of the brain, including myelin, a protective layer (composed of protein and fat) that surrounds some types of nerve fibers and increases the efficiency of nerve transmission. Myelin in the brain is sensitive to the damaging effects of free radicals and becomes damaged by the buildup of free radicals.[10] Once myelin has been damaged by free radicals, it becomes less stable and more vulnerable to further damage as we get older. Scientists now know that damage to myelin is one of the most important factors that accelerate the aging of the human brain.

Thyroid imbalance can increase your risk of impaired cognition as you become older because it has the same ability as aging to damage areas of the brain that are essential for normal cognition.[11] When your thyroid gland is overactive, oxygen consumption increases, and the number of free radicals overwhelms the cells' ability to clear them from the body.[12] With aging, the machinery in cells that is designed to clear these "bad guys" becomes less efficient. In essence, the "oxidative stress" resulting from too much thyroid hormone causes similar damage to our brain as aging. Long-standing hypothyroidism also has a damaging effect on many brain structures simply because thyroid hormone is essential for maintaining healthy brain cells. In fact, the development of these brain structures in the critical period of rapid growth during the fetal stage and immediately following birth also depends on normal thyroid levels.[13] During this time, thyroid hormone is essential for adequate formation of myelin. This explains why infants with congenital hypothyroidism suffer severe neurological problems and mental impairment.

How to Prevent and Cure
Residual Cognitive Impairment

When Cheryl came to me with impaired cognition after a significant thyroid imbalance, she was more frightened than most such patients. Her mother and maternal aunt had just been diagnosed with Alzheimer's disease. She had learned that Alzheimer's disease runs in families and that she could become a victim of this condition in the future. But the health program that Cheryl now follows—which includes a well-balanced diet, antioxidant supplementation, hormone treatment, and control of her blood pressure—not only helped her recover from some of the cognitive deficits she endured but also will slow down the anticipated deterioration brought on by aging. Furthermore, it will prevent Alzheimer's disease or slow it down if she were to become afflicted by it.

All of us should practice preventive measures to preserve a healthy, functioning brain and try to prevent the decline in cognitive abilities that occurs with aging. But if you have experienced a significant imbalance that left some residual deficits, you need to be more vigilant.

If you are predisposed to Alzheimer's disease or have a medical condition that could cause damage to your brain, a prolonged deprivation of thyroid hormone may accelerate dementia. Even if the damage caused by hypothyroidism is not quite severe, it may represent a setback. It will make you more vulnerable to developing dementia later in life. Long-standing depression and stress also cause deterioration of cognition.

Several measures are now recognized to help prevent further deterioration of brain function. The first step is to pay more attention to the many lifestyle factors that can affect your brain function. Supplementing your diet with adequate amounts of antioxidants is one of the most important measures. Vitamin C, zinc, vitamin E, and glutamate could prevent the damage and loss of brain cells due to the buildup of free radicals. (See Chapter 18 for more on antioxidants.)

You also need to reduce your risk of cerebrovascular disease and strokes, which are known to accelerate the dementia process. Atherosclerosis, or hardening of the arteries, typically increases with age. When this process affects the arteries in the brain, it can lead to poor blood supply, strokes, and ultimately loss of brain cells. Hardening of the arteries of the brain is a major factor in impairment of cognition and even dementia in older persons.[14] Researchers have found that more than 50 percent of patients older than eighty-five had hardening of the arteries in the brain. It is likely that many people with dementia, including those with Alzheimer's disease, have atherosclerosis as a contributing factor to their dementia.

If you have experienced a severe thyroid imbalance, you should control the vascular risks that could predispose you to hardening of the arteries and poor blood supply to the brain. To achieve this, you need to exercise and take antioxidant multivitamin supplements containing folate and vitamins B_6 and B_{12}. Controlling your blood pressure is essential. High blood pressure can damage blood vessels of the brain, heart, and kidneys. The longer your blood pressure stays high, the more damage it can cause. One study showed that patients already suffering from vascular dementia who received a treatment that lowered their systolic blood pressure to the 135–150 mm Hg range experienced either an improvement in their cognitive deficit or a delay in the worsening of their dementia.[15] Research has recently linked cardiovascular risk to accumulation of homocysteine, an amino acid.[16] The B-complex vitamins just mentioned will help reduce the accumulation of homocysteine and lower your risk of having low brain blood flow.

You also need to lower your cholesterol and triglycerides by diet and medication if necessary. High cholesterol is an important risk factor for cardiovascular disease in both men and women. For example, in women a cholesterol level of more than 265 milligrams per deciliter doubles the risk of cardiovascular problems compared to that of women whose cholesterol level is less than 205 milligrams per deciliter. Raise your HDL cholesterol to more than 60 milligrams per deciliter by eating less fat and less cholesterol and by exercising. Lower your triglycerides by eating less sugar. Avoid alcohol if you have high triglyceride levels. Your triglyceride level should be less than 190 milligrams per deciliter. Do not lower your cholesterol too much, however. Very low cholesterol can reduce brain serotonin, thereby causing depression and aggressive behavior. It can damage brain cells and cause impaired cognition as well. Try to keep your total cholesterol less than 200 milligrams per deciliter for the vascular benefit and higher than 150 milligrams per deciliter to avoid low mood and impaired cognition.

Several common health problems can act alone or in concert with others to precipitate or contribute to the development of cardiovascular disease (see the following list). Long-standing untreated hypothyroidism is one of these factors. Hypothyroidism can raise blood pressure, increase LDL cholesterol and even triglycerides, and lead to excess weight and thus a sedentary lifestyle. Even low-grade hypothyroidism has recently been shown to elevate LDL cholesterol. In Great Britain in the early 1970s, research already showed that people with Hashimoto's thyroiditis had a higher rate of cardio-vascular disease even after exclusion of other risk factors, such as weight, high blood pressure, and high cholesterol.[17] Because of the high frequency of low-grade hypothyroidism in menopausal women, and its effects on cho-lesterol, it is likely that long-standing low-grade hypothyroidism contributes to the occurrence of coronary artery disease among these women.

RISK FACTORS FOR CARDIOVASCULAR DISEASE
- High blood pressure
- High blood levels of cholesterol and triglycerides
- Smoking
- Diabetes
- Long-standing hypothyroidism
- Excess weight
- History of heart disease in other family members
- Sedentary lifestyle
- High insulin (syndrome X)
- Menopause

For people who suffer from a thyroid imbalance and possible damages from its consequences, it is essential to pay serious attention to the other additive risk factors.

High insulin levels can result from eating too much refined sugar and from developing insulin resistance. This occurs in people who are capable of producing insulin but whose organs do not respond well to insulin, causing the hormone to work less efficiently. High insulin levels increase the vascular risk. They also promote the retention of salt in the body and cause nar-rowing of the arteries in organs. Because insulin does not work efficiently, patients with "syndrome X" have a tendency to develop diabetes; they also have hypertension and high fat levels in their bloodstream. The key here is to lose weight and to lower sugar intake. A healthy, well-balanced diet is low in animal fat, dairy fat, and refined sugar. Avoid too much butter, whole milk, and eggs. Always include fish, fresh vegetables and fruits, legumes, whole grains, and beans in your diet. Vegetable oils such as olive, sunflower, and safflower are preferable to coconut or palm oil.

The Mental Benefits of Estrogens

If you are a perimenopausal or postmenopausal woman, you might have had some difficulty deciding whether estrogen therapy is the right choice for you. You might have been informed that taking estrogen lowers your cardiovascular risk and helps prevent bone loss and osteoporosis, but the emerging research showing that estrogen increases your risk for breast cancer also might frighten you.

I believe that the breast cancer risk has been overpublicized. The problems come from misinterpretation of the "relative risk," which is an expression of risk applied to a large population, versus the "absolute risk," which would apply to one particular person. The relative risk of breast cancer from estrogen therapy is certainly of some significance. When it comes right down to it, however, the "absolute risk" for getting breast cancer as a result of estrogen treatment, although real, is minimal.

Both mortality and cardiovascular disease are lowered by estrogen therapy. Not as widely publicized, however, are estrogen's beneficial effects on cognitive abilities. Scientific evidence for the use of estrogen not only to prevent impaired cognition but also to prevent and treat dementia is expanding. Research has shown that, in rats whose ovaries have been surgically removed, estrogen improves learning performance.[18] The beneficial effect of estrogen is so striking that women prone to Alzheimer's disease who do not take estrogen are likely to lose cognition more rapidly than women who take estrogen. I therefore encourage women who have experienced hypothyroidism to take estrogen when they become menopausal. If they don't, lack of estrogen will compound the residual impairment generated by an imbalance even if the latter occurred earlier in life.

The loss of estrogens that occurs at menopause could be an important factor in the occurrence of brain damage due to Alzheimer's disease. One study showed that estrogen therapy in postmenopausal women postpones the occurrence of Alzheimer's disease.[19] Estrogens interact with brain cells that are the most damaged in patients with Alzheimer's disease. Estrogens stimulate brain cells to produce more of the neurotransmitter acetylcholine, which plays an important role in memory and cognition. The hormone helps keep acetylcholine-containing cells intact and healthy and also helps blood flow in the brain.

Lack of estrogen after menopause is perhaps one of the reasons why dementia affects two to three times more women than men. Estrogen replacement improves several cognitive abilities of postmenopausal women not suffering from dementia—in particular, skills pertaining to verbal memory.[20] The duration of therapy as well as the dose determine the preventive effects. A 1.25 milligram dose of Premarin is more effective than a 0.625 milligram dose.

Estrogen improves not only cognitive abilities but also mood and overall well-being. Estrogen treatment in postmenopausal women has a tempering effect on stress. A woman who takes estrogen produces less cortisol in response to stress and is therefore subjected to fewer of the deleterious effects of cortisol on brain cells and memory.[21] Estrogens probably protect brain cells from the damaging effects of high cortisol levels resulting from stress.

In young postmenopausal women, estrogen improves well-being and reduces anxiety and depression. It does so by increasing serotonin levels. Women who suffer from even minute thyroid hormone deficits in brain cells risk a worsening of depression by not taking estrogen. By increasing serotonin in the brain, estrogens help relieve residual depression from hypothyroidism in postmenopausal women. Thyroid hormone treatment by itself may not resolve the depression. Only when estrogens are added is the depression improved.

Premarin contains several forms of estrogen that are of greater benefit to the brain than the pure estradiol found in the estrogen patches. For this reason, Premarin remains my favorite estrogen prescription for thyroid patients entering menopause. For older men suffering from low testosterone levels, testosterone patches (i.e., androderm or Testoderm) represent an important adjunct.

The lingering effects of thyroid imbalance in postmenopausal women may not go away unless doctors implement a well-balanced sex hormone regimen. In some women, adding a small amount of testosterone helps to improve both cognition and mood.[22]

While taking estrogen, avoid eating more than three servings of tofu or other soy foods per week. Soy contains vegetable estrogens, or "phytoestrogens," a class of estrogens deriving from plants that have either estrogen-promoting or estrogen-weakening properties. Phytoestrogens can interfere with the beneficial effects of estrogen on your mood and cognition when consumed more than three times a week.[23]

Not every woman can take estrogen replacement. Estrogen can cause adverse effects, including blood clots in the veins, water retention, high blood pressure, and cancer of the uterus.

If you have had a hysterectomy and want to take estrogen, it should be taken alone without progesterone. If you have an intact uterus, however, taking estrogen alone can increase your risk of uterine cancer. The reason is that estrogen causes a thickening and proliferation of the internal lining of the uterus (endometrium), which over time can cause a predisposition to cancer. This thickening and proliferation can be viewed as a build-up of the endometrium. It is prevented by taking progesterone, which causes shedding of the buildup. For this reason, you will be prescribed progesterone either in a cyclic fashion, such as Provera ten days each month, or in conjunction with Premarin continuously.

The drawback of progesterone treatment, however, is its interference with your brain chemistry.[24] Progesterone lowers serotonin in the brain, resulting in more symptoms of depression. Women taking estrogens and progesterone may have more symptoms of depression than women taking estrogens alone. Also, the higher the dose of progesterone, the greater the likelihood that women will experience depressed mood. On the other hand, progesterone helps relieve hot flashes.

The hormonal regimen I recommend to my thyroid patients depends on the severity of the hot flashes, whether low mood is a problem, and whether they become emotional, anxious, and fatigued when they take progesterone. Those who experience mood effects do better taking the progesterone at 2.5 milligrams a day for seven days every two to three months. This is enough to prevent uterine buildup and reduce the risk of uterine cancer. If the hot flashes are disturbing but the low mood is less of an issue, it may be more appropriate to take 5 milligrams of progesterone a day for seven to ten days a month.

The Circle of Wellness

The "Circle of Wellness" that I provide to my patients is a model that anyone can use to minimize cognitive deterioration with aging (see the accompanying illustration). Patients suffering from thyroid imbalance should recognize the importance of early diagnosis to minimize any permanent residual damage to cognition. They should also make sure their thyroid remains in balance throughout their lives. Even that may not be enough. If a significant blow to the brain has occurred as a result of the imbalance, people should do everything they can to minimize other deleterious effects on the brain.

CIRCLE OF WELLNESS FOR THYROID PATIENTS

START:
Get diagnosed early.

Take estrogen
replacement therapy
to:
• Improve cognition
• Prevent dementia
• Improve mood

Avoid too much or too
little iodine, which
causes changes in
thyroid function.

Take antioxidants to:
• Help thyroid
  hormone work
  efficiently
• Protect yourself
  from age-related
  brain damage
• Protect your
  thyroid from
  autoimmune
  reactions and
  damage

Control blood
pressure: high
blood pressure
causes vascular
disease and
accelerates
cognitive
impairment.

Correct the imbalance promptly:
avoid a treatment roller coaster.

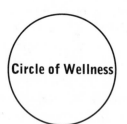

Circle of Wellness

Control
cholesterol levels:
• High cholesterol
  causes vascular
  disease.
• Too-low
  cholesterol impairs
  cognition and
  causes depression,
  suicide, and
  violence.

Maintain thyroid balance:
TSH = 0.5–2
milli–international units per liter

Avoid lingering
depression and stress
through:
• Stress management
• T4/T3 protocol
• Course of antidepressant
  if needed
• Counseling and psychotherapy

Get support and
understanding:
• From family
• From friends
• At work

Control weight
through:
• Mindful exercise
• Low-fat/high-protein,
  serotonin-enhancing diet
  (low in refined
  sugars, high in
  complex
  carbohydrates)

What some of my patients like Cheryl now know is that they need to take steps to preserve healthy brain structures as much as possible for the years to come. By failing to do so, they will place themselves at a much higher risk for further deterioration of their cognitive ability and possibly even dementia.

It is crucial for people afflicted with a thyroid condition to understand that the more a thyroid imbalance alters brain function, the greater their chances of having some residual effects, such as not feeling as well as before. Fight these residual effects using mind-body medicine that can help you alleviate some of the emotional effects.

Important Points to Remember

- If you've been successfully treated for a thyroid imbalance but have continued to be emotional, moody, tired, or exhausted, or have continued to have achy feelings throughout your body or other symptoms of an underactive thyroid, you are not alone! It is just the aftermath of the effects of the imbalance on your brain chemistry. Some of your symptoms can be explained by a deficit of T3 (the most active form of thyroid hormone) not provided by the synthetic T4 pill used for the treatment of hypothyroidism.
- To fight these symptoms, use mind-body techniques and aerobic exercise, maintain thyroid balance, and if necessary, use T4/T3 combination treatment and an antidepressant.
- The damaging effects of a severe thyroid imbalance on your brain may lead to impaired cognition and memory problems that resemble the effects of aging. You need to pay attention to your lifestyle, take antioxidants, lower your cholesterol, control your blood pressure, and avoid refined sugars.
- Pay attention to sex hormones if you are postmenopausal. Take estrogens, preferably Premarin, and consider small amounts of androgens to improve your mood and cognition. You need progesterone if you have a uterus.
- If you have a familial predisposition to Alzheimer's disease, you need to be more vigilant. Remember, estrogens slow the deterioration of cognition due to Alzheimer's disease.

17

THE NEW T4/T3 PROTOCOL:

"It Made Me Feel Better All Over"

A few years ago, I was invited to a Christmas party at the home of a friend. Although I had known Alan for several years, I had never met his wife, Jennifer. When I arrived at the party, I noticed immediately that Jennifer had bulgy eyes, a symptom of the overactive thyroid condition Graves' disease. Not only did her eyes protrude, but she also appeared depressed and withdrawn. She didn't mingle easily and often snapped at her husband throughout the evening, clearly quite unhappy that she had to be at this party.

Later, I learned from Alan that Jennifer had been diagnosed with Graves' disease two years earlier. What actually drove her to seek a doctor's help were her anger, extreme anxiety, and wild mood swings, which were taking a toll on their marriage.

Alan also explained that her emotional problems hadn't completely disappeared after her thyroid condition was treated. In fact, she never went back to "being herself." As a result of the treatment of her overactive thyroid, Jennifer had become hypothyroid and was receiving thyroid hormone treatment in the form of synthetic thyroxine (T4). Several physicians told her that her thyroid hormone levels were normal and there was nothing more they could do for her. One even suggested that she go see a counselor. Jennifer did take a course of an antidepressant but stopped the medication after three months when she realized that it had produced no significant improvement in the way she felt.

Later, when I took over Jennifer's care, she gradually returned to normal through an innovative treatment program that corrected the brain chemistry imbalance resulting from her thyroid condition. The program included the practice of a relaxation technique, but more important, it involved a dramatic change in the nature of her thyroid hormone treatment, from the use of a T4-only drug to a protocol I've devised that combines synthetic T4 (levothyroxine) and T3, the most potent and biologically active form of thyroid hormone. I believe that this protocol holds tremendous promise for a large number of people who, for whatever reason, are suffering from an underactive thyroid and need thyroid hormone treatment. I regard this new T4/T3 treatment as a state-of-the-art treatment for hypothyroidism and a viable alternative to the most widely accepted current medical approach, which has been to prescribe T4, a portion of which is then converted to T3 by bodily organs, including the brain.[1]

"I think that there are a lot of women like me," Jennifer told me, "who have to deal with the problems I faced every day without ever realizing that an effective treatment exists. And that's too bad, because thyroid conditions can totally alter not only your personality but your physical appearance, and lord knows that's a tough burden to bear in today's society."

Lifting the Cloud

It was quite obvious from the symptoms Jennifer described that, while suffering from a glandular disorder, she had gone through an unpleasant journey of disturbed mood and emotions that were never validated for her. Jennifer told me recently:

> Before I started on the new T4/T3 treatment, I was constantly wondering, Is this what it's going to be like for the rest of my life?
>
> Since then, the cloud has lifted. I'm once again able to process things in my mind normally and quickly. I have had, I would say, a 95 percent improvement in my symptoms. The tingling in my hands and feet is not as bad. I retain water less than before. I have more energy. I've gone back to work. I'm more outgoing and have a brighter outlook. I'm finally reclaiming myself. I really feel good, and I have hope!

When I began my career in the field of thyroid disease, my goal in treating patients with an underactive thyroid was to help them reach and maintain normal blood levels of thyroid hormones and TSH, the pituitary hormone that regulates thyroid gland function. I still remember those days when I faced countless patients who had achieved this goal but who nevertheless continued to complain of tiredness, dry skin, an inability to function, and other symptoms. I would vehemently reply to their complaints, "These problems are not from your thyroid." Although I was puzzled by these persistent symptoms, I felt in a way that I had accomplished my job. More often than not, when I searched for coexistent conditions, my efforts were in vain. My frustration continued to build, and I felt ineffective at providing the answers and cures that many of my hypothyroid patients were expecting of me.

In those early days, doctors began to be concerned about bone loss and osteoporosis in people being treated with too much thyroid hormone. Early treatments used desiccated animal thyroid. It is natural and provides both thyroid hormones (T4 and T3) but not in a composition close enough to the human chemicals to achieve stable levels.[2] The result was often daily surges of blood levels of T3 out of proportion to the normal pattern of human blood levels. Such patients were also at risk for significant bone loss. As many physicians did at the time, I switched to the newest treatment for hypothyroidism whenever possible: I took these patients off the desiccated thyroid and put them on synthetic T4.

Surprisingly to me, this was seldom entirely successful. Once switched from these natural T4/T3 tablets to T4 tablets, patients complained of sluggishness, decreased memory, impaired concentration, and a host of symptoms of ill-being. This was in spite of having reached normal blood levels of thyroid hormone and TSH. In fact, seldom was I able to convince a patient to remain on levothyroxine: they all wanted to go back on the old pill.

Because of these observations, I quickly came to realize that there must be a role for some form of T4/T3 combination therapy in many patients with underactive thyroid. Isn't this the reason why many doctors continue to prescribe desiccated thyroid to their hypothyroid patients? Isn't this the reason why synthetic combinations of T4 and T3 such as Liotrix have been manufactured for years? These combinations, however, have seldom been used since the 1970s, primarily because they also result in abnormal surges of T3 levels in the bloodstream. What levothyroxine-treated patients were missing was some T3, in the right amount and close to how the human gland produces it.

Adding T3 in the treatment of hypothyroidism is beneficial because the body and mind depend on this most potent form of thyroid hormone, which is also the main form of the hormone that works in brain cells. Therefore, even a minute T3 deficit, which may be present in many patients taking levothyroxine as a thyroid hormone replacement treatment, may impair the person's functioning. It is also true, however, that one person missing a minute amount of T3 may be symptom-free whereas another person may experience some effects.

Though pharmaceutical companies have tried to combine the two hormones, the results have not duplicated nature. In humans, 20 percent of T3 needed by the body is produced directly by the thyroid gland. The correct replacement is usually judged by monitoring what the pituitary senses and releases (TSH). But as we come to a better understanding of the complex chemistry and regulation of thyroid hormones in the body, we realize that these regulations in the pituitary gland, the brain, and other organs are somewhat different. The assumption was that, by giving only T4, doctors could normalize thyroid hormone levels in the body. This turns out not to be true in all cases. By giving patients only T4 to normalize TSH, some still miss a small amount of T3 that is normally provided by the thyroid gland. It is possible that, even though blood test results are normal and the conversion of T4 to T3 within organs is taken into account, some form of brain or perhaps even "general body" hypothyroidism, due to lack of T3, still exists. Having a normal TSH level does not necessarily mean that your brain and organs are receiving exactly the amount of T3 needed. Obviously, understanding what is missing in the brains and bodies of my hypothyroid patients became a prime concern.

I knew that T3 works as an antidepressant but that the doses used conventionally by psychiatrists were far higher than the physiological replacement doses (see Chapter 6). I also knew that the persistent suffering of treated hypothyroid patients is often of two kinds. Many people continue to suffer from symptoms of low metabolism. They have difficulty losing weight, and they complain of hair loss, dry skin, brittle nails, muscle cramps, and a host of physical symptoms. These symptoms indicate that the body is not receiving exactly the right amount of T3 from the conversion of T4. Many people suffer from some degree of depression, also probably due to some extent to low T3 in the brain. To some extent, none of the lingering effects of thyroid imbalance, discussed in the previous chapter, may be related to minor deficits of T3 in the brain.

This line of thinking brought all patients who required T4 treatment under the same umbrella, even those who had Graves' disease like Jennifer and those who had their thyroid gland surgically removed because of another thyroid disorder. The purpose of the treatment is to duplicate very closely how much T3 the brain and body require for normal functioning.

While searching for the right amount of T3 to be combined with T4, I determined that in general an average person needs 10 micrograms of synthetic T3 to achieve the best symptom relief. This amount is in fact very close to the amount that a normal thyroid gland produces each day for most people (6–10 micrograms). The protocol consists of treating patients with thyroxine first. Once they have reached and maintained normal and stable blood levels of TSH, I subtract 37–38 micrograms of thyroxine from the original amount and replace it with 10 micrograms of T3 in 2 divided doses (5 micrograms in the morning to be taken with the new reduced dose of thyroxine, and 5 micrograms at 2 P.M.). The following table gives you the most common conversions I use in my protocol:

Initial thyroxine dose (in micrograms)	New dose of thyroxine (in micrograms) to be taken with Cytomel (5 mcg, twice a day)
88	50
100	62.5
112	75
125	88
137	100
150	112

Jennifer, for instance, was orginally taking 100 micrograms of thyroxine. The new treatment that caused dramatic improvement in the way she was feeling was 62.5 micrograms of thyroxine ($^1/_2$ tablet of 125 micrograms) and 5 micrograms of Cytomel, twice a day.

This treatment combination allows both thyroid hormone and TSH levels to remain normal and stable. This way of treating persistent sufferers mimics closely what a normal thyroid gland provides to the body and the brain. Upon retesting several weeks after this conversion, all levels, including the pituitary-derived hormone TSH, are usually normal, and T3 never reaches abnormal levels. When you are retested, your T3 and TSH levels should be measured two to three hours after you take your morning dose of thyroid hormone.

Synthetic T3 at a dose of 10 micrograms a day achieves the desired benefits for most patients, even those who have required high doses of thyroxine. Only occasional patients, who initially required more than 175 micrograms of thyroxine, will need a higher dose of T3, (i.e., 5 micrograms 3 times a day), if they continue to have symptoms while taking 10 micrograms of T3.

"I Feel Beautiful Again"

Erin, a forty-four-year-old woman, had been diagnosed with hypothyroidism five years previously and had had a hysterectomy. Despite numerous adjustments of her T4 dose, she did not feel as good as she would have liked. Her symptoms had progressed, and three years ago, she got to a point at which she could no longer function. Because she continued to suffer from tiredness, trouble concentrating, and a host of other symptoms, her physician kept increasing the dose of thyroid hormone to make her feel better. Erin had no energy and had tingling in her hands that the doctors could not explain. She said:

One doctor kept telling me that there wasn't anything wrong. He would tell me that I was fine, I think because he really didn't know what to do. I got to the point where I thought there was something terribly wrong with me, although I had no idea what it was. I could feel that my body and my mind were not functioning properly for my age.

At one time, the doctor said I was hypoglycemic and put me on six little meals a day. It still didn't improve the way I felt.

Like most patients suffering from the lingering effects of a thyroid imbalance, Erin did not even suspect she might be depressed. But when I asked Erin about her symptoms, she confessed that she had most of the symptoms of depression. She was very irritable. "I went through a period where people would ask me a simple question, like 'Do you like my new haircut?' Instead of politely saying they looked nice whether they did or not, I would say something like, 'You know, it doesn't suit your face shape,' or 'It's horrible and makes you look bad.' Then I would be embarrassed at what had come out of my mouth."

Erin no longer suffers from depression or anger. Her physical symptoms have resolved since she began the T4/T3 protocol. She says:

Now I'm happier and more stable. I feel like I have a life again. I have more energy. I am not angry. I don't think I'm depressed at all. I'm able to do stuff for other people that for a long time I couldn't do. For a while, I couldn't give of myself, and now I'm much more involved in my church and in social activities.

As far as my relationship with my husband, he loves this change because I'm back to being my normal self again. I greet him with a smile and want to know about his day. Before, I wasn't able to do even that. I think I was so wrapped up in my own problems that I couldn't think about him. Now, we are back to where we sit down and we have our talks and spend time together.

At work, I'm more able not to be angry when the telephone rings at the wrong time or things don't work out as planned. I don't get as frustrated as I did.

As a result of this protocol, Erin lost ten pounds when she first started. Her skin felt better, and she stopped losing hair. The swelling around her face and her bloated look went away. "When I look in the mirror," she says, "I feel beautiful again. This treatment totally revolutionized my life."

When T4 Simply Does Not Do It

Another patient, a teacher named Priscilla, taught me the extent to which her cognitive impairment was the result of the small amounts of T3 that she was missing. Her experiences illustrate the fact that T4/T3 treatment relieves symptoms that can develop even in people who have not had depression or emotional problems as a result of a thyroid imbalance. Her case also illustrates that administering thyroxine to replace what a normal gland produces and delivers to the brain and body does not duplicate nature. The conversion of synthetic T4 to T3 simply does not yield the T3 needed even when the pituitary TSH has become normal.

Priscilla had a complete thyroidectomy for a large goiter. She was given T4 for her hypothyroidism and reached normal blood levels of thyroid hormones and TSH. Prior to the thyroidectomy, Priscilla had had no symptoms. She had been happy and energetic, but her problems started weeks after the surgery. In her words:

> I just couldn't seem to get the correct dosage. One doctor thought I was going through depression. He never really could get the dose straightened out either. I couldn't seem to get well.
>
> The doctors told me that everything was normal, although I certainly didn't feel normal. I was losing hair, I was nervous, I wanted to do destructive things. I thought I was crazy.
>
> It was an effort even to drive to a doctor's appointment. Unless I had the directions written down, I couldn't remember how to get there. Or I didn't feel like I could do it unless my husband came along, and I had been very independent before then. I became very scattered and couldn't stay focused on anything. Even in the house, it would be difficult to decide on which things to throw away and which things to keep. Everything would just seem to be a big mess. I was very disorganized.
>
> I had been teaching for twenty-five years, but it got to the point where I couldn't remember where I put files, and I couldn't remember what it was I wanted to do next. I'd become annoyed or upset with colleagues and just explode at times.

After removal of her thyroid gland, Priscilla's doctor gave her the exact amount of T4 needed to achieve a normal TSH level. But despite normal blood tests, she was missing a small amount of the active form of the hormone T3. As with low serotonin in the brain, this triggered depression, which became self-perpetuating.

The small deficit in T3 had also caused Priscilla's dry skin, puffiness, and low metabolism. When I changed her T4 treatment to the T4/T3 combination regimen, her emotional and physical symptoms rapidly resolved. Whereas most antidepressants take six to eight weeks to become effective, many people begin to notice an improvement in the way they feel as soon as one week after starting the T4/T3 treatment. Priscilla described the improvement in her symptoms as follows:

On the combination treatment, I was better able to handle situations. I could once again deal with children and colleagues at school. My emotions became more stable. I have been able to face challenges in life, and I've been able to challenge myself—taking classes, for example. I've noticed a big difference in how I feel about myself, how I dress and do my makeup, things that I was letting go because it was such an effort. I enjoy exercising again and want to do extra activities and go places.

Before T3, I felt like I was outside of myself, sometimes even just watching what's going on and not being able to figure out why I couldn't be a part of it. I feel like this protocol has put me back in touch with me, a person who's creative and energetic—the person I was before. I have a lot more self-esteem and self-control.

Priscilla's case has taught me that part of the problem when people rely on the T4 pill to obtain normal amounts of T3 in their body and brain is that the T4 pill simply does not provide the 100 percent correct amount of T3 needed for normal functioning.

Switching from the Natural Hormone
to the T4/T3 Protocol

The trend of switching patients treated with desiccated thyroid (that is, Armour thyroid) to the synthetic levothyroxine pill to avoid variability in thyroid hormone levels has continued over the years.[3] Patients who have taken desiccated thyroid for a long time, however, often resist being switched to levothyroxine tablets. Even though they achieve normal thyroid levels and their TSH level becomes normal and stable with thyroxine, many of these patients experience tiredness, sluggishness, and an inability to function the way they used to. They frequently claim that they felt much better when they were taking the "old natural pill." Counseling and offering medical explanations about why they *should* feel better fail to convince these patients that they need to continue taking the more modern thyroid pill containing only T4. After being on levothyroxine tablets for at most a couple of months, many of them wish to go back to their original form of treatment.

Patients treated with desiccated thyroid who go through periods of high T3 levels in the brain for a long time could theoretically experience a withdrawal syndrome once the desiccated thyroid is stopped and replaced by levothyroxine. In such patients, if one uses the combination of levothyroxine and a small amount of T3 delivered in two divided doses, as explained above, symptoms of brain hypothyroidism—including tiredness, exhaustion, and depression—often resolve. This approach has allowed me to success-fully switch many patients from desiccated thyroid to the synthetic pills.

A few patients, for reasons that remain unclear to me, either have refused to be switched or have tried my protocol for a few weeks and then asked to go back to the desiccated thyroid. Some of these people strongly believe that the natural hormones are better than the synthetic ones. In such patients, quite often, relief of symptoms is achieved at the expense of having a low TSH level and a significant rise of T3 levels for several hours after taking the pill. This rise in T3 causes a mental boost in many patients but can also produce heart problems and bone loss. The solution that will enable such patients to feel better with less adverse consequences from the animal-derived thyroid medication is to split the dose and take half in the morning and the other half in the early part of the afternoon. This will provide more even levels of T3 than taking the whole dose once a day.

The T4/T3 Protocol for Fibromyalgia

If you have been diagnosed with fibromyalgia, you might have heard about the use of T3 for the treatment of your condition. You might even have been tried on a course of T3. Several studies have reported that people suffering from fibromyalgia who have had normal thyroids can improve or even be cured when they are treated with 75 to 150 micrograms of T3 in conjunction with taking nutritional supplements, eating a wholesome diet, and exer-cising.[4] In one report, 75 percent of patients improved when they followed this treatment program, and nearly 40 percent were cured.[5] The doses used, however, generally exceed the amount of thyroid hormone that the thyroid gland produces naturally, which almost inevitably makes the patients hyper-thyroid. This is the same thing that happens to people treated for depression with high doses of T3 given once a day (see Chapter 6).

Like most other doctors, I find such a regimen inappropriate because it results in an excess of thyroid hormone, which often generates significant anxiety symptoms. It also places the patient at high risk for having rapid heartbeat and heart rhythm problems.

Nevertheless, doctors should not totally reject the logic behind using T3 in fibromyalgia. Patients with fibromyalgia have low serotonin levels, which have led to the use of tricyclic antidepressants and even Prozac for the treat-ment of this condition. The advocates of T3 treatment believe that the hor-mone may be doing an inefficient job maintaining adequate serotonin levels in the brain, and it is unable to promote normal metabolism in bodily tissues.[6]

This concept is probably valid because physicians often see patients who experience fibromyalgia as a result of hypothyroidism, and the fibromyalgia resolves with thyroid hormone replacement. (See Chapter 10 for more on fibromyalgia.) In short, fibromyalgia could be viewed as a manifestation of body and brain hypothyroidism. It has now become routine to distinguish between "hypothyroid fibromyalgia" (in which the thyroid is underactive) and "euthyroid fibromyalgia" (in which the thyroid is functioning normally), depending on whether blood tests show hypothyroidism. If you accept the idea that people suffering from euthyroid fibromyalgia have a problem with inefficient thyroid hormone, then indeed the ideal treatment for fibromyalgia should include T3.

For this reason, I have also used T3 for the treatment of several cases of fibromyalgia that have persisted despite adequate doses of levothyroxine that maintained normal thyroid test results. The only way I can achieve normal tissue thyroid hormone levels in these patients is to use a T4/T3 combination therapy in which T3 is given in small amounts in divided doses.

Michelle was the first patient whose fibromyalgia I successfully treated with the T4/T3 combination protocol. She was thirty-seven years old when she started feeling tired and noticing hair loss and brittle nails. She gained weight and was feeling sleepy. Gradually, she began suffering from pains in her shoulders, the middle of her back, and her arms. She eventually started going to doctors when her symptoms worsened.

Michelle actually suggested the diagnosis of hypothyroid fibromyalgia to one of the physicians. She said, "I was reading and trying to find out some information on why I felt so tired and was experiencing all those other symptoms. I knew about thyroid problems, so I started investigating them more, and that's when I decided to go to an endocrinologist."

For four years after Michelle was diagnosed with an underactive thyroid, she continued to suffer from many symptoms that clearly indicated fibromyalgia, despite receiving an adequate dose of thyroxine. Here's how she described these symptoms:

The pain in my shoulders at the top and right in the middle of my back was severe enough to wake me up in the middle of the night. I couldn't sleep because my joints hurt all the time. I was taking eight Advils a day, and they didn't help. I was exercising, which only seemed to make it worse. Sometimes the pain would shoot down my back, and I'd have tingling in my fingers, and sometimes it would come down my arm or up my neck.

I had a friend who thought it was arthritis, and that's when I went to a series of specialists. After three years of going in and out, one doctor told me I had back problems. He gave me a neck brace, and I received physical therapy three times a week for three weeks, and that didn't do any good. Another doctor told me that I probably had bruised some muscles in my back due to stress. One doctor told me that it was probably marital problems and stress.

Finally, I went to another doctor who, within five minutes, was touching the tender points in my back and my shoulders and took some X rays and diagnosed me with fibromyalgia.

When I saw Michelle, she was taking L-thyroxine for her underactive thyroid. Instead, I prescribed a T4/T3 combination treatment using small doses of T3 given three times a day. Not only did the lingering symptoms disappear, but her fibromyalgia also improved dramatically. Michelle also started practicing a relaxation technique and receiving massage therapy. Michelle said:

> They were remarkable changes. When I was just being treated with the T4 for my thyroid, I got to the point where I could hardly drag myself out of bed, and I really didn't want to be social anymore. Within a few weeks of starting on the T4/T3 protocol, I began to recognize a remarkable difference in the way I felt. I no longer wanted to sleep twenty-four hours a day. I could get up and function like a normal person. I no longer suffered from joint pain and body aches. That was exciting to me because I had felt so bad for so many years, I didn't think I would ever feel good again.

Michelle had suffered from hypothyroid fibromyalgia. Even in patients with fibromyalgia who have normal thyroid tests and have not experienced an underactive thyroid, this treatment may be beneficial. Remember, part of the problem may be an inefficiency of thyroid hormone. The body and brain need plenty of T3 to overcome this inefficiency. Administering T3 in appropriate amounts will not result in thyroid hormone excess in most people and will provide more consistent and stable levels of T3 throughout the day.

T4/T3 in Conjunction with Antidepressants

Thyroid hormone pharmacotherapy may help many people suffering from depression who have a brain deficit of T3 not completely corrected by Prozac and the other selective serotonin reuptake inhibitors (SSRIs). The initial success I've had with the T4/T3 protocol in people who have been prescribed antidepressants for lingering depression that resulted from a thyroid imbalance is astonishing. T3 given in small, divided doses has an almost miraculous effect on the brain chemistry. The beauty of this treatment is that, with small doses administered the way I've described, blood levels of T4, T3, and TSH stay within the normal range.

As discussed in the previous chapter, it is not unusual for hypothyroid persons to experience depression and require an antidepressant. Later, however, when their blood tests have been normal for some time, attempts to stop the antidepressant may cause the depression to return or become worse. In some patients, the antidepressant alone is not enough. When the patient is switched from T4 to the T4/T3 combination, the depression is resolved. It is as if the SSRI was not working properly because the brain chemistry mix was missing a small amount of T3 that was not being provided by the T4 pill.

Pat, a thirty-two-year-old pharmacist, recalls being diagnosed with hypothyroidism when she experienced a major depression that required hospitalization. She had had a previous episode of depression twelve years earlier when she was in college and broke up with her boyfriend. Her psychiatrist put Pat on Prozac along with thyroxine, and she regained normal thyroid function four months later. She continued to have a low-grade depression and anxiety, however, despite taking the maximum dose of Prozac and enough thyroid hormone to maintain normal blood levels.

Like most patients with residual suffering, Pat found the solution in the T4/T3 combination treatment. When she came to see me, she wondered whether it was her thyroid that was causing her depressive symptoms to persist. Adding T3 to her T4 treatment in conjunction with the Prozac transformed her mood and energy spectacularly. This treatment clearly augmented the other aspects of her depression treatment. Again, it is likely that the Prozac-levothyroxine treatment was not fully effective in curing the depression because Pat had a T3 deficit in her brain.

The small amount of T3 given in divided doses does not typically cause T3 levels in the blood to rise above the normal range. Nevertheless, before switching to a T4/T3 combination treatment, make sure that your doctor checks you for heart problems. That's because patients with heart disease may have heart rhythm problems or other heart complications that could be adversely affected by the minimal increases in the levels of T3. I have rarely used this combination treatment in people older than fifty-five because they have an increased risk of heart disease. If you are suffering from severe anxiety, T3 treatment may make your anxiety worse. Nevertheless, adding alprazolam for several weeks and then gradually decreasing the alprazolam will prevent the worsening of anxiety symptoms. Combine this protocol with a relaxation technique, diet, and exercise and you will be able to work on your weight more efficiently than ever before. Use the questionnaires provided in Chapters 3 and 5 before and during treatment so you can assess how well you are doing on this treatment program.

No longer do my patients with persistent symptoms who are being treated with T4 and have normal blood tests leave my office with the verdict that nothing else can be done for their suffering. My patients who had been taking desiccated thyroid now accept a more refined protocol that allows them to feel better than when they were taking the desiccated pill. Their thyroid hormone blood levels are normal and stable, and they don't have to accept bone loss as the price for feeling good. Even patients taking T4 for hypothyroidism who have been symptom-free may experience an improvement in well-being as a result of this treatment. Many confirm that it makes them feel more energetic and alert.

For the past five years, the T4/T3 protocol I use has worked in more than 90 percent of patients who have tried it, whether they were hypothyroid to begin with or had become hypothyroid following the treatment of Graves' disease or surgical removal of the thyroid. In my patients with lingering depression, standardized tests of depression show marked mood improvements after T4/T3 therapy. Scores for anxiety symptoms and cumulative physical thyroid-related symptoms go down, reflecting the change from a tired and disconnected person to a happy, symptomless one. One of my many patients who no longer needed Prozac and Zoloft after being switched to T4/T3 treatment told me, "I have not felt this way for God knows how long! Every day I think that this is going to stop working. I have great fears. But it has not. God bless you for bringing my life back together. Nothing worked for me ever before!"

Important Points to Remember

- Hypothyroid patients treated with T4-only drugs may suffer lingering effects because they're missing the right amount of T3, the most potent form of thyroid hormone as well as the main form that works in brain cells.
- Switching from T4 treatment to the T4/T3 combination regimen can begin to resolve emotional and physical symptoms, including depression, as soon as a week after the treatment is started.
- T4/T3 combination therapy may help maintain normal thyroid levels and improve symptoms in people suffering from persistent cases of fibromyalgia.

18

LIVING A
THYROID-FRIENDLY LIFE:

Healthful Choices Day by Day

Besides getting the right medical attention, thyroid patients also need to follow a lifestyle that includes eating healthy foods, taking the right supplements, following an exercise regimen, and practicing relaxation techniques. All of these activities are important for you to reach and maintain optimal physical and mental health, even though some doctors may lead you to believe that regular monitoring of thyroid hormone levels and making adjustments in drug dosages is all you need. But given what we now know of the significant mind-body effects of thyroid disease, you have seen for yourself in the preceding chapters that a combination of therapies is important.

We've seen the role of stress in triggering or perpetuating thyroid disease. But lifestyle factors also influence the likelihood of your developing a thyroid imbalance, including your diet and whether you exercise. These factors also determine to some extent how severe and consequential a thyroid imbalance will be. Genes account for only half of the risk of having an autoimmune thyroid disease such as Hashimoto's thyroiditis or Graves' disease. Your genes may make you susceptible to developing a thyroid condition, but whether or not you actually develop one is also linked to how you live your daily life.

It is certainly easier to prevent the onset of an autoimmune attack on the thyroid than to treat an imbalance once the attack has occurred. But even when the imbalance has already occurred, you can minimize and even halt some of its adverse effects on your health by following a thyroid-friendly lifestyle. Any such lifestyle must also take into account other health conditions that you have and any other medications you are taking that can contribute to the mental and physical effects of a thyroid imbalance.

The Best Diet for People
with a Thyroid Imbalance

What to eat and not eat is an obsession in our society. For some people, dieting is one way to control or avoid excess weight. For others, eating the right foods is a way to prevent disease. Many people also try to select foods that promote a stable, happy mood. But whatever the goal, people want to live a longer, healthier, and more fulfilled life.

Healthy nutrition for thyroid patients and for persons at high risk for having a thyroid imbalance combines all these goals: maintaining proper weight, preventing disease, and achieving a stable mood. In Chapter 7, I explained how and why thyroid patients often struggle with weight problems. Without a well-balanced diet, thyroid patients will never be able to win the weight battle. Furthermore, given the high rate of depression and anxiety among thyroid patients, no diet, however healthy, that fails to take into account the effect of food on mood can be truly thyroid-friendly. Healthy nutrition for patients at risk for having a thyroid disorder also means disease prevention. As with other major health conditions, including leading causes of death in the United States (coronary artery disease, high blood pressure, diabetes, and cancer), thyroid disease can be prevented by proper nutrition.

A thyroid-friendly diet should also be a diet friendly to the immune system, one that is likely to prevent or temper an autoimmune attack on the thyroid. This same diet should control the risk factors that can lead to brain damage and deterioration of cognition. The only diet I've identified that will give you all these benefits is:

- High in protein
- High in complex carbohydrates
- Low in fat
- Low in refined sugar

Research has shown that a high-protein, low-fat diet helps prevent the occurrence of autoimmune disease. Such a diet also appears to slow down the progress of autoimmune conditions.[1] Eating too much fat will harm your immune system and help precipitate an autoimmune attack on several organs, which could include your thyroid. A high-protein, high–complex carbohydrate, low-fat, and low–refined sugar diet helps you control not only your weight but also your cholesterol and blood pressure, to ensure your overall health. It helps you prevent damage to your brain from poor blood supply and strokes, too (see Chapter 16 for more information on how diet affects cardiovascular health).

I embraced the concept of a low–refined sugar diet years before the recent book *Sugar Busters!*[2] became a bestseller, but now that this book is widely available, I recommend that you use it as a good guide for healthy eating. I became an advocate of a low–refined sugar diet when I realized that many of my patients were unable to lose weight unless they reduced simple sugars in their diet. Refined sugars and simple sugars in general cause sugar to enter the bloodstream faster and produce a higher rise of blood sugar (blood glucose) levels than any other foods. The higher the blood glucose levels after food is consumed, the higher the resulting levels of insulin. Insulin is a hormone stimulated by glucose and released by the pancreas that makes sugar enter the cells to be stored in fat and used as energy. A great deal of recent research points to high insulin levels as the culprit for countless adverse effects, including weight gain, high blood pressure, and hardening of the arteries.

The magnitude of rise in blood glucose is expressed as the "glycemic index." The higher the rise of blood glucose after a particular food is eaten, the higher the glycemic index.

If you are suffering from the symptoms of after-meal fatigue and anxiety, difficulty concentrating, rapid heartbeat, and sweatiness, you may be experiencing a rapid drop of blood sugar after a rapid rise. Many people attribute these symptoms to hypoglycemia, whereas a rapid drop (following a rapid rise) could in fact trigger such symptoms without the cause being hypoglycemia (see Chapter 10). After a patient has reached normal thyroid levels, he or she may continue to suffer from symptoms after a meal.

The factors that determine a food's glycemic index are not limited solely to its simple sugar content. Other factors may include the amount of fat, protein, and fiber, as well as the methods of processing and cooking. For example, high amounts of fat increase a food's glycemic index, whereas high amounts of protein and fiber may lower it. To avoid annoying symptoms and low mood, eat more of the foods that result in a low glycemic index.

In general, complex carbohydrates such as whole grains, barley, nuts, pumpernickel bread, pastas, and dried legumes have a lower glycemic index than foods rich in simple sugars such as white bread, potatoes, plain crackers, chips, and breakfast cereals. Meals high in protein will delay the rise in blood sugar and cause fewer symptoms. If you have significant blood sugar–related symptoms, do not overcook your meals. Research has shown that eating raw starch flattens the blood sugar response because of its slow absorption from the gastrointestinal tract, whereas eating cooked cornstarch results in a higher sugar response than uncooked cornstarch.[3] Also, avoid sweet potatoes, sweet corn, boiled new potatoes, polished rice, oatmeal, cookies, biscuits, and buckwheat—all of which have an intermediate glycemic index. While following the dietary recommendations provided in *Sugar Busters!*, avoid as well foods containing animal fats.

A soy-based diet like that traditionally eaten by the Japanese is good for thyroid patients. A soy-based diet is well-balanced, high in complex carbohydrates and protein, and low in fat. Soy also has a beneficial effect on cholesterol and triglyceride levels. Consumption of soy protein reduces LDL cholesterol even if people continue to consume other foods containing saturated fat. You can choose from a wide variety of soy-based foods, including frozen desserts, soy cheeses, soy flour, and cholesterol-free soy milk products. But do not consume more than three servings a week of soy-based foods because of the possible effects of phytoestrogens on mood and cognition (see Chapter 16). Also make sure soy-based foods are cooked to avoid interference with the function of your thyroid.

Avoid eating raw foods containing goitrogens, substances that can impair the manufacture of thyroid hormone. Food such as turnips, cabbage, mustard, soybeans, peanuts, pine nuts, and millet are rich in goitrogens. Cooking usually neutralizes goitrogens, however, so it is quite safe to eat these foods after adequate cooking.

The Essential Dietary Fats

Fats in the body serve as a source of energy, but that's hardly their only, or even their most important, function. Various fats play roles in bodily processes as diverse as producing hormones and promoting intelligence: some 60 percent of the brain consists of lipids. Your thyroid also needs certain kinds of fats to work properly. Like other parts of the body, however, it doesn't need the most common kinds of fat that most people eat.

These useless dietary fats are principally saturated fats (they come mainly from meat, dairy, and other animal sources and are solid at room temperature) and hydrogenated fats. This latter type of fat is a modern invention that allows unsaturated oils, for example, to be changed in a way that extends products' shelf life. Thus, hydrogenated vegetable oils have become ubiquitous in everything from margarine to cookies. Unfortunately, hydrogenated fats serve no beneficial functions in the body, and eating a diet high in hydrogenated and saturated fats reduces rather than extends human life.

The essential fatty acids are the fats that you may not be providing in adequate amounts to your thyroid and the rest of your body. Essential fatty acids play a crucial role in the structure of cell membranes, the formation of various hormonelike substances in the body, proper functioning of the cardiovascular system, and other aspects of health. They're called essential because the body cannot manufacture them on its own: they have to be supplied by consuming foods or supplements. Essential fatty acids are polyunsaturated and are classified in a number of groups, the best known of which are the omega-3s and omega-6s. The chief omega-6 essential fatty acid is called linoleic acid, and the chief omega-3 is alpha linolenic acid. Consuming olive oil and other vegetable oils will increase your intake of these essential free fatty acids.

Two omega-3 free fatty acids have attracted the most attention for their health benefits:

1. Eicosapentaenoic acid (EPA)
2. Docosahexaenoic acid (DHA)

The primary dietary sources for these two essential fatty acids are various deep-sea fish, such as mackerel, shark, halibut, albacore tuna, herring, sardines, and cod. Eating the flesh of these oily fish or taking the popular fish oil supplements is widely recognized to help prevent heart disease. Animal research also suggests that a diet rich in EPA can prevent the occurrence of lupuslike autoimmune disease,[4] and it may also help prevent autoimmune attacks on the thyroid. Some doctors advocate using EPA in the treatment of rheumatoid arthritis and psoriasis. The beneficial effects of fish oil are expanding to include prevention of cancer, such as colon cancer. Concerns have been raised about the effects of encapsulated fish oils on diabetics because some (but not all) studies link these supplements to an increase in blood sugar levels. Also, avoid them if you are pregnant or if there is a concern about bleeding problems. My advice is to try to get your omega-3 fatty acids from eating fresh fish.

The amounts and types of fats you eat can also play a pivotal role in managing your weight. Eating more saturated fat is likely to make you gain weight—even if you don't increase your total caloric intake. Recent research that looked at energy and fat balance in hypothyroid animals fed a fat-rich or a low-fat diet showed that eating more fat resulted in a disproportionate gain in weight, even if the total number of calories is the same.[5] If you are hypothyroid, avoid consuming large amounts of saturated fat, since it goes straight to your fat stores.

This is how it works. Your body can adjust its metabolism when you eat proteins and carbohydrates. It cannot do this when you eat fat, however. When you increase your caloric intake of carbohydrates or proteins, your cells can speed up metabolism and burn up more of the excess calories, but your body has a poor ability to regulate fat balance.[6] Various hormones play a role in regulating energy balance, including thyroid hormone, insulin, adrenaline, and leptin.

The burning of fat is increased by starvation, aerobic exercise, and low levels of insulin (insulin contributes to the storage of fat calories). Fat metabolism also requires adequate amounts of thyroid hormone. A lack of active forms of thyroid hormone in bodily tissues will reduce the efficiency of the oxidation of fat, resulting in the fat's being stored and inevitably leading to a positive fat balance—and most likely, weight gain.

Animal research has shown that rats with normal thyroid glands increase their T3 levels in response to eating a high-fat diet, preventing them from becoming obese.[7] Perhaps an inadequate rise in T3 levels could be contributing to an increase in fat storage in some people with weight problems.

Leptin not only has a potent enhancing effect on metabolism but also decreases appetite and caloric intake. It is possible that the minute deficit of T3 in patients treated with thyroxine makes leptin less efficient in enhancing metabolism.

Antioxidants: Protecting the Thyroid from Harmful Free Radicals

Body cells need oxygen to function properly, but the result of the oxygen consumption is the production of oxygen-rich by-products. These oxygenated compounds, called free radicals, are toxic to cells. For instance, a buildup of free radicals produced from bodily metabolism has the propensity to weaken the immune system and the body's ability to fight disease. Free radicals damage cells and their surroundings. They harm genes, which tell cells what to do and not do. Genetic damage from too many free radicals can result in a "loss of identity" for the cells, which damages their functioning and could promote cancer.

Antioxidants are natural compounds that have the ability to bind and neutralize free radicals in the body. Providing antioxidants in the diet minimizes the buildup of the "bad guys" and improves the cells' health. Antioxidants prevent free radicals from damaging important cellular components, including genetic material. In fact, antioxidants can help prevent cancer, and some of them—such as beta-carotene and vitamins C and E—help prevent thyroid cancer.[8] Some antioxidants found in nature not only clear the body's toxic by-products but are essential for maintaining a healthy thyroid gland and an adequate supply of thyroid hormone. Taking adequate antioxidant supplements enhances the thyroid gland's production of thyroid hormones. These supplements include the trace elements selenium and zinc, and vitamins A, B2 (riboflavin), B3 (niacin), B6 (pyridoxine), C, and E. (See the "Optimal Daily Supplement Levels" list in the next section of this chapter.)

A deficiency in selenium, for example, can allow the damaging effects of free radicals to increase inflammation and destruction of the thyroid gland. Severe hypothyroidism causing significant mental impairment is quite common in central Africa and has been shown to be related to a combined selenium and iodine deficiency.[9]

A lack of selenium is also associated with thyroid-related infantile cretinism, which can occur as a result of a deficient blood supply to the placenta, such as can happen when the mother suffers from a severe infection of the reproductive tract.[10] These conditions cause a release of chemicals that are toxic to the cells as well as the spread of bacteria that utilize selenium. The resulting selenium deficiency then leads to low thyroid hormone levels in the fetus during brain development.

Various bacteria in the natural environment and in the environment of our bodies compete for selenium, which they require. Therefore, when certain bacteria pollute the environment, they can consume the selenium available to humans and make us deficient in this trace element essential for proper functioning of the thyroid. Infections with bacteria such as *Escherichia coli* can not only cause selenium deficiency but also release substances that can inhibit the manufacture of thyroid hormone.

According to an old study of people in the Himalayas, goiter was found in 45 percent of people living in a downstream village compared to only 12 percent of the people living in an upstream village.[11] When the researcher had volunteers drink either boiled water or unboiled river water, he noticed that people began to have goiters one month after they began drinking unboiled water. The occurrence of goiter was in fact due to poor sanitation, resulting in an increase in the downstream water's bacterial content, which, in turn, depleted the supply of selenium.

Zinc is another important trace element that is essential for the normal production of thyroid hormone. A study found low levels of zinc in children with Down's syndrome.[12] These children are also frequently hypothyroid, as indicated by high TSH levels. Administering zinc supplements to these children for four months corrected the underactive thyroid. The low zinc levels in Down's syndrome children are not due to poor nutrition but are thought to be the result of low intestinal absorption. Guinea pigs that are fed a diet low in zinc typically suffer from damage to the thyroid gland.[13]

The Thyroid-Friendly Nutrients

For thyroid hormone to work properly, several chemicals, nutrients, and enzymes in the cells must work in concert. Of these nutrients, selenium and zinc are also important constituents of the cell chemistry that allows thyroid hormone to work properly in the cells.

Several antioxidants are being touted for their ability to enhance metabolism and help you lose weight. The basis for the beneficial effect on weight is the antioxidants' ability to prevent the accumulation of free radicals that could slow metabolic activity. Low zinc levels have been found in obese people, and some physicians have suggested using zinc in the treatment of obesity.[14] No research, however, clearly demonstrates that antioxidants make you lose weight if you don't also exercise and eat a well-balanced diet.

Antioxidant supplementation is beneficial even if its effects on metabolism are minor. The rate of aging depends in part on what we eat. Clearly, reducing free radicals allows the cells to live longer and be healthier. Slowing the destruction of cells with a well-balanced diet that contains adequate amounts of antioxidants, thus allowing you to maintain normal thyroid levels in your system, will definitely slow premature aging. Slow cellular functions are features of low thyroid and aging. Some researchers believe that aging is a form of tissue hypothyroidism. Advancing age leads to a cellular deficit in zinc and selenium, which may produce lower thyroid hormone action similar to hypothyroidism.[15]

Hyperthyroid patients should take adequate zinc supplements. Although research has shown that both hypothyroidism and hyperthyroidism result in zinc deficiency, this deficiency is more significant in hyperthyroidism because of the increased elimination of zinc in the urine caused by thyroid hormone excess. Zinc also plays a role in the functioning of the immune system, and excess or deficiency might influence the development of autoimmune disease.[16]

For thyroid hormones to work properly in body cells, adequate supplies of antioxidants are essential. Selenium is a crucial component of the enzyme that converts T4 to T3 in the body.[17] Without it, T3 cannot be produced in the right amounts, and organs will function as if they were hypothyroid even though blood levels are normal. Thus, adequate selenium intake is essential for thyroid hormone to regulate the function of various organs. People suffering from a selenium deficiency (which is quite common among those older than sixty) will experience an improvement in the conversion of T4 to T3 when they take selenium supplements. A long-standing deficit in selenium will reduce the availability of T3, causing tissue hypothyroidism even though TSH levels are normal. Selenium supplements are likely to prevent tissue hypothyroidism and will therefore slow down some of the effects of aging. It is possible that the muscle damage and decreased muscle performance associated with selenium deficiency partly result from the damaging effects of free radicals on the muscle. Also, in people deficient in selenium, the muscle performs as if it were in a hypothyroid state.

Be cautious, however, when taking selenium supplements. Too much may cause many undesirable effects, including fatigue, abdominal pain, diarrhea, nerve damage, and even infertility. Too much selenium can also damage your thyroid. Selenium taken in a dose of 50 micrograms daily is adequate to provide significant antioxidant activity.

In hyperthyroidism, excessive production of free radicals overwhelming the cells' ability to neutralize them has been implicated in the progression of degenerative diseases. Research has shown that, when the thyroid is overactive, the consumption of oxygen is higher, leading to an accumulation of oxygenated compounds that are toxic to cells.[18] This accumulation has been called oxidative stress. To help cells clear these damaging oxidants, antioxidant supplements such as vitamins C and E and mixed carotenoids might prevent cellular damage in many parts of the body, including muscles.

Patients with an overactive thyroid need to increase their consumption of vitamin B$_6$ (pyridoxine) and vitamin B$_1$ (thiamine). Pyridoxine is important in the conversion of tryptophan to serotonin in the brain. Pyridoxine as part of a B-complex or multinutrient supplement may be quite helpful for patients being treated for an overactive thyroid and for those who have regained normal thyroid levels with treatment.

Vitamin A is required for the body to convert T4 to T3 in appropriate amounts. Too much preformed, animal-derived vitamin A can build up to toxic levels in the liver. Plant-based vitamin A precursors such as beta carotene and other carotenoids are nontoxic and are among the most potent antioxidants found in foods. Rich sources that I recommend are dark, leafy green vegetables.

Vitamin E can lower the risk of coronary artery disease and strokes, in part by preventing oxidized LDL cholesterol from damaging the cells in blood vessels. It also helps the thyroid.

Although an optimal diet includes plenty of fresh fruits and vegetables (see the accompanying table), these by themselves may not contain enough of the vitamins and antioxidants that you need. Unfortunately, most fruits and vegetables that you buy at the supermarket have been processed, stored, and refrigerated. Many reach your table several weeks to a few months after harvest. Because the vitamins and antioxidants in fresh foods are unstable, processing techniques and the time lag between harvest and consumption conspire to reduce the amounts of these essential nutrients. In particular, the selenium content of foods is easily lost during processing, storage, and cooking.

FOODS RICH IN ESSENTIAL NUTRIENTS FOR THYROID PATIENTS

Selenium*	Beta Carotene	Vitamin C	Vitamin E	Zinc
Whole grains	Kale	Citrus	Whole grains	Fish
Tuna	Sweet potatoes	Red peppers, sweet	Almonds	Lean beef
Organ meats	Carrots		Soybeans	Herring
Mushrooms	Butternut squash	Orange juice	Sunflower seeds	Maple syrup
Egg noodles	Spinach	Broccoli	Beans	Soybeans
Halibut	Cantaloupe	Cantaloupe	Liver	Turkey
Beef (no fat)	Broccoli	Melons	Cereals	Wheat bran
Soybeans	Asparagus	Green peppers, sweet	Vegetable oil	Whole grains
Oatmeal	Pumpkin		Leafy green vegetables	Sunflower seeds
Wheat germ	Liver	Cauliflower	Asparagus	
Sunflower seeds	Lettuce	Strawberries		

*Plant and land-animal sources of selenium are very dependent on the selenium content of soil.

How much of the various vitamin and antioxidant supplements should you take every day? The following list summarizes my recommendations:

OPTIMAL DAILY SUPPLEMENT LEVELS
- Vitamin C: 250–1,000 milligrams
- Vitamin E: 200–800 international units
- Beta carotene and mixed carotenoids: 1,000–5,000 international units of vitamin A activity
- Selenium: 50–100 micrograms
- Zinc: 15–20 milligrams
- Riboflavin (vitamin B$_2$): 1.5 milligrams
- Niacin (vitamin B$_3$): 15–20 milligrams
- Pyridoxine (vitamin B$_6$): 25–50 milligrams
- Folic acid: 400–600 micrograms

If you are suffering from an overactive thyroid, I recommend that you take the vitamins and antioxidants even when your thyroid levels are still high. If, on the other hand, you are hypothyroid, it is probably safer to start taking the supplements when your levels have become normal or close to normal. Add this to avoid buildup of these supplements in your system.

Although we know little about the various constituents of herbal products and their potential beneficial or detrimental effects on the thyroid, you ought to be aware that there could be such effects. For instance, the popular culinary herb thyme contains an essential oil that may reduce thyroid activity.[19] Thyme oil—found in mouthwashes and decongestants and used by some to treat tiredness, depression, digestion problems, and muscle aches and pains—can also cause nausea, vomiting, and cardiac and respiratory problems when used in large amounts. A 1985 study of freeze-dried extracts from four plants, including the common relaxant herb lemon balm (*Melissa officinalis*), which is used to treat viral infections, documented potential thyroid-related effects.[20] The extracts were shown to diminish the activity of thyroid-stimulating immunoglobulin, the antibody that causes an overactive thyroid in Graves' disease.

Thyroid hormone is synthesized by plants as well as by animals that do not possess a thyroid gland.[21] This suggests that thyroid hormone can pass through the food chain. If this is the case, thyroid hormone may be like vitamin D, a chemical with vitamin- and hormone-like functions that is both manufactured in the body (the skin can form vitamin D through an interaction with sunlight) and derived from food.

More research is needed to determine how plant compounds affect the thyroid and whether plants might directly provide significant levels of thyroid hormone, but in the meantime, if you are using herbs, do not abuse them. Their effects and side effects remain to be discovered.

Iodine: A Double-Edged Sword

The trace mineral iodine is an essential component for the manufacture of thyroid hormone by a healthy gland. To function normally, the thyroid requires 150 micrograms a day, which is far surpassed in most Americans' daily diets. In the United States, iodine consumption ranges between 300 and 700 micrograms a day. For the vast majority of Americans, advice such as "Supplement your diet with iodine to assist your thyroid" has no scientific basis and is actually harmful. Because high iodine intake can cause or precipitate autoimmune attacks on the thyroid, researchers are speculating that the increasingly high frequency of autoimmune thyroid disease being observed in the United States and Japan is partly the result of overly high iodine consumption.[22] Research has clearly established that the high dietary iodine content in some areas of the world has resulted in a rise in the prevalence of thyroiditis and thyroid cancer.[23]

Too much iodine in your diet will cause iodine to be trapped by a large protein found in the thyroid gland called thyroglobulin. The process of manufacturing thyroid hormone takes place in this protein. High amounts of iodinated thyroglobulin prompt the immune system to react and to cause an inflammation in the thyroid, characteristic of Hashimoto's thyroiditis. Animal research has demonstrated that the severity of autoimmune thyroiditis is increased by high iodine intake. High iodine intake can also cause iodine to be stored in fat tissue. The constant release of iodine into the bloodstream from the fat stores can then cause an underactive or overactive thyroid among healthy people as well as those with a preexisting thyroid disease.

Recently, NASA physicians consulted me because they had observed low-grade hypothyroidism in a few people participating in a ground study. The imbalance occurred within a few weeks of the subjects' beginning to consume high amounts of iodine. The amount of iodine given to these people was 4 grams per liter, comparable to the amount delivered to astronauts in flight, who consume recycled water with iodine added to keep it sterile. In Russia, silver is used instead of iodine. In some of the ground subjects, the consequences of the high iodine intake might eventually have included an autoimmune attack on the thyroid gland. One of these people had a persistent low-grade overactive thyroid after having been low-grade hypothyroid. Alarmed by my warnings about the potential consequences of thyroid imbalance for both astronauts and ground subjects, NASA decided to change its sterilization system and stop the high-iodine diet.

Inadvertent intake or administration of products high in iodine can trigger a thyroid imbalance among patients with Hashimoto's thyroiditis and Graves' disease. Too much iodine can cause hypothyroidism in certain patients with Graves' disease, particularly those who had regained normal thyroid function after treatment. Clearly, consuming high amounts of iodine from taking sea kelp supplements (sea vegetables are a particularly rich source of iodine) or using large amounts of iodized salt may represent a health hazard for thyroid patients.

Iodine excess from certain medications and contrast agents used in X-ray procedures also places thyroid patients at risk for thyroid dysfunction. For example, chronic ingestion of expectorant solution containing inorganic iodine for treating lung disease has been shown to cause goiter and hypothyroidism. Even iodinated glycerol, which was thought to be a safe alternative and contains no organic iodine, has been shown to result in hypothyroidism. Amiodarone, a medication commonly used to correct life-threatening heart rhythm problems, contains large amounts of iodine (75 milligrams per tablet). Approximately 20 percent of people taking amiodarone become hypothyroid, and 2 percent develop hyperthyroidism. In parts of the world where iodine deficiency remains a problem, amiodarone causes more hyperthyroidism and less hypothyroidism than it does in the United States.

Marcie, a thirty-five-year-old housewife whose sister had been diagnosed with Hashimoto's thyroiditis and an underactive thyroid a few years previously, visited a physician because of weight gain and fatigue. Disappointed that her thyroid tests were normal, and being left with no explanation for her symptoms, she began reading nutritional books, one of which recommended 2,000 to 3,000 milligrams of kelp every day as essential for a healthy thyroid. Marcie took the suggested supplements, thinking that ingesting too much iodine would reduce her likelihood of having a thyroid problem like her sister's and might alleviate her symptoms. As a result, however, she became afflicted by an overactive thyroid due to Graves' disease, which necessitated the destruction of her gland.

Among common foods, seafoods contain the highest amounts of iodine. These include lobsters, crabs, oysters, and other shellfish. Plant and dairy products may have some iodine if they are derived from areas that have iodine in the soil. (Soil in ocean coastal areas usually has higher iodine levels than soil in inland areas.) Other foods that contain high amounts of iodine are breads and eggs. Iodized salt, which contains 70 micrograms per gram of salt, is the most common source of iodine for most Americans.

People like Marcie with a known genetic predisposition to an autoimmune thyroid disease should avoid excess iodine. If any of your relatives have thyroid disease, minimize the use of iodized salt insofar as possible. Although the general recommendation is that dietary consumption should not exceed 1 milligram of iodized salt per day, I advise not consuming more than 500 to 600 micrograms a day.

Whereas too much iodine is harmful to the thyroid gland and can result in an under- or overactive thyroid, too little iodine in the diet can result in goiter and an underactive thyroid. When the level of iodine in the blood and in the gland is low, it causes the thyroid cells to enlarge and proliferate as a result of stimulation by the pituitary TSH (thyroid-stimulating hormone). Nearly 200 million people worldwide suffer from iodine deficiency and resulting goiters. In some parts of the world where the iodine content of the soil and thus the food is very low, and fish are not prominent in the diet, more than 50 percent of the population has goiter. Because the functioning of the thyroid gland in a developing fetus relies on the iodine supplied by a pregnant woman, women living in an iodine-deficient area may deliver babies with brain impairment. This condition is easily preventable by taking supplemental iodine.

In the United States, iodine deficiency has been rare since 1924, when table salt producers started to add iodine. Ironically, this same measure that was originally taken to prevent iodine deficiency and goiter might be one of the reasons for the rise in the frequency of autoimmune thyroid disease in people having the genetic predisposition. Nevertheless, some people do suffer from mild iodine deficiency. Clearly, a balance must be reached. You need to avoid both iodine deficiency and iodine excess.

Calcium and Vitamin D

An overactive thyroid will cause a significant amount of bone loss over time. Hypothyroid patients overcorrected with thyroid hormone are also at risk for losing bone. The risk is even greater if you are postmenopausal. Being subjected to high thyroid hormone levels for a prolonged period of time is especially worrisome if you have other risk factors for osteoporosis. These include being thin or a Caucasian woman, suffering from diabetes, smoking, or having a family history of osteoporosis.

For this reason, you should make sure you take enough calcium. In addition to dairy foods (which unfortunately are rich in animal fats), the following foods are rich in calcium:

Sardines	1 ounce	123 milligrams
Orange juice (calcium-enriched)	1 ounce	36 milligrams
Orange juice (regular)	1 ounce	3 milligrams
Salmon (with bones)	1 ounce	56 milligrams
Collard greens	1 cup	360 milligrams
Broccoli	1 cup	180 milligrams
Bread	1 slice	20 milligrams

If you consume too little dietary calcium and cannot eat dairy products because you have lactose intolerance or need to follow a low-fat diet, supplement your diet with at least 1,000 milligrams of elemental calcium (for instance, in the form of calcium carbonate) per day. Even consuming dairy products may not provide enough calcium to meet your recommended daily requirement. Calcium supplementation is the solution for most people. Calcium supplements can cause constipation, however. To alleviate or prevent constipation while taking calcium supplements, be sure to exercise and drink six to eight 16-ounce glasses of water a day. The exercise will also help protect you from further severe bone loss.

Optimal Diet: Putting It All Together

Healthy nutrition is essential for controlling weight, preventing degenerative diseases, maintaining a positive mood, and extending longevity. It is probably even more crucial for thyroid patients than for anyone else, because thyroid hormone is one of the major factors that allow the body to adjust its metabolism to the kind of food we eat in order to prevent weight gain. The accompanying table summarizes what I think are the best and most important features of a thyroid-friendly diet.

SUMMARY OF IMPORTANT BENEFICIAL EFFECTS OF RECOMMENDED NUTRITION FOR THYROID PATIENTS

Components of Healthy Nutrition	General Beneficial Effects
Well-balanced diet Low in fat, high in protein High in complex carbohydrates, low in simple sugars	Weight control Cholesterol control Decrease in autoimmune reaction Enhancement of tryptophan-serotonin (complex carbohydrates) Reduction in cravings
Antioxidants (selenium, zinc, vitamin E, beta carotene, vitamin C)	Prevention of thyroid cancer Weight control Decrease in degenerative damage Prevention of thyroid damage and autoimmune reactions to the thyroid Increased efficiency of thyroid hormone
Vitamins B_1, B_6, B_{12}, and folate	Increased conversion of tryptophan to serotonin (improves mood) Prevention of deficiencies that can cause dementia

SUMMARY OF IMPORTANT BENEFICIAL EFFECTS OF RECOMMENDED NUTRITION FOR THYROID PATIENTS

Component of Healthy Nutrition	General Beneficial Effects
Essential Fatty Acids	Decrease in autoimmune attacks
	Cardiovascular system benefits
	Maintenance of cell membrane integrity

The Benefits of Exercise

Thyroid patients often ask me whether they can engage in physical exercise. I don't recommend strenuous exercise while you are still hypothyroid or hyperthyroid. You risk muscle damage from the exercise when there is a thyroid hormone deficit. Strenuous exercise during hyperthyroidism should be avoided, too, because the performance of many parts of the body—such as the heart, muscles, and respiratory system—is somewhat impaired. When thyroid hormone levels have become normal, however, I highly recommend physical exercise, not only for weight control but also because exercise produces psychological benefits related to mood and self-esteem. These are crucial for patients who have experienced a thyroid imbalance.

Regular exercise relieves tension, anger, and confusion. Exercise training is effective in improving mood, alleviating depression and anxiety, and also reducing the perception of stress. Studies have shown that mindful exercise (a combination of slow, graceful movements and peaceful mental imagery) is much more effective for women than for men in enhancing feelings of well-being. I encourage men or women to perform tai chi, yoga, or other forms of mindful exercise. This seems to enhance the improvement in mood. Along with some form of weight-bearing exercise for bones and muscles, mindful exercise and other mind-body techniques can have a significant effect on enhancing thyroid patients' self-esteem.

Jon Kabat-Zinn, founder and director of the Stress Reduction Clinic at the University of Massachusetts Medical Center, has said, "Yoga does far more than get you relaxed and help your body to become stronger and more flexible. It is another way in which you can learn about yourself and come to experience yourself as whole, regardless of your physical condition or level of fitness."[24]

Recently, Dr. David Brown compared the effect of an exercise-training program three times a week using moderate-intensity walking (65 to 75 percent of heart rate reserve), low-intensity walking (45 to 55 percent of heart rate reserve), low-intensity walking in conjunction with the relaxation response (from wearing a portable cassette player and headphones), and mindful exercise (tai chi) for forty-five minutes three times a week.[25] He showed that the use of mindfulness in conjunction with exercise has a greater effect on psychological well-being than just walking. In meditation and relaxation techniques, thoughts are structured and focused on a sound, word, prayer, or phrase. Negative thoughts are overridden by focused thinking. Such techniques are suitable for people suffering from depression, anxiety, chronic fatigue syndrome, and heart disease, as well as for older people who may not be able to engage in vigorous exercise.

MIND-BODY TECHNIQUES
Biofeedback
Dance/movement therapy
Guided imagery
Art therapy
Meditation
Music therapy
Yoga
Tai chi
Self-help support groups

During a thyroid imbalance and prior to reaching normal blood tests, I recommend only mild aerobic exercise such as walking fifteen to twenty minutes daily. This strengthens the heart and lungs and allows you to adjust to the new demands of your body as thyroid levels normalize. Avoid rigorous anaerobic, muscle-building exercise in this phase of treatment because metabolism in the muscle is either too slow or too rapid, and it may impose demands on muscles that cannot be met without damaging them.

There are three main reasons why a wellness program designed to provide optimal physical and mental health for thyroid patients should include exercise:

1. Exercise or regular physical activity boosts endorphin levels and alleviates low mood.
2. Exercise increases muscle mass, which in the long run will raise metabolism. It is thus essential for weight control for both hypothyroid and hyperthyroid patients once blood levels have become normal.
3. Exercise improves heart function and prevents damage to blood vessels in the body and brain. Reducing your risk of vascular disease is an

investment in your future. It will help you minimize the risk of impaired cognition brought on with aging.

Assuming that you are not suffering from any kind of heart condition, follow an exercise program that fulfills these three long-term goals, implementing the program in three consecutive phases.

Phase one: This is an initiation phase, during which you perform endurance exercise three days a week for only thirty to sixty minutes. It can include:

Walking
Stair-stepping
Swimming
Cross-country skiing
Bicycle riding
Jogging
Treadmill exercise
Cycling
Rowing

You should stretch for five to ten minutes prior to each session and take a cool-down period of five to ten minutes of walking or stretching after each session.

Phase two: This can begin during the second month, when you are ready to increase the frequency of endurance exercise from three to six days a week. This step-up period should extend from one to two months. You can increase to four days a week the first week, five days a week the second week, and six days a week the third week. While gradually increasing the frequency of endurance exercise, you should begin a strength-training program. A good target for strength training is thirty minutes a day, three days a week.

Phase three: This comes later, when you are ready to follow a maintenance program, and combines endurance exercise six days a week and strength training three days a week.

Aerobic exercise strengthens the heart and makes it more efficient. It improves mood and helps you burn calories and fat. It is the cornerstone of any exercise program that will help you to take control of your health once again. If you are forty or older or have any history of heart disease, you need to check with your physician. He or she might recommend a heart stress test prior to commencing the exercise program, to estimate your level of fitness and determine whether you have heart disease. Stress tests are a good idea for most people who had hypothyroidism that remained undiagnosed for a long time.

Medications That Can Affect Your Thyroid

Thyroid patients often wonder whether taking various over-the-counter medications will affect their thyroid function. Whether you are hypo- or hyperthyroid, you should not be overly concerned about taking most cold remedies and decongestants—as long as your blood thyroid levels are relatively stable. Some cold remedies containing pseudoephedrine may cause a hyperthyroid person to have more symptoms of thyroid hormone excess, such as trembling, nervousness, sleep problems, and rapid heartbeat. Taking a decongestant that contains pseudoephedrine may also be a concern if you are hyperthyroid and have a heart condition. You should also avoid antihistamines that cause a drowsy effect if you have hypothyroidism and your thyroid levels are still low. Note as well that whether you have an underactive or overactive thyroid, too much caffeine may increase your anxiety symptoms and cause your heart to beat even faster.

Avoid sleeping pills and sedatives when your thyroid levels are low. It is not unusual for sedatives to precipitate myxedema coma, a dangerous condition related to very low thyroid, especially in older people. Because low thyroid slows the clearance of these medications from your body, they may make you drowsy.

Thyroid patients taking warfarin (Coumadin), a blood thinner used to treat phlebitis and some forms of cerebrovascular disease, should be aware that their thyroid levels will affect the dosage needed to maintain the desired level of anticoagulant effect. If the thyroid levels become high or low, they will need a change in the dose of warfarin.

Thyroid hormone levels also affect the levels of many other medications. Those that need to be adjusted when you have a thyroid imbalance include beta-blockers and digitalis (which is used for congestive heart failure). Theophylline, an antiasthma drug, may also need to be adjusted. A number of medications taken for asthma may heighten the effect of thyroid hormone. Some antiasthma medications should be avoided when your thyroid levels are high.

People who develop mild hypothyroidism from taking the heart drug amiodarone should have their TSH monitored. Doctors should not, however, prescribe thyroid hormone replacement unless the degree of thyroid underactivity is significant (TSH higher than 20). In many patients, the hypothyroidism is transient, and TSH will become normal over time, even when they continue to take the medication.

Hyperthyroidism from amiodarone use represents a more complex problem, since excess thyroid hormone can cause irregularities in heart rhythm and makes amiodarone less effective in controlling this problem.[26] Hyperthyroidism due to amiodarone should be promptly corrected. Two distinct types of hyperthyroidism are caused by amiodarone, however. Type I is the result of an increase in iodine uptake by the gland or an increase in the amount of thyroid hormone manufactured. Type II is due to the medication's having a toxic effect on the gland, which results in damaged thyroid cells' leaking thyroid hormone into the bloodstream (similar to what happens in silent thyroiditis and subacute thyroiditis; see Chapter 4). It is important for your physician to determine which is the predominant mechanism for the hyperthyroidism, since the required treatment differs. Other medications such as interferon and interleukin-2 can also trigger an autoimmune attack on the thyroid, resulting in thyroid dysfunction.

Many persons with lingering depression require a course of antidepressants (see Chapter 16), which may result in an increase in the thyroid hormone dosage.[27] Patients with a known thyroid disorder who are given antidepressants must be tested more frequently and the dose of thyroid medication adjusted. Otherwise, the antidepressant may be less effective in treating the depression.

Lithium can result in hypothyroidism, too, since it inhibits the release of thyroid hormone from the thyroid gland and causes the gland to retain iodine. Research has shown that lithium can promote an autoimmune attack of the Hashimoto's thyroiditis type on the thyroid. It can also exacerbate Hashimoto's thyroiditis and cause more damage to the gland. A significant number of people who take lithium for mood swing disorders have evidence of an underactive thyroid. More rarely, lithium can induce an overactive thyroid related to an autoimmune attack on the thyroid. Hyperthyroidism may rarely occur after patients discontinue lithium, as if stopping the lithium had caused overactivity as a rebound phenomenon.

In someone with preexisting Hashimoto's thyroiditis, the addition of lithium may cause an even more profound state of hypothyroidism and may confound the mental problems associated with the bipolar disorder. For this reason, manic-depressive patients treated with lithium often have thyroid testing on a regular basis. Even if the underlying thyroid gland is normal, lithium can cause mild or low-grade hypothyroidism, which should be treated with thyroid hormone to minimize the adverse effects of low-grade hypothyroidism on the mood swings. Treatment with thyroid hormone may help persons with manic-depression and lithium-induced low-grade hypothyroidism avoid manic episodes.

Alcohol and Nicotine:
Enemies of the Thyroid

Heavy alcohol consumption and depression often go hand in hand. Alcohol interferes with normal thyroid balance because depressed and alcoholic hypothyroid persons push their self-neglect to such a point that they may stop taking their medication or take it irregularly, thereby precipitating another vicious cycle. Alcohol consumption also contributes to excess caloric intake and increases the risk of weight gain.

Smoking harms most of your vital organs, and the thyroid gland is no exception. Smoking concentrates in your body compounds that weaken the thyroid—for example, 2,3-hydroxypyridine, which impairs the conversion of T4 to T3. Smoking can worsen Graves' disease and thyroid eye disease and may contribute to autoimmune attacks on the thyroid.[28] Even the severity of an autoimmune attack on the thyroid is more pronounced among pregnant women who smoked heavily prior to pregnancy.

Improper Use of
Thyroid Hormone for Weight Control

Thyroid hormone has quite often been prescribed to weight-clinic patients without preliminary thyroid testing, a practice that could be dangerous to patients with heart disease or a tendency toward emotional instability. The doses prescribed frequently exceed what a normal thyroid gland produces. People that are overweight who are given T3 and who are also placed on a low-calorie diet have a greater loss of weight than persons on a diet alone. Therefore, thyroid hormone treatment may be effective in producing the desired weight loss, but as a consequence these patients develop thyroid hormone excess and symptoms of hyperthyroidism. While the person may be initially happy with the weight loss, he or she may experience anxiety, mood swings, anger, difficulty concentrating, and even weakness. In other people this may cause an amphetamine-like effect and a state of hypomania. I have also witnessed inadvertent thyroid hormone treatment of patients with dormant Graves' disease trigger a state of permanent hyperthyroidism that has resulted in significant mental suffering.

Another drawback of using thyroid hormone for weight control is that T3 increases muscle breakdown to a greater extent during dieting. This is a high price to pay for a temporary weight loss. Long-term results of T3 are often disappointing—most people regain the weight.

In recent years the availability of natural desiccated thyroid preparations, sold over the counter, in natural food stores, or even by mail order, has become a health hazard to the public and may be responsible for thyroid hormone overdose. For instance, people who took Enzo-Caps, a diet pill sold as a nonprescription capsule made from "natural food products" of papaya, garlic, and kelp, became hyperthyroid.[29] Analysis of the Enzo-Caps showed that the T3 and T4 content of a single capsule was equivalent to what is found in 60 to 120 mg of desiccated thyroid. Similarly, several years ago 100 women from various areas of Japan became unintentionally hyper-thyroid as a result of taking a weight-reducing pill, Basetsuper, containing thyroid hormone.[30] A third of these women experienced psychiatric problems. Two women needed to be admitted to a mental institution, where doctors diagnosed an addiction to the medication. I therefore urge you to pay attention to exactly what you are taking when you attend a diet clinic or you decide to use supplements for weight control.

Important Points to Remember

- The best diet to help thyroid patients with mood, weight control, and disease prevention is a diet low in refined sugar and animal fat and rich in complex carbohydrates and protein.
- Make sure you are taking the right amount of antioxidant supplements and vitamins. They will reduce damage to the thyroid gland and make thyroid hormone work more efficiently in your body. The supplements will help you preserve a healthy body and a healthy brain.
- You need to achieve the right balance in your iodine intake. Too much can be harmful to your thyroid; too little can make your gland underperform.

19

LIVING WITH
THYROID EYE DISEASE

Thyroid eye disease, formerly known as Graves' eye disease, is one of the most dreaded thyroid conditions because of its potential emotional, personal, and professional effects on a person's life. In the minds of many people, having Graves' disease is associated with having bulgy eyes. When I notice people with bulgy eyes, I find myself also looking at their necks to see whether they have a goiter, their hands to see whether they are shaky, and their behavior to see whether they are nervous and fidgety. Recently, while in a coffee shop, I could not refrain from asking a middle-aged woman with all of these symptoms if she knew she had a thyroid condition. I was relieved to hear that she had just been diagnosed with Graves' disease two weeks previously and was currently taking medication.

I should note, however, that only half of those with Graves' disease have bulgy eyes, and some people with Hashimoto's thyroiditis who have either normal or below-normal thyroid function may have this thyroid-related eye disease.

Support groups dealing exclusively with thyroid eye disease have formed in the United States and other countries to help patients understand their disease and cope with their suffering. Despite these organizations' efforts to help people become better informed about thyroid eye disease, fear generated by the unknown continues to be rampant among patients with Graves' disease. However, in less than 20 percent of patients with Graves' eye disease is the condition severe enough to require aggressive intervention. Technological advances in corrective surgery as well as other treatments have improved the prospects of these patients.

The Affinity between
the Eyes and the Thyroid

Eye problems range along a continuum from minimal to severe in thyroid eye disease.[1] If researchers did a diagnostic study, such as an ultrasound or a magnetic resonance imaging (MRI) of the eye orbits (bony sockets), they would find that more than 90 percent of people with Graves' disease have some involvement, not of the eyes themselves but of the fat surrounding the eyes and the muscles that are responsible for the movement of the eyes. There is typically an enlargement due to inflammation of the muscles. Nearly 40 to 45 percent of people with Graves' disease have evidence of minimal involvement of the tissue surrounding the eyes but show no symptoms. Of the more than 50 percent remaining, the eye disease can range from mild to very severe.

Although thyroid eye disease is not a direct consequence of the thyroid condition, it occurs as a result of the immune system's having produced antibodies that target the eye muscles and structures situated around the eyes. The reason for the production of such antibodies in persons with thyroid disease is related to similarities in the structure of the eye muscles and the thyroid gland.[2] Because of these similarities, the immune system attacks the eyes as well as the thyroid. Therefore, the eye disease may be viewed as an incidental process occurring in autoimmune thyroid disease. Some patients with Graves' disease, however, have eye symptoms even though their thyroid function is normal. In such patients, the eye disease progresses on its own and may be the only actual problem the patient experiences. A number of these persons, when followed for months or years, may subsequently develop some kind of thyroid dysfunction, either hypothyroidism or hyperthyroidism.

Thyroid eye disease is more common in women than men simply because Graves' disease is primarily a woman's condition. Severe cases, however, tend to occur in older persons and men.[3]

Thyroid eye disease may have one or more of three major components:

1. An inflammation of soft tissue that can affect the conjunctiva (a protective fine layer of mucosa normally covering the sclera of the eye and inner parts of the eyelids) and structures surrounding the eyes, causing redness, a sensation of sand in the eyes, increased tearing, and visible swelling around the eyes
2. Swelling in the fat tissue surrounding the eyes, which accounts for the protrusion and bulginess of the eyes
3. Inflammation and loss of function in one or several of the four small muscles that are normally responsible for the movement of the eyes

How a person reacts to being diagnosed with thyroid eye disease is affected to some extent by the timing of the onset of the eye problem in relation to the thyroid imbalance. The onset of thyroid eye disease could occur simultaneously with the onset of hyperthyroidism, or it could occur months or years before or after. People who have just been diagnosed with hyperthyroidism due to Graves' disease but do not currently have the eye disease typically ask, "What about my eyes? Will I ever have bulgy eyes?" As is the case with most questions pertaining to thyroid eye disease, the physician's answer is often, "I don't know!" If you have been diagnosed with an overactive thyroid due to Graves' disease, you need to educate yourself about what to watch for should you develop eye disease.

Some of the most important eye changes in Graves' disease are the retraction of the upper eyelids, resulting in a wide-eyed look (because more of the visible portion of the eye is uncovered when the person looks straight ahead) and infrequent blinking. The condition is also responsible for the upper eyelid's inability to smoothly follow downward movements of the eyes when the person is asked to look down. (Doctors call this "lid lag.") In addition, when the patient looks straight ahead without staring, one can see a white band of sclera (connective tissue) above the border of the cornea (the central colored circle of the eye). This retraction of the upper eyelid resulting in the impression of staring and a widening of the eyes, often due to hyperthyroidism, frequently cause cosmetic concerns when they are noticed by patients or their family and friends. Appearance issues become an even greater concern when bulgy eyes develop, resulting from swelling in the fat tissue surrounding the eyes.

Other types of changes not only have cosmetic implications but also cause the patient significant discomfort. These include changes inherent to the inflammatory reaction of the soft tissue of the orbit, such as increased tearing, a feeling of having a foreign body in the eye, and a sensation of tense eyes. The eyelids become swollen and pockets of fluid form below the eyes, the conjunctiva becomes red, and blood vessels become apparent, as occurs in allergic reactions involving the eyes. This redness and blood congestion in the visible structures surrounding the eyes result in part from increased pressure within the orbits. In some patients, exposure to warm temperatures and radiation from the sun cause eye irritation and prevent them from performing outdoor activities in warm weather.

The most disabling symptom of the condition is double vision, resulting from inflammation and thickening of the eye muscles. Of all possible eye movement abnormalities, the most common one involves the upward movements of the eyes. Finally, when the disease has progressed significantly, the protrusion of the eyes may cause the cornea to be exposed continuously even during sleep, thus making it susceptible to damage from foreign bodies.

This may result in infection or perforation of the cornea, potentially causing loss of vision and even loss of the eye. Another dreaded effect is the compression of the optic nerve, which is likely to restrict vision. It is due to muscle swelling and enlargement as well as swelling of the orbit content.

The following lists summarize the symptoms of thyroid eye disease:

MOST COMMON SYMPTOMS
- Aversion to light
- Redness of eyes
- Protruding eyes
- Swelling of upper eyelids
- Blurred vision
- Watery eyes
- Sore eyes
- Gritty sensation in eyes
- Aches behind the eyes
- Dry eyes
- Poor night vision
- Eye pain when the person moves around
- Flashing lights

LESS COMMON SYMPTOMS
- Double vision
- Reduced sight in one eye or (more rarely) both eyes
- Reduced color brightness
- Swelling of lower eyelids

Which Comes First:
The Eyes or the Thyroid?

Some Graves' disease patients initially develop symptoms of hyperthyroidism with virtually no eye symptoms. Months or years after their thyroid condition has been treated, however, eye symptoms such as bulging or irritation of the conjunctiva or even eye muscle malfunctioning may develop.[4] These symptoms may be attributed to other problems or may come as an unhappy surprise. Although you shouldn't become unduly alarmed about your chances of being afflicted with this condition in the future, you do need to learn about possible symptoms of thyroid eye disease.

Theresa, aged forty-nine, had experienced no eye symptoms whatsoever in the twelve years since she had received radioactive iodine treatment for hyperthyroidism due to Graves' disease. Suddenly, she started having redness in her eyes, as well as puffiness, and her eyes began to bulge. Not suspecting that her eye symptoms were related to her thyroid condition, she went to see an ophthalmologist, who made the connection.

Theresa was devastated. She was also infuriated that no one had explained to her that this could happen even twelve years after the radioiodine treatment. "When I started having the eye problem," she said, "I was concerned about my appearance. The eyes were getting larger but not grotesquely buggy at the beginning. I was aware of some eye changes, but I didn't know what they meant."

Theresa was happy to hear that her eye disease was not severe. In fact, her eye condition later improved with treatment.

If eye disease occurs at the same time as the thyroid imbalance, the diagnosis is easy. The patient is frequently frightened, however, by the presence of eye problems. The fears are exaggerated because of the anxiety and loss of control or depression frequently generated by the thyroid imbalance. The loss of self-esteem that can be provoked by the thyroid imbalance is exacerbated by the appearance or functional impairment of the eyes and may make the thyroid patient feel unable to function mentally or physically.

In some patients, the onset of hyperthyroidism and eye disease is simultaneous, but the hyperthyroidism symptoms are minimal, so that the only discomfort experienced is related to the eyes. The suffering of such patients can be compounded by dismissal, misdiagnosis, or a lack of understanding, which could continue for a long time before doctors make the correct diagnosis and initiate treatment of the eye problems. The patient and even physicians frequently implicate allergies. Barbara Bush indicated in her memoirs that she attributed her eye symptoms to allergies for some time before she was diagnosed with Graves' disease.[5]

Paulette, like many patients with Graves' disease, suffered from eye symptoms but had no symptoms of a thyroid imbalance. She wandered from physician to physician for almost a year and was diagnosed with allergies even though she was experiencing worsening eye disease. She said:

> When I finally found out what was wrong with me, it had taken exactly one year and a lot of treatments at an allergy clinic that I was referred to. The doctor there who was giving me allergy shots kept telling me that my eyes were becoming red and itchy from allergies. I was told I was allergic to a lot of things, especially cats, but that was not my problem.

Although the patient and his or her immediate family may not notice the eye changes, strangers who see the person for the first time may notice these changes and even comment on them. Laura, the wife of a physician, suffered from undiagnosed hyperthyroidism due to Graves' disease for more than a year and was angry that her husband had failed to notice the changes that strangers immediately spotted.

Laura said, "People would ask, 'What is wrong with your eyes?' Even people I didn't know. One day, someone took a close-up picture of me, and when I saw it, I was stunned. How could my husband have let me go to work like this? No wonder people ask me what's wrong with my eyes! Now I'm self-conscious about it."

Because few ophthalmologists are trained to recognize or manage thyroid eye disease, patients suffering from eye problems due to undiagnosed Graves' disease may remain undiagnosed for some time even when they are seen and evaluated by eye doctors.

Twenty-nine-year-old Elizabeth, an attractive, successful architect, was under the care of an ophthalmologist when she showed signs of thyroid eye disease. She was seeing the ophthalmologist to have a radial keratotomy, a surgical procedure involving the cornea aimed at correcting myopia to avoid the necessity of wearing glasses. Before she went to see the ophthalmologist, she had recently complained of changes in her vision. She could not see as clearly as she had before and wanted to correct her focusing problem to eliminate the need for glasses. Prior to the scheduled surgery, Elizabeth started experiencing more symptoms in her right eye, which became swollen and developed a pocket. She said:

> It was like a water bubble. I could push it, and it was squishy. I could feel the pressure on it, and I started getting headaches. I thought maybe I had contracted an infection or the eyedrops had done it. I did not notice the eyelid receding, though my eye looked puffy and bruised. I told the ophthalmologist, "I know I'm scheduled for surgery, but my eye is doing something." He looked in my eye and saw no infection, so he recommended going ahead with the surgery.
>
> The surgery caused swelling for maybe two weeks. When I went back for my visit, I started complaining that my eye was drooping. I thought this was part of the recovery. He kept saying to come back for checkups. He kept saying this was not one of the reactions. I went to an ear, nose, and throat doctor, and he said he didn't know either.
>
> My face was distorting. All I could see in the mirror was that I was getting uglier every day.

For six months, Elizabeth went from doctor to doctor. A couple of eye doctors said the condition might be sinus-related. Finally, Elizabeth went to see an internist for other symptoms, and he suspected Graves' disease.

In Elizabeth's case, the ophthalmologist did not consider that her initial eye symptoms could be caused by Graves' eye disease. In fact, the eye surgery could have worsened the eye problem. Any trauma to the eye, including surgical trauma, may exacerbate or even trigger the autoimmune reaction to the eye in a patient with pre-existing Graves' eye disease and may make eye problems worse.

The Diverse Effects
of Thyroid Eye Disease

The onset of eye symptoms may have numerous effects on a person's job performance, lifestyle, self-esteem, and even mood. Anita, for instance, had almost quit her architectural design job as a result of thyroid eye disease. Her eye disease manifested itself as a severe inflammation and bulging, but she did not suffer from eye muscle problems. Thus, she did not see double unless pressure in her eyes increased due to improper positioning of her head while sleeping. Her suffering was due primarily to the swelling around the eyes and the pressure in her eyes, which affected her vision.

In some patients, Graves' eye disease does not cause inflammation or bulginess but primarily attacks the muscles that allow the eyes to move around smoothly. The sudden onset of the resulting double vision is one of the most frightening manifestations of Graves' eye disease. The afflicted person may experience many difficulties during this time that will be compounded if doctors don't make a prompt diagnosis.

Mark, aged fifty-four, had had a stable job for twenty-two years in the same company when he began suffering from anxiety, depression, and total turmoil in his life as a result of eye muscle malfunction. He did not experience any symptoms of swelling or inflammation around his eyes, however. Because double vision was the only symptom of an eye problem, physicians were searching for a neurological condition, and it took some time for the diagnosis of Graves' eye disease to be made.

Mark was unable to relax and began to experience sleeping problems. He became intolerant and irritable. His anger peaked when he realized he could not do simple things like changing a lightbulb or pushing a button. His wife said that he became a totally different person.

An ophthalmologist at a major medical school who saw Paul finally diagnosed the condition and initiated plans for treatment, which included eye muscle surgery and external radiation. Months later, Mark's functional ability returned.

Without adequate family support, patients with severe Graves' eye disease find it difficult to cope with the disease and its effects on functioning both at home and at work. Spouses and partners are often called on to play a major role in understanding the disease process and its treatment, as the person with the condition is frequently stressed by the situation and may not comprehend what the doctor is trying to explain. The spouse should be involved as much as possible in the case and, in turn, should reassure his or her partner about the outcome. This will minimize the anger and mood swings generated by the effects of eye disease. These feelings, which are also symptoms of thyroid imbalance, are exaggerated when eye impairment or disfiguration from Graves' eye disease occurs.

More Questions Than Answers

Once eye disease is diagnosed, the patient is usually faced with a situation in which answers may not be forthcoming because of uncertainty about the effectiveness of treatment and a lack of knowledge about the natural history of the disease. Many patients become frustrated and angry because they cannot get straightforward answers to such questions as:

- "What might happen later?"
- "Is it reversible?"
- "Could it be corrected totally without further damage to my eyes?"

Vanessa suffered from symptoms of thyroid eye disease for about six months before she was diagnosed. She had red, bulgy eyes and a fixed stare. After she was told that most of her eye problems were due to Graves' disease, Vanessa joined a thyroid support group to learn more about her condition. Her endocrinologist did not give her definite answers or provide her with literature describing outcomes and treatment options. The ophthalmologist to whom she was referred told her, "Let's wait and see." Attending thyroid support meetings helped her cope better because she found out that she was not the only one dealing with this situation. She said:

> Nobody seems to have answers. In the support group meetings, I meet a lot of people who have been misdiagnosed for a lot of years.
>
> At first, before going to the support group, I was so bitter and angry. It's a disease to be angry at. It's like righteous justification. We should be angry for having to go through this. Some of the people I see are so disfigured it makes me want to cry. I say, "That could be me in a year or two."
>
> I think now I'm willing to fight, though I still don't understand this complicated disease. I now realize that I was not really in tune with my health until it became bad.

The lack of adequate and reassuring information contributed to Vanessa's anxiety when she saw other people disfigured from Graves' disease.

Only after her endocrinologist explained to her that, in general, only a small percentage of people afflicted with thyroid eye disease reach a severe stage did she feel better. Vanessa said, "Talking with my husband and other patients with Graves' disease helped me to cope better with this. Now I don't feel as awkward and different as before. Most of the time, I just feel that I have an eye disease, and I am hopeful it will get better."

Promising Treatments for Thyroid Eye Disease

Graves' patients view thyroid eye disease with dread, and unfortunately, some people afflicted with severe eye disease may find their personal and professional lives significantly affected and become depressed. Such patients can take comfort in the following information:

- Having Graves' disease and even thyroid eye disease does not necessarily mean that your eye condition will become severe, disfiguring, or disabling. In only 5 to 10 percent of patients with thyroid eye disease is the condition severe enough to warrant aggressive treatment interventions.
- Many patients with Graves-related eye changes will experience a spontaneous improvement or near resolution of those changes over time; only a small percentage (nearly 20 percent) may have worsening eye disease, and even then, it could subsequently improve on its own.[6]
- Generally speaking, from the time the eye disease begins, a worsening or progression of the eye symptoms may occur over a period of six to twenty-four months.[7] After this initial period (often referred to as the hot phase), the eye symptoms often remain stable for a period of one to three years. Later, many patients experience a gradual improvement and often an incomplete resolution of the symptoms. For instance, one study showed that lid retraction disappeared in 60 percent of people several years after the beginning of the eye problems[8] and that eye muscle problems improved in 38 percent of patients. Bulgy eyes, however, tend to persist: less than 10 percent of people with bulgy eyes will have an improvement in the condition without receiving treatment.
- For those with significant eye changes, several treatments can improve or even correct the most severe eye effects. When such patients understand from the outset that the treatment process may be lengthy, it helps to minimize frustration, anger, and despair. It is also important for patients to be confident that treatments are available, not only to prevent loss of vision and to restore and maintain normal eye function but also to correct cosmetic disfigurement.[9]

For example, eyedrops that counteract the effect of the increased contraction of the eyelid may help eyelid retraction. Increasing the humidity in the home and work environment will help alleviate the dryness of the eyes caused by constant exposure due to the retraction of the lid. It is helpful for the patient to wear sunglasses when outdoors and to use eyedrops of artificial tears (methylcellulose 1 percent solution) during the day, as well as emollients to lubricate the eyes at bedtime.

I often recommend that my patients elevate the head of their bed or use two or three pillows to reduce eye swelling upon awakening in the morning.

Cosmetic upper eyelid surgery, performed when the patient's thyroid imbalance has been corrected and normal thyroid function has stabilized, provides excellent results when done by well-trained specialists.

For patients experiencing discomfort (a sensation of having sand or dirt in their eyes) and disfigurement from soft tissue inflammation around the eyes, a more aggressive treatment is needed. It consists of either a course of corticosteroid drugs, external radiation treatment to the orbits, or surgery to decrease the swelling in the orbits. An experienced ophthalmologist may recommend one or more of these treatments after performing a complete and thorough evaluation. In general, for patients having severe inflammation around the eyes, a course of corticosteroids is the most effective form of treatment and is given initially as 60 to 80 milligrams of prednisone a day for two to four weeks. Then the dose can be gradually reduced by 2.5 to 10 milligrams each week over a period of several weeks if the eye symptoms do not flare up. The corticosteroids seldom improve the bulgy eyes or muscle problems, however.

Patients who experience worsening bulginess but no major inflammation and those who have significant functional impairment of the eyes are generally treated with external radiation given in several sessions over two weeks. After external radiation, two-thirds of patients have a noticeable if not dramatic improvement in the soft tissue swelling.[10] The improvement is often noticeable as early as six weeks after the treatment, and after three months, the eyes may be much less bulgy. Inflammation of the optic nerve also improves after external radiation. Although external radiation does not help with the muscle dysfunction, it is often recommended before eye muscle surgery is performed. Other medications that are also helpful are cyclosporin, with or without corticosteroids.

External radiation usually produces significant improvements and is especially helpful when the optic nerve is affected by the swelling. Some patients who are initially treated with corticosteroids but fail to improve may be given external radiation as well. The best results are seen when corticosteroids and external radiation are used together. Doctors frequently recommend this when both significant bulginess and inflammation are present.

In addition to corticosteroids and external radiation, surgery of the orbit to remove portions of bone walls and decrease the pressure existing in the orbits may be recommended for cosmetic reasons or because vision is affected. This type of surgery is performed when the first two treatment options have failed to achieve an improvement or when vision becomes compromised as a result of exposure of the cornea or pressure on the optic nerves.

Even though physicians may offer different recommendations, it appears that external radiation treatment and corticosteroids are the main initial forms of treatment. However, nearly one-third of patients who require corticosteroids, radiation, or both will also need some form of surgery, either an eyelid correction or a decompression procedure.

Because of the lack of specific treatments to cure thyroid eye disease and completely eliminate the autoimmune attack on the eye, patients afflicted with thyroid eye disease continue to be treated with these unpleasant methods. The good news is that, by and large, these treatments achieve significant cosmetic and functional improvements. The assurance that help is available should serve to dispel much of the fear and anxiety that patients experience upon being diagnosed with thyroid eye disease.

How to Ensure
the Best Possible Outcome

Patients with Graves' disease, with or without eye disease, often ask what they can do to prevent or stabilize their eye problems. The answer is that anything that either has been proved to affect eye changes or is justifiably suspected of affecting eye changes should be considered.

First, any thyroid imbalance should be corrected as promptly as possible. Researchers have clearly shown that thyroid imbalances promote a worsening of eye symptoms.[11] Severe hyperthyroidism may be associated with a higher risk of having more severe eye disease. In addition, occurrence of hypothyroidism during the treatment of Graves' disease may cause a worsening of eye symptoms. Therefore, both thyroid specialists and patients must take care to ensure that normal thyroid function is maintained throughout the course of treatment, especially in those patients with more severe eye disease. A block-replace regimen, utilizing an antithyroid medication such as methimazole (which seems to have a beneficial effect on an autoimmune attack) in conjunction with levothyroxine (so that the patient has a stable, normal thyroid function), is often recommended for patients having hyperthyroidism. This regimen, administered for the first year to patients with moderate to severe eye disease, will help prevent the deleterious effects of a thyroid imbalance on the eye disease.

Second, for patients with significant eye disease, deactivating the thyroid gland, by exposing it to radioactive iodine, should be avoided the first year until the eye disease is more stable. This is because radioactive iodine treatment can exacerbate the eye disease by enhancing the autoimmune attack. Instead, it is advisable during this critical period to use an antithyroid medication to counteract the effect of hyperthyroidism and potentially diminish the autoimmune attack.

For patients with eye disease who experience side effects from methimazole, corticosteroid treatment begun when radioactive iodine treatment is administered may prevent a worsening of the eye disease.[12]

As we saw in Chapter 2, stress is a major trigger of Graves' disease and of the autoimmune attack responsible for hyperthyroidism.[13] Although not much has been written about the effect of stress on thyroid eye disease, it is inconceivable that stress could affect the thyroid condition but not the eyes. Extensive research suggests that the mechanism and the underlying trigger are the same for both eye disease and the thyroid condition. Thus, persons with even minimal thyroid eye disease should learn as much as possible about how to cope with stress effectively. The thyroid condition and the eye disease, themselves sources of stress, may overburden the patients, who can then easily lose control due to worrying and functional impairment. Again, strong support is crucial to help patients cope with the stress. People afflicted with thyroid eye disease need to educate themselves quickly, and learning about the promising treatment options that are available should serve to reinforce their sense of optimism. Remember, a positive attitude can promote a successful outcome.

Research has shown that smoking may make thyroid eye disease worse.[14] The negative effects of smoking are primarily related to increased inflammation of the eye. Thyroid specialists and ophthalmologists urge patients with Graves' disease to quit smoking. Such an emphasis on the adverse effects of smoking generates a great deal of anxiety among Graves' disease patients. Although I by no means encourage smoking, I feel that it is sometimes overly stressful for a person who has just been diagnosed with Graves' disease and is frequently suffering from a multitude of mental effects—including anxiety, low self-esteem, and depression—to quit smoking immediately. One patient of mine who tried to quit smoking during this vulnerable period experienced unmanageable anxiety. Finding this situation unbearable, she resumed her smoking habit only five days after quitting. Therefore, in this phase of the disease, patients should only attempt to quit smoking if they can do so without experiencing exaggerated anxiety and stress, which in themselves are potential triggers of worsening eye disease. For those who cannot quit smoking while experiencing the effects of an overactive thyroid, I suggest wearing suitable glasses that can protect their eyes from the detrimental effects of smoke. As soon as thyroid levels become normal, every effort to stop smoking should be made.

Despite the fact that we do not yet have a cure that entirely eliminates the root of thyroid eye disease, Graves' disease patients afflicted with eye problems need no longer resign themselves to despair and disability. A good understanding of their condition and the availability of effective treatments have changed the outlook for patients suffering from this condition. If you have thyroid eye disease and require treatment, ask your physician to refer you to an ophthalmologist with expertise in this field. You are likely to find the help you need in most institutions affiliated with medical schools.

20

THYROID CANCER:

Curable but Anguishing

In recent years, an increase in the frequency of certain types of cancer—such as lung, breast, and prostate—associated with a high risk of poor outcome has made people more fearful and aware of this dreaded condition. In the 1990–92 period, based on one study, the estimated frequency of thyroid cancer in the United States was approximately 6 in 100,000 women and 3 in 100,000 men.[1] Although thyroid cancer is less common than many other forms of cancer, the thyroid cancer rate has increased markedly in recent years. This is primarily due to the routine practice between the 1920s and 1950s of treating various head and neck conditions with high doses of radiation. Thyroid cancer has also been associated with radioactive fallout.

When a physician tells a patient that he or she has a thyroid gland growth that could be cancer, the person commonly reacts with fear, anxiety, and even shock. If the growth does turn out to be malignant, the patient reacts with the denial, anger, and depression typical of patients with many other types of cancer. Thyroid cancer, however, is one of the most curable cancers. Even so, people with thyroid cancer may go through significant hassle and worries. In some cases, it may take years of repeated treatments to eradicate the cancer cells completely. Even after the cancer is eradicated, people often go through lifelong monitoring, and some live with fears of recurrence.

In general, there is no clear-cut consensus among physicians about the best way to treat thyroid cancer. Even thyroid experts who deal with thyroid cancer patients on a routine basis do not follow exactly the same approaches to treatment. Thyroid cancer has been quite difficult to study, and the guidelines for treatment have been based primarily on retrospective studies. Researchers recently conducted a survey of members of the American Thyroid Association[2] to determine how doctors treat papillary thyroid cancer, the most common type of thyroid cancer. The survey confirmed that thyroid specialists take a range of approaches to the same problem.

Not surprisingly, when a patient seeks a second opinion, the treatment approach often differs from what the first physician suggested. The patient's confusion may then be augmented by the lack of information and education concerning the management of thyroid cancer. This bewilders many patients. A thyroid cancer patient whom I saw for a second opinion complained, "I had to borrow a medical book from a friend to find any useful information. Not knowing brought a lot of anxiety."

The Many Faces of Thyroid Cancer

Thyroid cancer comes in two main forms. The aforementioned papillary cancer, which is associated with the best outcome, accounts for 70 percent of all cases of thyroid cancer. Papillary cancer also tends to occur at a younger age. The other main variant of thyroid cancer is follicular cancer, which accounts for 20 to 25 percent of all cases of thyroid cancer. It is more aggressive than papillary cancer, and the outcome is in general worse. It tends to occur in older people.

Fortunately, poorly differentiated thyroid cancer (anaplastic cancer), which is one of the most aggressive cancers that affect mankind, is very rare. The source of this type of cancer can be in some cases an untreated or poorly treated differentiated cancer. Nearly 5 percent of thyroid cancers are called medullary thyroid cancers. At times they are familial and can coexist with tumors of other endocrine glands (multiple endocrine neoplasia) such as the parathyroid gland and adrenal glands. Medullary thyroid cancer derives from a different type of thyroid cells called C cells. These cells produce a hormone called calcitonin, which is also used as a marker for these cancers.

Because anaplastic thyroid cancer and medullary thyroid cancer are much less common and require different treatment, I'll focus on the papillary and follicular types in this chapter. The treatments for these two types of cancer are in general the same. Surgical removal of the thyroid gland is the first and most important component of the treatment. The follicular type, however, requires more aggressive surgery and even lymph node dissection for better outcome. One of the main factors suggesting a better outcome is an age of younger than forty years for men and younger than fifty years for women, even when the cancer has already spread.[3] The outcome is generally better in children and adolescents,[4] in women, and in people whose cancer is small at the time of diagnosis (less than 3 centimeters).[5] After initial surgery, patients are often treated with radioactive iodine typically followed by regular whole-body scanning and measurement of thyroglobulin levels (a marker in the blood that helps to determine whether there is residual thyroid activity). An indication that the treatment has probably effectively inactivated the disease is a low thyroglobulin level and a negative scan during follow-up.[6]

Treatment with radioactive iodine is effective after surgical removal of the thyroid because thyroid cells selectively concentrate iodine in the thyroid. Doctors specializing in nuclear medicine formulate a liquid containing a form of iodine that is radioactive. The patient drinks this liquid, allowing the radioactive iodine to travel to the thyroid and kill any remaining active thyroid cells, normal or abnormal, including cancerous ones. Some patients may require more than one or two treatments to eradicate the cancer. Doctors often administer the treatment six to eight weeks after the initial surgery and repeat it once or several times, if necessary, at intervals of six months to a year.

Dealing with Lumps

Doctors usually diagnose thyroid cancer when the patient has a lump, or what doctors call a nodule. Sometimes the lump is noticeable on the neck, and sometimes doctors find it by touching (palpating) the thyroid gland. In many cases, the nodule might have been present for a long time before it is discovered. Physicians tend to overreassure patients whom they have diagnosed with thyroid nodules and thyroid cancer. Although expressions such as "Oh, if you had to get cancer, that's the kind I would want you to have" or "Nobody dies of thyroid cancer. You'll live forever, and you won't have any problems" are quite appropriate, they may cause the patient to be unconcerned about the condition, which could lead to unhappy surprises down the line.

Lumps in the thyroid that can be detected by a manual examination of the thyroid are very common and occur in as much as 5 percent of the population, with women being affected more often than men. The frequency of small nodules (less than 1 centimeter in diameter) is much higher than nodules detected by palpation. Much more than 10 percent of people have small nodules.[7] These nodules are detected by ultrasound and at times incidentally by a procedure such as a magnetic resonance imaging (MRI) or computerized axial tomography (CAT) scan of the neck ordered for other reasons. Most of these small nodules are benign.

There are two basic types of nodules. Hot or warm nodules do not carry a significant risk of cancer, pick up significant amounts of iodine, and may even become autonomous from the rest of the thyroid gland and lead to hyperthyroidism over time. Cold nodules that do not pick up iodine appear as nonfunctioning areas on thyroid scans. They are often benign: only 10 to 15 percent of them are cancerous. Nearly 85 percent of all nodules are cold, and the remaining are warm or hot.

To evaluate patients with thyroid nodules, some physicians obtain a thyroid scan. Nowadays, however, doctors perform this procedure less frequently. Most order a TSH test instead. Only if the TSH level is low (indicating the possibility of a hot nodule) do they order a thyroid scan. If the TSH is normal, then doctors assume it is a cold nodule. To avoid performing surgery on everybody found to have a thyroid nodule, physicians recommend a procedure known as a fine-needle aspiration biopsy.[8] Doctors withdraw cells via a very thin needle stuck (three to five times) into the nodule. This helps to determine whether the nodule is benign or cancerous. The procedure can be done blindly, but increasingly it is performed with the help of an ultrasound machine to make sure that the needle is indeed within the nodule. If your nodule is smaller than 2.5 centimeters, using ultrasound guidance will give more conclusive results than doing a blind biopsy. In good hands, this procedure is quite reliable.

This procedure is not foolproof, unfortunately.[9] As many as 20 to 30 percent of the readings are inconclusive or fail to distinguish between benign and cancerous lesions. And many of these readings indicate a follicular lesion. The reading, however, does not have the ability to differentiate between a benign follicular tumor and a follicular cancer. No consensus exists as to whether all patients with inconclusive readings should undergo surgery. Quite often, the physician explains the options and leaves the decision up to the patient. Research has shown that men with a follicular lesion larger than 3 centimeters have an 80 percent chance of having cancer, whereas women with small follicular lesions have a much lower risk.[10] To avoid unhappy surprises, however, it may be prudent to have surgery if the readings show a follicular lesion.

Rosa had just turned thirty-eight when, after a neck injury from an auto accident, she was incidentally found to have a nodule measuring 2 centimeters. The doctor performed a fine-needle biopsy, and the reading was a follicular lesion. He told Rosa that, although it could be cancer, the likelihood of its being malignant was not high and he would look at it again in one year. He also added, "If you want it removed, I can refer you to a surgeon. It's a personal choice. You need to decide whether you can live with it or whether to deal with it now."

Rosa had to make the decision. She said, "I was very scared, but I kept thinking that, since this had been discovered, it must be a blessing in disguise. I kept going back and forth. One day I would think everything was going to be okay. Then I would have periods when I would get depressed and scared and think about my three-year-old daughter."

Rosa worried for many months. Then she came to see me for a second opinion. Rosa elected to have surgery, and the nodule turned out to be benign. She no longer worries about the possibility of having thyroid cancer. She had only one lobe of the thyroid removed, and I put her on 75 micrograms a day of thyroxine to prevent an underactive thyroid and the growth of nodules in the future.

A similar dilemma often occurs when the nodule is small. Since these lumps are quite common and are usually benign, doctors do not recommend surgery or fine-needle aspiration biopsy. Your doctor may repeat the ultrasound six months to a year later, to see whether the nodule has grown. If the nodule increases in size and becomes larger than 1 centimeter, doctors often recommend a biopsy. Nevertheless, if you have a history of radiation when you were a child or if you have a family history of thyroid cancer, you ought to have an ultrasound-guided biopsy immediately.

Recently, I diagnosed papillary cancer in a few patients who had small nodules (7 to 8 millimeters in size). Small cancers are common, and according to research, many remain small for a long time. If you have a papillary thyroid cancer smaller than 1 centimeter, your doctor may recommend removing just the cancerous lobe, followed by thyroid hormone treatment. Some small cancers are aggressive, however; and some will come back if only half the gland is removed. For this reason, I tend to recommend near-total thyroidectomies for small cancers.

Several factors indicate a heightened likelihood of cancer in patients diagnosed with thyroid nodules, regardless of their size:

- Nodules that grow over time
- Being male, since nodules by and large are more common in women
- Symptoms of hoarseness, difficulty swallowing, or spitting blood
- History of external radiation or exposure to radioactive fallout from nuclear accidents
- Family history of colon cancer and familial intestinal polyposis (genetic link)

A common source of problems in diagnosing thyroid cancer is the lack of awareness that even if a person has a normal reading on the first fine-needle aspiration biopsy, the lesion may nonetheless contain cancer cells. Some 3 to 4 percent of persons who have a benign reading on the initial biopsy turn out to have thyroid cancer down the line. For this reason, when the initial reading suggests a benign nodule, some doctors recommend that the biopsy be repeated a few months later. The repeat biopsy is unfortunately not done routinely, and some patients may continue to harbor their malignancy for months or years before thyroid cancer is diagnosed and the patients' thyroid glands are finally removed.

Andrea went to see her internist because of a bad sore throat. He discovered a lump in her thyroid and referred her to an endocrinologist, who performed a fine-needle aspiration biopsy of the growth. Andrea was reassured that the nodule was benign. She was started on thyroid hormone treatment, which can reduce the size of the nodule in some patients. She thought that this was the end of her trouble.

Almost three years later, she saw another endocrinologist because she had gained weight and had heard that thyroid malfunctions can cause weight gain. This doctor recommended that she have her thyroid gland surgically removed. While recuperating from the operation, Andrea was advised that she had thyroid cancer in the nodule. It was of the papillary type. Andrea became very upset and overwhelmed by the news.

She could not believe that the nodule had been detected nearly three years ago, that she had been assured it was benign, and that nothing had been done about treating it. After further treatment of her cancer with a single dose of radioactive iodine, Andrea was cured, and she has done well since. The lesson here is that, if you are told that your thyroid nodule is benign, have your doctor repeat the biopsy six months later.

Not All Doctors Treat Benign
Thyroid Nodules the Same Way

Some doctors recommend thyroid hormone treatment to suppress or reduce TSH levels in order to make a nodule shrink after the fine-needle aspiration biopsy has shown that the lump is benign. Recent research has concluded, however, that this treatment is effective in only a small percentage of patients.[11] Many benign nodules can eventually shrink without any treatment. Thyroid hormone treatment does seem to prevent other nodules from growing, however, but to achieve this beneficial effect, the thyroid hormone treatment is likely to cause an excess of thyroid hormone in your system, which can affect your bones, heart, mood, and emotions. For this reason, I seldom recommend thyroid hormone treatment for benign nodules. If a nodule grows and raises concerns, surgery may be the best route.

An Emotional and
Physical Roller Coaster

Doctors diagnosed Louise with thyroid cancer three to four years after she had been diagnosed with hypothyroidism. She was taking thyroid hormone replacement for her hypothyroidism when, during her yearly follow-up visit with her endocrinologist, he told her that she had a lump. According to Louise, "He said, 'I don't think it is anything—no big deal.' He was going on vacation and said that, when he came back, he would do an ultrasound."

Louise asked the endocrinologist to do the ultrasound before he went on vacation. "He did the ultrasound, and he started calling it a nodule. Then he said, 'When I come back from vacation, I'll do a fine-needle aspiration biopsy, and we'll see what it is.' "

Louise was very disturbed by her endocrinologist's apparently casual attitude and went to see an endocrinologist recommended by a friend. The second endocrinologist did a fine-needle aspiration biopsy and advised her that the nodule was benign. He increased her dose of thyroid hormone to suppress the nodule.

One year later, Louise moved to a different city, where another endocrinologist repeated the fine-needle aspiration biopsy. The next day, the endocrinologist called to tell her that cancer had been found and she required surgery.

Louise rushed to see a surgeon, who told her she needed to have her thyroid removed but also reassured her that everything would be fine. When the surgery was completed, the surgeon came out and told her mother and husband that the nodule was benign and that he had therefore removed only one lobe of the thyroid gland. He said this happens quite often. Louise was told the good news in the recovery room. Louise and her family all felt as if a weight had been lifted from their shoulders.

Thirty minutes later, the surgeon came back and wanted to speak to Louise's husband. He explained to him that when the pathologist had actually dissected the tumor, he found another tumor, which was malignant. By the time this was discovered, Louise had already been sewn up.

The surgeon reassured Louise that, because the tumor was not very big, there was nothing to worry about and for all intents and purposes she was cured. He did not recommend radiation. He basically said she was fine and told her to go home. Because of what had happened to her, Louise's happiness was tempered by a little suspicion. "How could you go from telling me it was malignant to telling me it was benign and now saying that it is malignant but go home, you're fine?"

A few weeks later, Louise had her internist request the slides and send them to a teaching institution for a second opinion. The results of the interpretation were rather different from the original one. The second opinion indicated multifocal cancer—multiple areas of cancer in the thyroid. (When thyroid cancer is multifocal, it often requires more aggressive treatment.) This was even more confusing. Now Louise completely lost faith in the physicians taking care of her.

When Louise came to see me, I recommended surgical removal of the remaining lobe, which, sure enough, turned out to be cancerous. Louise was devastated by the news. Her fears mounted, and she became overtly depressed. She said:

It was an emotional and physical roller coaster. Sometimes I think I'm lucky that I can still remember my name after all this. You think you're losing your mind at times. I'm very upset that my condition wasn't dealt with properly in the first place. I feel like this whole thing has been a nightmare. I'm always going to live with that memory. I don't know that you are ever cured from all of this.

After the second surgery, I followed Louise's progress closely. Each year for four consecutive years, I administered radioactive iodine treatment. This treatment finally cured her cancer.

The scenario just described is typical for many thyroid cancer patients. Although sometimes their treatment is hampered by differences of opinion, most often it is hampered by lack of knowledge and expertise on the part of some physicians who care for these patients.

Who Should Care for Your Thyroid Cancer?

Oncologists (cancer specialists) typically do not have an adequate handle on the management of thyroid cancer. In fact, most oncologists are seldom called on to manage thyroid cancer since chemotherapy has no role in its treatment. Some mainstream endocrinologists do not have much experience with managing thyroid cancer patients either. Unless they work in a referral center or in a setting where they are exposed to many patients with thyroid cancer, they often offer stereotypical recommendations that may or may not be applicable and appropriate for an individual patient.

Furthermore, thyroid surgery is delicate and difficult to perform. The surgeon chosen to do the procedure must be sufficiently experienced with thyroid surgery and have adequate knowledge about the management of thyroid cancer. The surgeon needs to work closely with the referring endocrinologist to plan an optimal treatment. If this does not occur, mismanagement or a delay in appropriate therapy may result.

Some nuclear medicine doctors tend to take over the care of thyroid cancer patients because they deal with this condition more frequently than mainstream endocrinologists. However, they lack the experience and expertise about pathological types that would enable them to make specific recommendations for individual cases.

A surgeon referred one patient I know with thyroid cancer to a nuclear medicine doctor to continue her care. The nuclear medicine doctor directed the radioactive iodine treatment and the administration of thyroid hormone. Two years later, this patient turned out to have a substantial amount of thyroid cancer in her neck area. She had suffered from many symptoms of thyroid hormone excess as well. The nuclear medicine doctor simply does not know how to fully evaluate and treat patients with thyroid cancer.

Patients diagnosed with thyroid cancer should therefore do a meticulous search for an endocrinologist who specializes in thyroid diseases and who has had a great deal of experience with managing thyroid cancer. The endocrinologist who takes on the care of a patient with thyroid cancer should closely monitor the treatments given by other specialists. Thus, he or she should be the main coordinator of the various therapies and interventions performed on the patient, such as:

- Surgery, including the extent of the procedure (whether to remove all or part of the thyroid)
- The appropriateness of the pathology report
- Recommending second opinions based on reading the pathology slides from thyroid specimens
- Interacting with radiation therapists if external radiation is recommended
- Interacting with the nuclear medicine doctor

It is especially critical for the endocrinologist and the surgeon who is performing the initial surgery to coordinate their efforts. If this does not happen, a great deal of mismanagement may occur. This could lead to significant suffering, anxiety, and frustration and might prolong the course of the cancer.

Vera's case illustrates how a lack of communication between the endocrinologist and the surgeon may be responsible for serious management problems and subsequent suffering. Vera was in tears when she came all the way from New Mexico to see me and tell her story. She said:

> When I felt a big bulge in my neck, I went to a doctor, who sent me to an endocrinologist. He said that it needed to be operated on because it could be cancer. I went right away to surgery. I didn't know at the time that thyroid cancer is very curable. I worried a lot and cried all the time. I was afraid to be alone dealing with this. I was depressed because I thought I was going to die, and I still think I might die. I always think that the only thing I want is to live long enough to have my son reach eighteen before I go.
>
> When they took me out of the recovery area to my room, my husband told me it was cancer. The surgeon came to talk to me and informed me that he took only the lobe where the cancer was and he hadn't removed the whole thyroid. I couldn't understand why. I did not know whether the surgeon had a lot of experience with thyroid surgery, but the endocrinologist told me that the surgeon was good.

Vera's voice was hoarse due to a vocal cord injury from the surgery, and she started crying when I told her that she needed to have the other lobe of the thyroid removed. After the second surgery, which showed involvement of the other lobe and of the lymph nodes, Vera received several whole-body scans six to twelve months apart to see whether there were any residual complications. Each time, she required a high-dose radioactive iodine treatment.

A sizable thyroid cancer (larger than 1 centimeter) should be treated by having the thyroid gland completely removed by a skilled surgeon who has performed numerous thyroid surgeries. Currently, some surgeons are performing such surgery on an outpatient basis, although there is controversy over whether outpatient thyroid surgery is safe.[12] The surgery may be difficult and may involve complications such as damage to the nerve that controls speech and voice. Surgeons can also damage or inadvertently remove the parathyroid glands, which are located behind the thyroid gland and help to control calcium and phosphorus levels in the body. A person who suffers severe damage or removal of the parathyroid glands will experience low calcium problems that may require lifelong treatment with calcium and vitamin D. The most common symptoms of low calcium levels are tingling and numbness around the mouth and fingers as well as muscle spasms affecting the hands. Therefore, to avoid adverse outcomes, have your endocrinologist refer you to a surgeon who has had a lot of experience with thyroid surgery.

Again, it is important to ask about the surgeon's track record. The surgeon should have done at least ten to fifteen thyroid surgeries a year for two to three consecutive years.

Preparing for the
Radioactive Iodine Treatment

After a surgeon performs a total thyroidectomy, most of the time he or she will schedule six to eight weeks later a scan of your entire body using radioactive iodine. You will then be admitted to the hospital to receive radioactive iodine treatment. You no longer have a fully functioning thyroid gland, and during the intervening six to eight weeks, you are allowed to become hypothyroid on purpose so that your TSH becomes higher than 40 milli–international units per liter. It takes that long for thyroid hormones to drop to very low levels. A high TSH is necessary because it makes the thyroid cells (normal or cancerous) pick up the maximum amount of radioactive iodine, which would destroy them.

For the few weeks that you are hypothyroid, you are likely to experience numerous physical and emotional symptoms. Many patients become depressed and quickly start observing strange things happening to their body. They feel out of control or become angry and irritated about trivial things, upset at the whole world. Patients frequently do not want to go out and do not want to see or be seen by others. Their anger is generated both by the thyroid hormone deficit in the brain and by the rapid transformation of their bodies, which alters their self-esteem and their normal functioning.

Danielle, aged thirty-four, had a thyroidectomy and was told to return for the scan six weeks later. For a while, she felt nothing happening, and then, all of a sudden, she became a different person. Here's how she described the experience:

> It is like you are floating above your body and mind. You have no control over them, and it is frightening. I hate the physical changes that happened so quickly. All of a sudden, my face puffed up, and I gained lots of weight. I became lethargic. There was nothing in the world that was worse than looking into a mirror and seeing the change that happened to my face. It is like the mirror tells you what is happening on the inside of your body.
>
> It was a depressing feeling. Everything is happening to you, but there is nothing you can do to change it.

Michael, another patient with thyroid cancer, described his first experience with acute hypothyroidism. The physical effects were so overwhelming that he had to rely on his wife to supervise his business operations. "Over the two-month period after the surgery," he said, "I started putting on weight. My motorcycle helmet no longer fit my head because it was so swollen. My eyes were so swollen I couldn't put my contacts in. My ring finger started to swell, and it took me an hour of soaking to get a ring off. None of my clothes fit. My shoes didn't fit. These little things are really what aggravated me."

To minimize and shorten the torture of rapid hypothyroidism, I typically prescribe Cytomel (T3) for the first three weeks after surgery. I then stop the Cytomel for the next three weeks. After the Cytomel is stopped, the TSH rises to the desired level (in excess of 40 milli–international units per liter), and you will be ready for the scan and treatment. To avoid an imbalance of long duration, start taking Cytomel on day three after surgery at a dose of 10 micrograms twice a day for one week. Then increase the dose to 12.5 micrograms twice a day if you weigh less than 115 pounds, if you are older than fifty-five, or if you have a history of heart disease. Otherwise, increase the dose to 25 micrograms twice a day for two more weeks and then stop the Cytomel. While taking T3, you will continue to function normally and may not experience any symptoms. After stopping the Cytomel, however, you may feel the annoying symptoms of hypothyroidism.

As soon as you stop the T3, I recommend that you follow a special diet consisting of low-iodine foods. (The section entitled "Iodine: A Double-

Edged Sword" in Chapter 18 lists iodine-rich foods and nutrients, which you should avoid during this period.) You need to avoid all dairy products, luncheon meats, bacon, sausage, fish and seafood, egg noodles, pastry, cookies, dressings, ketchup, crackers, pretzels, chips, and all canned foods. During this period, you can consume small portions of chicken, turkey, and veal. Fresh potatoes, pasta, homemade rice, fresh fruits, and fresh vegetables (except spinach) are also low in iodine. Make sure that what you eat is not salted and read the labels of everything you consume, including vitamin supplements. Continue this low-iodine diet until one week after you have received the radioactive iodine treatment. Depriving your system of iodine makes any remaining thyroid cells "hungry" for the iodine you will receive from the radioactive iodine treatment, which increases the likelihood of your being cured with just one radioactive iodine treatment.

A low-iodine diet will also make you consume less salt, which will reduce the swelling and fluid retention likely to occur when you become rapidly hypothyroid. The diet should be low in saturated fat to prevent your body from storing a lot of fat when you are made hypothyroid. During the three-week period, avoid drinking alcohol and taking sedatives. Be aware that problems with focus and alertness may affect your ability to drive safely. Inform your supervisor at work about the effects of rapid hypothyroidism. If possible, avoid going through this period of forced hypothyroidism during the holidays, as it may make you more depressed.

After you have been hypothyroid for three weeks, your doctor will order a TSH test. If your TSH level is high enough, you will be given a small amount of radioactive iodine (4 to 5 millicuries). A nuclear medicine doctor will take pictures of your neck area and the rest of your body forty-eight hours later. After the scan, you will be admitted to a hospital to receive radioactive iodine treatment.

The Loneliness of Radiation Treatment

People who are scheduled to receive radioactive iodine treatment are seldom given an adequate description beforehand of what they will experience. Emily remembers thinking:

> Nobody really educated me about the radiation. I always think how it is interesting that, when it is thyroid cancer, everybody thinks, "It's no big deal because people don't die from it, and if I had to choose cancer, that is what I would choose." I look at them, and I say, "Sorry, but I would choose no cancer." Cancer is cancer. The anxiety that comes with the treatment is significant. While everybody really minimizes the effect of thyroid cancer, I

think a lot of things would have been better if I had just really dealt with having cancer.

Physicians frequently tend to forget that these patients are profoundly hypothyroid when they return for the scan and treatment. Their perception of their surroundings is often distorted. The slightest thing can become a source of fear and apprehension. While receiving the treatment, they feel alienated when they are isolated in a room. Many patients wonder why everybody is so cautious about handling the radioactive solution, wearing gloves—and they have to drink it!

The first time Emily was hospitalized for radioactive iodine treatment, she found the experience doubly frightening because she had not been given an adequate description of what was about to occur. She knew that the liquid was radioactive and that there were good reasons for the precautions taken by the medical personnel. Emily said:

They made my husband stand out in the hallway, and I was the only person in the room. They put all this paper around. You can't walk on the floor, only on special material taped to it. You put on your gown, and they come with this cart and little bottles protected by iron. What is this going to do? Is it going to kill me? I wonder if somebody has checked if it's the right amount. They measure in the room. You don't want to have a mistake. I saw all these precautions with the radioactive iodine material. The person who was handling it looked like an outer-space alien. I was told, "Drink this. Just touch the edge of the cup!" I started crying, and I was really scared. I thought, "You want me to take this, and all you guys are out there and you're wearing all these gloves. What is happening to me?" I was hysterical. The nuclear medicine doctor was standing outside saying, "Don't cry, Emily, just drink it." I kept thinking, "I'm not sure this is what I want to do!" But then I kept thinking, "Do I want to have cancer? Do I want to stay hypothyroid?" No, so I took it.

They served food on disposable plates with disposable utensils. Everything that the patient touches has to be thrown away. You have to flush the toilet three times after you use it. You have to drink lots of water to go to the bathroom and take several showers to wash the radioactivity off your body.

I felt like some type of alien plagued with an unknown disease. This really depressed me. My mental state worsened when I was informed I could not be near my son, nor could he hug and kiss me for five days. This was probably the hardest part.

The Aftermath of the Radiation Treatment

Once you have received a radioactive iodine treatment, you will be given thyroid hormone in the form of L-thyroxine. You will gradually regain your physical health, and your mood will gradually improve. It takes about two weeks, however, before you feel a significant improvement and about three to four weeks for you to return to the way you were feeling.

Here's how Emily described the post-treatment period:

> I just couldn't get my appetite back. It is real hard when you are in that situation to know what are hypothyroid symptoms and what are radiation symptoms. The way it was explained to me, a lot of the fatigue goes hand in hand with both. It was two weeks before I felt something kicking in, and it was a good three or four weeks before I was back to normal.

To speed up your recovery from the hypothyroidism, you can start taking L-thyroxine the day after the radioactive iodine treatment. With several patients suffering from severe symptoms, I added 5 micrograms of T3 three times a day for ten days to further accelerate their recovery.

Some patients treated with radioactive iodine experience symptoms in the neck area, such as sore throat, swelling in the throat, or pain and tenderness in the neck. These symptoms occur primarily after the first radioactive iodine treatment and mostly in persons who did not have their thyroid gland completely removed surgically.[13] A nonsteroidal anti-inflammatory medication such as ibuprofen will help these symptoms. Many thyroid specialists request that the nuclear medicine doctor take a picture of the whole body three to seven days after the treatment (a "post-treatment scan"). You will not be asked to take more radioactive iodine for the scan. Since the amount of radioactive iodine that you receive for the treatment is much higher than the dose used for a regular scan, the post-treatment scan may show more areas of thyroid activity in your neck or other parts of your body. The results of this scan will be used as a baseline so that future scans can be compared to this one and the effects of the treatment can be thoroughly assessed.

The Need for Continued Monitoring

After the radioiodine treatment, doctors often give thyroid cancer patients doses of thyroid hormone slightly higher than what they would need in order to maintain a normal thyroid function. The purpose is to decrease the TSH levels to below normal, because TSH is known to stimulate thyroid cancer cells and may promote a recurrence of the cancer. Some doctors, however, prescribe a thyroid hormone dose much higher than is needed to produce this effect, and many patients end up suffering from symptoms of hyperthyroidism. Recently, I saw one patient who had been treated by an oncologist and was prescribed very high amounts of thyroid hormone, which resulted in a state of hyperthyroidism and abnormal behavior.

Depending on how aggressive and large the original tumor was, you will be asked to have a repeat scan six months or a year later. At that time, you will be asked to stop L-thyroxine, and you will be made hypothyroid for another whole-body scan, as you were the first time. Doctors also measure your thyroglobulin levels when you are off thyroid hormone to decide whether you need another treatment. If the whole body scan is negative, but the thyroglobulin level is still high, you may still have thyroid cancer cells in your neck and you may benefit from another radioactive iodine treatment.

This process is repeated yearly until thyroglobulin levels have become low and the scan has become negative. Thyroid cancer patients may suffer significantly from the anxiety produced by the severe, rapid, and profoundly acute hypothyroidism that results from stopping thyroid hormone treatment. This is often compounded by the considerable anxiety they experience while waiting for the result of the whole-body scan. Overall, it is a dreadful experience!

"The first time you do it, you don't know any better," said one patient about her experiences with becoming acutely hypothyroid. "You are dumb, and you don't know what is going to happen. The second time, you are really nervous; and the third time, you are almost suicidal because you know what is about to happen."

As you did before the first treatment, use T3 for three weeks so that you are off thyroid hormone for no more than three weeks. Follow the same dietary guidelines as for the first treatment. Your doctor can now use Thyrogen (recombinant TSH) injected in the muscle to obtain high TSH levels, which will produce more or less the same result as becoming hypothyroid.[14] This will allow maximal uptake of radioactive iodine by thyroid cells without your having to stop thyroid hormone treatment. The FDA has at this time approved Thyrogen only for the purpose of scanning. If, after injections of Thyrogen, the scan shows abnormal uptake, you will then have to stop taking thyroid hormone as you did the first time to receive another radioactive iodine treatment.

You need to know, however, that the scan performed after injection of Thyrogen may not always reveal activity that would have been detected by a scan obtained after stopping thyroid medication. For this reason, thyroglobulin levels are measured after the injection of Thyrogen. If thyroglobulin levels increase to 2 nanograms per milliliter or higher, this may mean you still have thyroid activity even if it is not detected by the scan. When your doctor reviews both the thyroglobulin levels after injection of Thyrogen and the results of the scan, the risk of overlooking persistent or recurrent disease becomes slim. The thyroglobulin level threshold of 2 nanograms per milliliter after the injection of Thyrogen may need to be changed as clinical experience with these methods expands. Side effects from Thyrogen include headaches, tiredness, and, only rarely, fever and flu symptoms.

If you have respiratory, cardiac, or emotional problems, your doctor will be allowed to use Thyrogen for the purpose of radioactive iodine treatment as well. This is called the "compassionate program" for Thyrogen use. Your doctor will then follow a protocol of treatment with Thyrogen that will allow you to be treated with radioactive iodine without stopping thyroid hormone medication.

Doctors also monitor thyroid cancer patients with other types of scans, including neck ultrasound, CAT scan of the neck, chest X rays, and thallium 201 scan. These procedures are extremely useful in conjunction with thyroglobulin levels, once any activity from the whole-body scan has ceased. Remember that a radioactive iodine whole-body scan is not foolproof. Some people with a negative iodine scan still have thyroid cancer.[15]

It is true that thyroid cancer is often curable. But don't forget, it can come back. You need to have your doctor periodically order the right tests even when you seem to be cured.

Fighting the Cancer

Some patients with thyroid cancer may require several treatments with radioactive iodine and even external radiation (which will be prescribed when there is lymph node involvement or recurrence in the neck). Despite several treatments, a few patients may continue to have cancer. The higher the cumulative dose of radioactive iodine, the greater the patient's risk of becoming afflicted with leukemia or cancers of the salivary glands, kidneys, colon, and reproductive organs in women.[16] For instance, leukemia may occur in five out of one thousand patients who receive at least 500 millicuries. Sucking on lemons reduces the risk of inflammation of the salivary glands and might reduce the risk of salivary gland cancer. I also often prescribe laxatives for a few days when the person is given the radioiodine to clean the radioactivity from the gastrointestinal system. This laxative treatment will reduce the risk of colon cancer.

The anxiety generated by the uncertainty of the outcome is similar to that experienced by patients afflicted with many other types of cancer. In thyroid cancer patients, the anxiety is prolonged because the treatments are given only once or twice a year. Some patients agonize about their outcome for an entire year before getting an answer. The worries, anxiety, and anger worsen as they get close to D-day—the date when they will be told whether the scan is still positive and whether they will need another radioiodine treatment. The emotional issues relating to the cancer are often exacerbated by the depression caused by stopping the thyroid medication.

Kelly, who has continued to have some residual thyroid tissue uptake in the neck despite three radioactive iodine treatments, had become slightly depressed because her cancer was not yet cured. When she was taking the thyroid hormone, she was able to work and function, and she tried to lead a normal life. She tried not to dwell on her cancer. She still had fears but kept herself busy. Whenever she stopped taking the medication, however, she began a journey into depression and misery.

In one of her office visits, she told me, "I hope and pray that my previous radioactive iodine treatments have taken care of the problem and I do not have to go through this protocol again. I just wish I could run away. I think I still have cancer and I am going to die. I don't want to leave my children. That's what bothers me the most. When I'm hypothyroid, I feel it is overwhelming." This is the period when thyroid cancer patients experience the most intense feelings and when they need a great deal of support from family and friends.

The Power of a Good Support System

In addition to support from family members (who should educate themselves about the disease), thyroid cancer patients should join support groups. Having close friends pray for you and with you can help. Positive thinking is very important. Thyroid cancer is a curable disease. Rather than joining groups dealing with cancer in general, however, it is much more beneficial to interact with people who have had thyroid cancer.

One patient I know became much more depressed when she attended a program dealing with cancer in general and found much more relief, support, and understanding when she met two thyroid cancer patients who were going through the same treatments that she was:

> I went to a popular cancer patient program. I was hoping they would teach me how to deal with the problem. When I got out of there, I was more depressed than at any other time. A doctor gave a lecture on the most common types of cancer, like breast cancer and prostate cancer—the cancers you hear about the most. I was upset. He talked about metastases in the bone, which was what I had, and then he started saying how hard it was to get rid of it and how painful it was going to be and how your bones are going to break. I was devastated. He was no help at all to people trying to cope with the situation. I never went back.

Spouses and partners of thyroid cancer patients may lose their patience and get frustrated. A support group where spouses and close relatives or their partners who have to live with thyroid cancer patients can talk to each other is helpful. Spouses should understand that changes in personality are normal and should be expected. A supportive spouse may periodically say, "Remember, this is what happens to you. The book says so. We're going to make it through this. There are only X number of days until the scan, and then you'll get back on your medication."

I cannot overemphasize the need for verbal support. Rapid and profound hypothyroidism renders patients more withdrawn. They want to be with someone who can anticipate their needs and understand that they require a lot of support. Afflicted people lack patience, lose control, and don't feel well. It is understandable that a spouse, unfamiliar with the mental and physical consequences of acute hypothyroidism, may not handle the impatience and anger very well. Emotions get stronger, emotional needs become greater, and patients realize their vulnerability. They tend to reach out more.

In general, thyroid cancer has a high cure rate, and the outcome is good, although, in some cases, the treatment may be lengthy. For everyone diagnosed with thyroid cancer, the follow-up period is indefinite. Understanding the general principles of treatment and knowing and understanding the basis for the mental suffering that could come with it will undoubtedly help you to cope better with this condition.

Important Points to Remember

- Although thyroid cancer is one of the most curable cancers, it can cause significant worries, and years of repeated treatments may be required to completely eradicate it.
- Physicians have not yet developed a consensus about the best way to treat thyroid cancer.
- The two main forms of thyroid cancer are papillary cancer, which tends to be associated with the best outcome, and follicular cancer, which is more aggressive.
- Thyroid cancer patients should find an endocrinologist who specializes in thyroid diseases and who has had a great deal of experience in managing thyroid cancer.
- Patients need to be well informed about the nature of radioiodine treatment and how they might react to it before they are scheduled to receive the treatment.
- Thyroid cancer can return even after apparently successful treatment, so patients should ask their doctors to test for it periodically.
- Putting together a powerful support team of family members and close friends can help your recovery immensely.

21

EIGHT STEPS
FOR THE FUTURE:

How to Promote a Better Understanding
of Thyroid, Mind, and Mood

Most people who seek medical help and are trying to feel better have no idea whether their physicians have a thorough knowledge of the complex field of thyroid disease. What really matters to patients is whether they feel better. They rightly expect that their physician will find the reason for the way they feel and correct it. Yet too many physicians do not recognize thyroid disease or know how to treat it or how to deal with the lingering effects of thyroid imbalance.

There is a critical need for the medical community to assess and revise its standards of care for thyroid patients and to better appreciate the effects of subtle thyroid abnormalities on overall health and emotions. The general public and people with thyroid imbalances also need to promote better overall care of the thyroid. How can all this be accomplished? Here are some suggestions for how you can begin to improve the quality of your care.

Educate yourself about your own thyroid. When patients become more knowledgeable, they can work with their physicians and become partners in their treatment and healing. Like other people with complex illnesses, many thyroid patients feel at the mercy of the medical system. Some patients suffering from a thyroid imbalance may see an endless parade of endocrinologists, nuclear medicine physicians, cardiologists, and other specialists. Ask your doctor to provide you with information during your office visits or how to obtain the information you need. Some of the information you find on the Internet is helpful, but in some instances it is not quite accurate. Many patients feel that they are shuffled along to the next specialist because of their multiple symptoms, which are in fact all related to the thyroid condition. It is especially important for you to understand the nature of symptoms such as anxiety and depression and how to cope with them. If you do, you will be less likely to be frightened by these symptoms if they return. By educating yourself through talking with other thyroid patients, reading books, and joining thyroid patient support groups, you can more fully understand the challenges you face in healing your disease.

Talk openly with your doctor about your experiences, symptoms, and treatments. Clear communication between you and your health care providers is priceless for successful treatment. You also want to make sure that your endocrinologist and primary care physician, as well as any social workers, psychiatrists, and other health care professionals involved in your care, also talk to each other. All health care providers treating you should discuss your problems to ensure that everyone understands your diagnosis and treatment.

If your spouse, partner, family member, or loved one has a thyroid condition, become better informed about the condition and more closely involved in its treatment. In my experience, thyroid patients who develop a good support system through family, friends, and coworkers cope much better.

For those who are newly diagnosed, family therapy and couple therapy may be a valuable support mechanism. You need to reach out for the support you need. Just as with treatment for mood disorders, family treatment for thyroid patients may be done in groups. Support group meetings offer opportunities for the family to share the difficulties of dealing with thyroid disease, which can include personality changes in the afflicted person. Because thyroid conditions such as Hashimoto's thyroiditis and Graves' disease can be considered genetic conditions, other family members (even children) may be afflicted in the future. It is extremely helpful for you and your family to feel that you are not the only ones dealing with the mental effects of a thyroid condition. In addition, meeting with other patients will give you an opportunity to learn about coping mechanisms that have worked successfully in other families.

Don't allow your doctor to dismiss your concerns or mislabel your condition. Throughout this book I have shown the similarities between symptoms of thyroid imbalance and symptoms of other conditions such as depression, anxiety disorders, hypoglycemia, chronic fatigue syndrome, and fibromyalgia. The similarities are so striking that you may receive the wrong diagnosis and the wrong treatment. Be persistent in having your doctor pursue an alternative diagnosis if your symptoms persist. If you educate yourself about your disease and common treatment options, however, you can become a more confident advocate for yourself.

Support public screenings and other efforts to make thyroid testing more commonplace. The public has been educated about cholesterol as a risk factor for coronary artery disease. People have learned that they should try to keep their total cholesterol level lower than 200 and that they need to have a proper ratio of the "good" HDL cholesterol to the "bad" LDL. In the same way, the public should be made more aware of the importance of tests to assess thyroid function. The American Association of Clinical Endocrinologists recently took a good step in this direction by promoting screening programs in several U.S. communities to detect unrecognized hypothyroidism. In Houston alone, these screenings enabled a significant number of individuals with previously undiagnosed thyroid conditions to get diagnosed and start treatment.[1]

A recent study published in the *Journal of the American Medical Association* showed that TSH screening every five years in women aged thirty-five and older is cost-effective because it allows the detection of unrecognized thyroid disease that may have significant health implications, including elevation of cholesterol and other problems.[2] This study, of course, did not take into account the toll that undiagnosed thyroid disease takes on personal relations and job performance. Given these additional costs, one realizes that more frequent TSH screening would undoubtedly prevent not only the negative effects on physical health but also a great deal of mental and emotional suffering.

Don't be shy about asking your primary care physician to refer you to an endocrinologist if necessary. A paradox in the current health care system that frustrates both endocrinologists and patients is that, as research and knowledge have expanded, enabling specialists to provide the best care for thyroid patients, the responsibility for detecting and managing thyroid conditions still falls mainly on primary care physicians. Often, these doctors cannot provide optimal care for thyroid imbalances because they generally have neither the time, the expertise, nor the interest in the complex and intricate field of thyroidology. The American College of Physicians, the American Medical Association, and many other physician organizations recognize endocrinologists as physicians with expertise in hormonal and metabolic disorders. Thyroid specialists (traditionally endocrinologists) are trained in diagnosing and treating disorders of hormones, the body's chemical messengers. They are the most suitable physicians to care for patients with complex hormonal and metabolic conditions. The most common endocrine disorders are thyroid imbalances, diabetes mellitus, and metabolic bone disease, including osteoporosis.

The Endocrine Society's Clinical Endocrinology Initiatives Committee recently issued recommendations relating to when primary care physicians should refer patients to endocrinologists.[3] With respect to thyroid disorders, some recommendations stipulate that patients with hyperthyroidism should be assessed and treated by an endocrinologist until they are stabilized.

Others who should be referred include patients with unusually complicated hypothyroidism, those with difficult-to-interpret thyroid function tests, and patients with thyroid eye disease. Referrals should also be made for evaluation, biopsy, and management of thyroid nodules as well as for patients with unexplained abnormal thyroid exams or thyroid function tests. The recommendation also includes patients with thyroid cancer as well as those with subacute thyroiditis or tender, painful thyroid glands.

Until primary care physicians become knowledgeable enough in the treatment of thyroid disease, insist on being referred to an endocrinologist with expertise in this field if you do not achieve the results you were expecting.

If you're enrolled in a managed care system, be assertive about having your thyroid-related needs met. Managed care emphasizes the use of primary care physicians rather than endocrinologists to care for thyroid patients, which may eventually lead to dismissal of symptoms or less-than-optimal treatment. Because of cost constraints, primary care physicians in managed care settings may not retest as frequently as they should.

In the managed care system, many endocrinologists have even become concerned about the survival of endocrinology as a specialty. Several managed care plans discourage referrals to specialists. In fact, in many plans, when a patient is referred, reimbursement for primary care services is often reduced. Another problem is that managed care programs often dictate that, when a referral is made, the patient must choose from a small pool of endocrinologists.

Shifting the care of thyroid patients from endocrinologists to primary care physicians and limiting referrals not only affect the quality of care but probably also increase overall costs. Selecting the wrong thyroid tests, misinterpreting the results, and monitoring test results either too often or not often enough may lead to even costlier health problems in the long run. According to a recent article on the potential inefficiencies of primary care in treating thyroid patients, marginal and subclinical diseases may be commonly dismissed in managed care environments.[4]

Agitate for improvements in physician training. Training program directors responsible for allocating teaching rotations need to implement a required systematic rotation in endocrinology. Family practitioners should have a thyroidologist teach them the art of examining a thyroid, emphasizing the importance of looking for thyroid problems and reiterating how to interpret thyroid function tests appropriately. They should also be given guidelines for referring patients to specialists, including doing so early if they are uncomfortable managing a patient.

Training and education in psychiatry for primary care physicians should be enhanced during residency. Psychiatrists also should receive adequate instruction about detecting thyroid disease and be encouraged to refer patients to thyroid specialists.

These steps will help you and your family avoid unnecessary suffering. They will also help everyone become more aware of how important the thyroid gland is for health and happiness.

NOTES

CHAPTER 1:

THYROID IMBALANCE: A HIDDEN EPIDEMIC

1. L. C. Wood, D. S. Cooper, and E. C. Ridgway. *Your Thyroid: A Home Reference*. 3rd ed. (New York: Ballantine Books, 1995), 215–219.

2. R. Arem and D. Escalante, "Subclinical Hypothyroidism: Epidemiology, Diagnosis, and Significance," *Advances in Internal Medicine* 41 (1996): 213–50.

3. S. I. Sherman, P. Nadkarni, and R. Arem, "Outcomes of a Community TSH Screening Program" (abstract presented at the Seventy-ninth Annual Meeting of the Endocrine Society, Minneapolis, June 11, 1997).

4. L. Wartofsky, "The Scope and Impact of Thyroid Disease," *Clinical Chemistry* 42, no. 1 (1996): 121–24.

5. R. J. Graves, "Newly Observed Affection of the Thyroid Gland in Females," *London Medical Surgical Journal* 7, part 2 (1835): 516.

6. Collections from the unpublished writings of the late C. H. Parry, London, Underwoods, 1825.

7. W. W. Gull, "On a Cretinoid State Supervening in Adult Life in Women," *Transitional Clinical Society* (London) 7 (1873): 180–85.

8. G. Lewis and S. Wessely, "The Epidemiology of Fatigue: More Questions Than Answers," *Journal of Epidemiology and Community Health* 46 (1992): 92–97.

9. D. B. Kamerow, "Anxiety and Depression in the Medical Setting: An Overview," *Medical Clinics of North America* 72 (1988): 745–51.

10. R. C. Kessler, K. A. McGonagle, S. Zhao, et al., "Lifetime and Twelve-Month Prevalence of DSM-III-R Psychiatric Disorders in the United States: Results from the National Comorbidity Study," *Archives of General Psychiatry* 51 (1994): 8–19.

11. D. A. Regier, R. M. A. Hirschfeld, F. K. Goodwin, et al., "The NIMH Depression Awareness, Recognition, and Treatment Program: Structure, Aims, and Scientific Basis," *American Journal of Psychiatry* 145 (1988): 1351–57.

12. K. B. Wells, R. D. Hays, M. A. Burnham, et al., "Detection of Depressive Disorders for Patients Receiving Prepaid or Free-for-Service Care: Results from the Medical Outcomes Study," *Journal of the American Medical Association* 262 (1989): 3298–3302.

13. W. Katon, M. Von Korff, E. Lin, et al., "Adequacy and Duration of Antidepressant Treatment in Primary Care," *Medical Care* 30 (1992): 67–76.
14. V. M. Victoroff, S. J. Mantel, A. Bailetti, et al., "Physical Examinations in Psychiatric Practice," *Ohio Hospital Commission of Psychiatry* 30 (1979): 536–40.
15. R. G. Kathol and J. W. Delahunt, "The Relationship of Anxiety and Depression to Symptoms of Hyperthyroidism Using Operational Criteria," *General Hospital Psychiatry* 8 (1986): 23–28.
16. B. A. Bartman and K. B. Weiss, "Women's Primary Care in the United States: A Study of Practice Variation among Physician Specialties," *Journal of Women's Health* 2, no. 3 (1993): 261–68.
17. L. Laurence and B. Weinhouse, *Outrageous Practices: The Alarming Truth about How Medicine Mistreats Women* (New York: Random House, 1994), 259–61.

CHAPTER 2:
STRESS AND THYROID IMBALANCE: WHICH COMES FIRST?

1. J. K. Levey, K. E. Bell, B. L. Lachar, et al., "Psychoneuroimmunology," in *Neuroimmunology for the Clinician*, edited by Loren A. Rolak and Yadollah Harati, 35–55 (Newton, Mass.: Butterworth-Heinemann, 1997).
2. D. N. Khansari, A. J. Murgo, and R. E. Faith, "Effects of Stress on the Immune System," *Immunology Today* 11 (1990): 170–75.
3. J. K. Kiecolt-Glaser, W. B. Malarkey, and M. Chee, "Negative Behavior during Marital Conflict Is Associated with Immunological Down-Regulation," *Psychosomatic Medicine* 55 (1993): 395–409.
4. S. Cohen, A. J. Tyrell, and A. P. Smith, "Psychological Stress and Susceptibility to the Common Cold," *New England Journal of Medicine* 325 (1991): 606–12.
5. G. Philippou and A. M. McGregor, "The Aetiology of Graves' Disease: What Is the Genetic Contribution?" *Clinical Endocrinology* 48 (1998): 393–95.
6. D. A. de Luis, C. Varela, H. de la Calle, et al., "*Helicobacter pylori* Infection Is Markedly Increased in Patients with Autoimmune Atrophic Thyroiditis," *Journal of Clinical Gastroenterology* 26, no. 4 (1998): 259–63.
7. Collections from the writings of the late C. H. Parry, London, Underwoods, 1825.
8. V. R. Radosavljevic, S. M. Jankovic, and J. M. Marinkovic, "Stressful Life Events in the Pathogenesis of Graves' Disease," *European Journal of Endocrinology* 134 (1996): 699–701.
9. K. Yoshiuchi, H. Kumano, S. Nomura, et al., "Stressful Life Events and Smoking Were Associated with Graves' Disease in Women, but Not in Men," *Psychosomatic Medicine* 60 (1998): 182–85.
10. B. Harris, S. Othman, J. A. Davies, et al., "Association between Postpartum Thyroid Dysfunction and Thyroid Antibodies and Depression," *British Medical Journal* 305, no. 6846 (1992): 152–56.
11. J. J. Haggerty, K. L. Evans, R. N. Golden, et al., "The Presence of Antithyroid Antibodies in Patients with Affective and Non-affective Psychiatric Disorders," *Biological Psychiatry* 27 (1990): 51–60.
12. K. C. Hyams, F. S. Wignall, and R. Roswell, "War Syndromes and Their Evaluation: From the U.S. Civil War to the Persian Gulf War," *Annals of Internal Medicine* 125 (1996): 398–405.
13. S. Wang, "Traumatic Stress and Attachment," *Acta Physiologica Scandinavica* 161, suppl. 640 (1997):164–69.
14. H. Brooks, "Hyperthyroidism in the Recruit," *American Journal of Medical Science* 156 (1918): 726–33.

15. R. Grelland, "Thyrotoxicosis at Ullevâl Hospital in the Years 1934–44 with a Special View of Frequency of the Disease," *Acta Medica Scandinavica* 125 (1946):108–38.

16. Abigail Trafford, "Me, Bush, and Graves' Disease: Many Thyroid Patients Face an Emotional Roller Coaster," *The Washington Post*, May 26, 1991, p. D1.

17. S. A. Ebner, M-C. Badonnel, L. K. Altman, et al., "Conjugal Graves' Disease," *Annals of Internal Medicine* 116 (1992): 479–81.

18. J. B. Jaspan, H. Luo, B. Ahmed, et al., "Evidence for a Retroviral Trigger in Graves' Disease," *Autoimmunity* 20 (1995): 135–42.

19. A. Fukao, M. Ito, and S. Hayashi, "The Effect of Psychological Factors on the Prognosis of Antithyroid Drug-Related Graves' Disease Patients" (abstract), *Thyroid* 5, suppl. 1 (1995): S-244.

20. H. M. Voth, P. S. Holzman, J. B. Katz, et al., "Thyroid 'Hot Spots': Their Relationship to Life Stress," *Psychosomatic Medicine* 32 (1970): 561–68.

21. E. Moschowitz, "The Nature of Graves' Disease," *Archives of Internal Medicine* 46 (1930): 610–29.

22. D. R. Brown, Y. Wang, and A. Ward, "Chronic Psychological Effects of Exercise and Exercise Plus Cognitive Strategies," *Medicine and Science in Sports and Exercise* 27, no. 5 (1995): 765–75.

CHAPTER 3:
HYPOTHYROIDISM: WHEN THE THYROID IS UNDERACTIVE

1. F. F. Cartwright, *Disease and History* (New York: Dorset Press, 1972), 105–106.

2. H. F. Stoll, "Chronic Invalidism with Marked Personality Changes Due to Myxedema," *Annals of Internal Medicine* 6 (1932): 806.

3. W. M. Easson and T. Kay, "Myxedema with Psychosis," *Archives of General Psychiatry* 14 (1966): 277–83.

4. R. Asher, "Myxedematous Madness," *British Medical Journal* 2 (1949): 555–62.

5. I. Klein and K. Ojamaa, "Thyroid Hormone and Blood Pressure Regulation," in *Hypertension: Pathophysiology, Diagnosis, and Management,* 2d ed., edited by J. H. Laragh and B. M. Brenner, 2247–62 (New York: Raven Press, 1995).

6. J. J. Series, E. M. Biggart, D. St. J. O'Reilly, et al., "Thyroid Dysfunction and Hypercholesterolaemia in the General Population of Glasgow, Scotland," *Clinica Chimica Acta* 172 (1988): 217–22.

7. E. Beghi, M. Delodovici, G. Boglium, et al., "Hypothyroidism and Polyneuropathy," *Journal of Neurology, Neurosurgery, and Psychiatry* 52 (1989): 1420–23.

8. M. A. Laylock and R. Pascuzzi, "The Neuromuscular Effects of Hypothyroidism," *Seminars in Neurology* 11, no. 3 (1991): 288–94.

9. R. Arem and D. Escalante, "Subclinical Hypothyroidism: Epidemiology, Diagnosis, and Significance," *Advances in Internal Medicine* 41 (1996): 213–50.

10. W.M.G. Tunbridge, M. Brewis, J. M. French, et al., "Natural History of Autoimmune Thyroiditis," *British Medical Journal* 282 (1981): 258–62.

11. D. Brown and D. Hoffman, "Russian Government Continues to Hide Details of Yeltsin's Medical Problems," *Washington Post* 116, no. 5 (February 20, 1996), 3.

12. Cable News Network, heart specialist: "Yeltsin didn't look sick," September 26, 1996.

13. Cable News Network: "Yeltsin's health problems cloud Russia's future. More than heart disease may be involved," September 21, 1996.

14. R. Arem and W. Patsch, "Lipoprotein and Apolipoprotein Levels in Subclinical Hypothyroidism," *Archives of Internal Medicine* 150 (1990): 2097–2100.

15. R. Fierro-Benitez, R. Casar, J. B. Stanburly, et al., "Long-Term Effects of Correction of Iodine Deficiency on Psychomotor and Intellectual Development," in *Proceedings of*

the Fifth Meeting of the PAHO/WHO Technical Group on Endemic Goiter, Cretinism, and Iodine Deficiency, edited by J. T. Dunn et al. (Washington, D.C.: Pan American Health Organization, 1986).

16. E. Nyström, K. Caidahl, G. Fager, et al., "A Double-Blind Cross-over 12-Month Study of L-Thyroxine Treatment of Women with 'Subclinical' Hypothyroidism," *Clinical Endocrinology* 29 (1988): 63–76.

17. J. J. Haggerty, J. C. Garbutt, D. L. Evans, et al., "Subclinical Hypothyroidism: A Review of Neuropsychiatric Aspects," *International Journal of Psychiatry in Medicine* 20, no. 2 (1990): 193–208.

18. F. Monzani, P. Del Guerra, N. Caraccio, et al., "Subclinical Hypothyroidism: Neurobehavioral Features and Beneficial Effect of L-Thyroxine Treatment," *Clinical Investigator* 71 (1993): 367–71.

19. J. V. Felicetta, "Thyroid Changes with Aging: Significance and Management," *Geriatrics* 42 (1987): 86–92.

20. M. Bahemuka and H. M. Hodkinson, "Screening for Hypothyroidism in Elderly Inpatients," *British Medical Journal* 2 (1975): 601–3.

21. D. L. Ewins, M. N. Rossot, J. Butler, et al., "Association between Autoimmune Thyroid Disease and Familial Alzheimer's Disease," *Clinical Endocrinology* 35 (1991): 93–96.

22. C. T. Sawin, D. Chopra, F. Azizi, et al., "The Aging Thyroid: Increased Prevalence of Elevated Serum Thyrotropin in the Elderly," *Journal of the American Medical Association* 242 (1979): 247–50.

23. F. Delange, "Neonatal Screening for Congenital Hypothyroidism: Results and Perspectives," *Hormone Research* 48 (1997): 51–61.

24. M. A. Jabbar, J. Larrea, and R. A. Shaw, "Abnormal Thyroid Function Tests in Infants with Congenital Hypothyroidism: The Influence of Soy-Based Formula," *Journal of the American College of Nutrition* 16, no. 3 (1997): 280–82.

25. H. E. Roberts, C. A. Moore, P. M. Fernhoff, et al., "Population Study of Congenital Hypothyroidism and Associated Birth Defects, Atlanta, 1979–1992," *American Journal of Medical Genetics* 71 (1997): 29–32.

26. P. J. Leedman, "Thyroid Disease and Hearing Disorders: New Genetic Links," *European Journal of Endocrinology* 135 (1996): 394–95.

27. T. Hua, "A Test That Failed: No System . . . Is Going to Pick Up Every Case," *Los Angeles Times* (Orange County), July 7, 1997, sec. B, 1–2.

CHAPTER 4:
HYPERTHYROIDISM: WHEN THE THYROID IS OVERACTIVE

1. H. F. Dunlap and F. P. Moersch, "Psychic Manifestations Associated with Hyperthyroidism," *American Journal of Psychiatry* 91 (1935): 1215–38.

2. M. Gomberg-Maitland and W. H. Frishman, "Thyroid Hormone and Cardiovascular Disease," *American Heart Journal* 135 (1998): 187–96.

3. S. Nagasaka, H. Sugimoto, T. Nakamura, et al., "Antithyroid Therapy Improves Bony Manifestations and Bone Metabolic Markers in Patients with Graves' Thyrotoxicosis," *Clinical Endocrinology* 47, no. 2 (1997): 215–21.

4. C. Giani, P. Fierabracci, R. Bonacci, et al., "Relationship between Breast Cancer and Thyroid Disease: Relevance of Autoimmune Thyroid Disorders in Breast Malignancy," *Journal of Clinical Endocrinology and Metabolism* 81 (1996): 990–94.

5. P-T. Trzepacz, I. Klein, M. Roberts, et al., "Graves' Disease: An Analysis of Thyroid Hormone Levels and Hyperthyroid Signs and Symptoms," *American Journal of Medicine* 87, no. 5 (1989): 558–61.

6. V. I. Reus, "Behavioral Aspects of Thyroid Disease in Women," *Psychiatric Clinics of North America* 12, no. 1 (1989): 153–63.

7. R. C. W. Hall, "Psychiatric Effects of Thyroid Hormone Disturbance," *Psychosomatics* 24, no. 1 (1983): 7–18.

8. P. H. Rockey and R. J. Griep, "Behavioral Dysfunction in Hyperthyroidism: Improvement with Treatment," *Archives of Internal Medicine* 140 (1980): 1194–97.

9. D. G. Folks and W. M. Petrie, "Thyrotoxicosis Presenting as Depression," letter to the *British Journal of Psychiatry* 140 (1982): 432–33.

10. J. W. Taylor, "Depression in Thyrotoxicosis," *American Journal of Psychiatry* 132, no. 5 (1975): 552–53.

11. P. F. Giannandrea, "The Depressed Hyperthyroid Patient," *General Hospital Psychiatry* 9 (1987): 71–74.

12. B. Schlote, B. Nowotny, L. Schaaf, et al., "Subclinical Hyperthyroidism: Physical and Mental State of Patients," *European Archives of Psychiatry and Clinical Neuroscience* 241 (1992): 357–64.

13. B. Uzzan, J. Campos, M. Cucherat, et al., "Effects on Bone Mass of Long-Term Treatment with Thyroid Hormones: A Meta-analysis," *Journal of Clinical Endocrinology and Metabolism* 81 (1996): 4278–89.

14. B. Biondi, S. Fazio, A. Cuocola, et al., "Impaired Cardiac Reserve and Exercise Capacity in Patients Receiving Long-Term Thyrotropin Suppressive Therapy with Levothyroxine," *Journal of Clinical Endocrinology and Metabolism* 81 (1996): 4224–29.

15. W. M. G. Tunbridge, D. C. Evered, R. Hall, et al., "The Spectrum of Thyroid Disease in a Community: The Whickham Survey," *Clinical Endocrinology* 7 (1977): 481–93.

16. C. Trivalle, J. Doucet, P. Chassagne, et al., "Differences in the Signs and Symptoms of Hyperthyroidism in Older and Younger Patients," *Journal of the American Geriatrics Society* 44 (1996): 50–53.

17. F. I. R. Martin and D. R. Deam, "Hyperthyroidism in Elderly Hospitalized Patients: Clinical Features and Treatment Outcomes," *Medical Journal of Australia* 164 (1996): 200–3.

18. E. C. Bartels and J. W. Kingsley Jr., "Hyperthyroidism in Patients over Sixty," *Geriatrics* 4 (1949): 333–40.

19. R. A. Nordyke, F. I. Gilbert, and A.S.M. Harada, "Graves' Disease: Influence of Age on Clinical Findings," *Archives of Internal Medicine* 148 (1988): 626–31.

CHAPTER 5:
THYROID IMBALANCE, DEPRESSION, ANXIETY, AND MOOD SWINGS

1. F. Monzani, P. Del Guerra, N. Caraccio, et al., "Subclinical Hypothyroidism: Neurobehavioral Features and Beneficial Effect of L-Thyroxine Treatment," *Clinical Investigator* 71 (1993): 367–71.

2. J. Scherer, "The Prevalence of Goiter in Psychiatric Outpatients Suffering from Affective Disorders," letter to the *American Journal of Psychiatry* 151 (1994): 453.

3. M. B. Dratman and J. T. Gordon, "Thyroid Hormones as Neurotransmitters," *Thyroid* 6, no. 6 (1996): 639–47.

4. C. Kirkegaard and J. Faber, "The Role of Thyroid Hormone in Depression," *European Journal of Endocrinology* 138 (1998): 1–9.

5. G. A. Mason, C. H. Walker, and A. J. Prange Jr., "L-Triiodothyronine: Is this Peripheral Hormone a Central Neurotransmitter?" *Neuropsychopharmacology* 8 (1993): 253–57.

6. P. C. Whybrow and A. J. Prange Jr., "A Hypothesis of Thyroid-Catecholamine-

Receptor Interaction: Its Relevance to Affective Illness," *Archives of General Psychiatry* 38 (1981): 106–13.

7. J. M. Gorman, *The New Psychiatry* (New York: St. Martin's Press, 1996).

8. J. Morrison, "DSM-IV Made Easy," *The Clinician's Guide to Diagnosis* (New York: Guilford Press, 1995).

9. M. S. Gold, A. L. C. Pottash, and I. Extein, " 'Symptomless' Autoimmune Thyroiditis in Depression," *Psychiatry Research* 6 (1982): 261–69.

10. C. B. Nemeroff, J. S. Simon, J. J. Haggerty, et al., "Antithyroid Antibodies in Depressed Patients," *American Journal of Psychiatry* 142 (1985): 840–43.

11. J. J. Haggerty, R. A. Stern, G. A. Mason, et al., "Subclinical Hypothyroidism: A Modifiable Risk Factor for Depression?" *American Journal of Psychiatry* 150, no. 3 (1993): 508–10.

12. C. Kirkegaard and J. Faber, "The Role of Thyroid Hormones in Depression," 1–9.

13. K. D. Denicoff, R. T. Joffe, M. C. Lakshmanan, et al., "Neuropsychiatric Manifestations of Altered Thyroid State," *American Journal of Psychiatry* 147, no. 1 (1990): 94–99.

14. R. H. Howland, "Thyroid Dysfunction in Refractory Depression: Implications for Pathophysiology and Treatment," *Journal of Clinical Psychiatry* 54, no. 2 (1993): 47–54.

15. D. Elfenbein, ed., *Living with Prozac and Other Selective Serotonin-Reuptake Inhibitors: Personal Accounts of Life on Antidepressants* (New York: HarperCollins, 1995).

16. P. J. Goodnick, I. L. Extein, and M. S. Gold, "TRH Test in the Treatment of Depression," Proceedings of the 143d Annual Meeting of the American Psychiatric Association, San Francisco, May 6–11, 1989, *New Research Abstracts*, 126.

17. R. C. Kessler, K. A. McGonagle, S. Zhao, et al., "Lifetime and 12-Month Prevalence of DSM-III-R Psychiatric Disorders in the United States. Results from the National Comorbidity Study," *Archives of General Psychiatry* 51 (1994): 8–19.

18. Kessler et al., "Prevalance of DSM-III-R Psychiatric Disorders," 8–19.

19. C. G. Lindemann, C. M. Zitrin, and D. Klein, "Thyroid Dysfunction in Phobic Patients," *Psychosomatics* 25 (1984): 603–6.

20. S. Matsubayashi, H. Tamai, Y. Matsumoto, et al. "Graves' Disease after the Onset of Panic Disorder," *Psychotherapy and Psychosomatics* 65 (1996): 277–80.

21. M. E. Lickey and B. Gordon, *Medicine and Mental Illness: The Use of Drugs in Psychiatry* (New York: Freeman, 1991).

22. J. M. Gorman, *The New Psychiatry,* 212.

23. R. W. Cowdry, T. A. Wehr, A. P. Zis, et al., "Thyroid Abnormalities Associated with Rapid-Cycling Bipolar Illness," *Archives of General Psychiatry* 40 (1983): 414–20; and M. Kusalic, "Grade II and Grade III Hypothyroidism in Rapid-Cycling Bipolar Patients," *Neuropsychobiology* 25 (1992): 177–81.

24. H. A. P. C. Oomen, A. J. M. Schipperijn, and H. A. Drexhage, "The Prevalence of Affective Disorder and in Particular of a Rapid Cycling of Bipolar Disorder in Patients with Abnormal Thyroid Function Tests," *Clinical Endocrinology* 45 (1996): 215–23.

CHAPTER 6:
MEDICINE FROM THE BODY: THYROID HORMONE AS AN ANTIDEPRESSANT

1. G. R. Murray, "Note on the Treatment of Myxoedema by Hypodermic Injections of an Extract of the Thyroid Gland of a Sheep," *British Medical Journal* 2 (1891): 796–97.

2. S. C. Kaufman, G. P. Gross, and G. L. Kennedy, "Thyroid Hormone Use: Trends in the United States from 1960 through 1988," *Thyroid* 1 (1991): 285–91.

3. R. T. Joffe, S. T. H. Sokolov, and W. Singer, "Thyroid Hormone Treatment of Depression," *Thyroid* 5, no. 3 (1995): 235–39.

4. A. Baumgartner, M. Eravci, G. Pinna, et al., "Thyroid Hormone Metabolism in the Rat Brain in an Animal Model of 'Behavioral Dependence' on Ethanol," *Neuroscience Letters* 227 (1997): 25–28.

5. P. Hauser, A. J. Zametkin, P. Martinez, et al., "Attention Deficit–Hyperactivity Disorder in People with Generalized Resistance to Thyroid Hormone," *New England Journal of Medicine* 328 no. 14 (1993): 997–1001.

6. T. Takeda, S. Suzuki, R-T. Liu, et al., "Triiodothyroacetic Acid Has Unique Potential for Therapy of Resistance to Thyroid Hormone," *Journal of Clinical Endocrinology and Metabolism* 80, no. 7 (1995): 2033–40.

7. B. Rozanov and M. B. Dratman, "Immunohistochemical Mapping of Brain Triiodothyronine Reveals Prominent Localization in Ventral Noradrenergic Systems," *Neuroscience* 74 no. 3 (1996): 897–915

8. J. A. Hatterer, J. Herbert, C. Hidaka, et al., "Transthyretin in Patients with Depression," *American Journal of Psychiatry* 150 (1993): 813–15.

9. C. Kirkegaard and J. Faber, "The Role of Thyroid Hormones in Depression," *European Journal of Endocrinology* 138 (1998): 1–9.

10. S. T. H. Sokolov, A. J. Levitt, and R. T. Joffe, "Thyroid Hormone Levels before Unsuccessful Antidepressant Therapy Are Associated with Later Response to T3 Augmentation," *Psychiatry Research* 69 (1997): 203–6.

11. W. N. Henley and T. J. Koehnle, "Thyroid Hormones and the Treatment of Depression: An Examination of Basic Hormonal Actions in the Mature Mammalian Brain," *Synapse* 27 (1997): 36–44.

12. R. T. Joffe, W. Singer, A. J. Levitt, et al., "A Placebo-Controlled Comparison of Lithium and Triiodothyronine Augmentation of Tricyclic Antidepressants in Unipolar Refractory Depression," *Archives of General Psychiatry* 50 (1993): 387–93.

13. S. Gupta, P. Masand, and J. F. Tanquary, "Thyroid Hormone Supplementation of Fluoxetine in the Treatment of Major Depression," *British Journal of Psychiatry* 159 (1991): 866–67.

14. E. E. Feldmesser-Reiss, "The Application of Triiodothyronine in the Treatment of Mental Disorders," *Journal of Nervous and Mental Disease* 127 (1958): 540–46.

15. A. Campos-Barros, A. Musa, A. Flechner, et al., "Evidence for Circadian Variations of Thyroid Hormone Concentrations and Type II 5'-Iodothyronine Deiodinase Activity in the Rat Central Nervous System," *Journal of Neurochemistry* 68 (1997): 795–803.

16. E. Souetre, E. Salvati, T. A. Wher, et al., "Twenty-four-Hour Profiles of Body Temperature and Plasma TSH in Bipolar Patients during Depression and during Remission and in Normal Control Subjects," *American Journal of Psychiatry* 145, no. 9 (1988): 1133–37.

17. N. Konno and K. Morikawa, "Seasonal Variation of Serum Thyrotropin Concentration and Thyrotropin Response to Thyrotropin-Releasing Hormone in Patients with Primary Hypothyroidism on Constant Replacement Dosage of Thyroxine," *Journal of Clinical Endocrinology and Metabolism* 54 (1982): 1118–24.

18. M. S. Bauer and P. C. Whybrow, "Rapid-Cycling Bipolar Affective Disorder," part 2, "Treatment of Refractory Rapid Cycling with High-Dose Levothyroxine: A Preliminary Study," *Archives of General Psychiatry* 47 (1990): 435–40.

19. L. Gyulai, J. Jaggi, M. S. Bauer, et al., "Bone Mineral Density and L-Thyroxine Treatment in Rapidly Cycling Bipolar Disorder," *Biological Psychiatry* 41 (1997): 503–6.

20. G. S. Kurland, M. W. Hamolsky, and A. S. Freedberg, "Studies in Non-myxedematous Hypometabolism," *Journal of Clinical Endocrinology* 15 (1955): 1354–66.

21. B. O. Barnes and L. Galton, *Hypothyroidism: The Unsuspected Illness* (New York: Harper and Row, 1976).

22. B. Barnes, "Basal Temperature versus Basal Metabolism," *Journal of the American Medical Association* 119 (1942): 1072–74.

23. E. D. Wilson, *Wilson's Syndrome: The Miracle of Feeling Well* (Orlando, Fla.: Cornerstone Publishing, 1991).

CHAPTER 7:
WEIGHT, APPETITE, AND METABOLISM: THE THYROID'S ACTIONS

1. R. J. Kuczmarski, K. M. Flegal, S. M. Campbell, et al., "Increasing Prevalence of Overweight among U.S. Adults: The National Health and Nutrition Examination Surveys, 1960–1991," *Journal of the American Medical Association* 272 no. 3 (1994): 205–11.

2. J. E. Morley, "Neuropeptide Regulation of Appetite and Weight," *Endocrine Reviews* 8, no. 3 (1987): 256–87.

3. J. E. Mitchell, D. E. Laine, J. E. Morley, et al., "Naloxone but Not CCK-8 Attenuates Binge-Eating in Patients with Bulimia Syndrome," *Biological Psychiatry* 21 (1986): 1399–1406.

4. S. F. Leibowitz and G. Shor-Posner, "Brain Serotonin and Eating Behavior," *Appetite* 7, suppl. (1986): 1–14.

5. C. Hart, *Secrets of Serotonin* (New York: St. Martin's Paperbacks, 1996).

6. G. A. Bray, D. H. Ryan, D. Gordon, et al., "A Double-Blind Randomized Placebo-Controlled Trial of Sibutramine," *Obesity Research* 4 (1996): 263–70.

7. C. Hart, *Secrets of Serotonin*, 24.

8. S. R. Gambert, T. L. Garthwaite, C. M. Pontzer, et al., "Thyroid Hormone Regulation of Central Nervous System (CNS) Beta-Endorphin and ACTH," *Hormone Metabolic Research* 12 (1980): 345–46.

9. S. Z. Donhoffer and J. Vonotzky, "The Effect of Thyroxine on Food Intake and Selection," *American Journal of Physiology* 150 (1947): 334–39.

10. Z. Orban, S. R. Bornstein, and G. P. Chrousos, "The Interaction between Leptin and the Hypothalamic-Pituitary-Thyroid Axis," *Hormone Metabolic Research* 30 (1998): 231–35.

11. J. N. Loeb, "Metabolic Changes in Hypothyroidism," in *Werner and Ingbar's The Thyroid,* 6th ed., edited by Lewis E. Braverman and R. D. Utiger, 1064–71 (Philadelphia: Lippincott, 1991).

12. S. I. Sherman, P. Nadkarni, and R. Arem, "Outcomes of a Community TSH Screening Program" (abstract presented at the Seventy-ninth Annual Meeting of the Endocrine Society, Minneapolis, June 11, 1997).

13. D. Cooper, R. Halpern, L. Wood, et al., "L-Thyroxine Therapy in Subclinical Hypothyroidism," *Annals of Internal Medicine* 101 (1984): 18–24.

14. G. N. Burrow, J. K. Oppenheimer, and R. Volpe, "Graves' Disease," in *Thyroid Function and Disease,* edited by Robert Volpe, 214–60 (Philadelphia: Saunders, 1990).

15. S. Jansson, G. Berg, G. Lindstedt, et al., "Overweight: A Common Problem among Women Treated for Hyperthyroidism," *Postgraduate Medical Journal* 69 (1993): 107–11.

16. F. Celsing, S. H. Westing, U. Adamson, et al., "Muscle Strength in Hyperthyroid

Patients before and after Medical Treatment," *Clinical Physiology* 10 (1990): 545–50.

17. U.S. Department of Agriculture, U.S. Department of Health and Human Services, "Nutrition and Your Health: Dietary Guidelines for Americans" (Washington, D.C.: U.S. Department of Agriculture, 1995).

CHAPTER 8:
HORMONES OF DESIRE: THE THYROID AND YOUR SEX LIFE

1. B. J. Kumar, M. L. Khurana, A. C. Ammini, et al., "Reproductive Endocrine Functions in Men with Primary Hypothyroidism: Effect of Thyroxine Replacement," *Hormone Research* 34 (1990): 215–18.

2. R. W. Hudson and A. L. Edwards, "Testicular Function in Hyperthyroidism," *Journal of Andrology* 13 (1992): 117–24.

3. C. Longcope, "The Male and Female Reproductive Systems in Hypothyroidism," in *Werner and Ingbar's The Thyroid,* 6th ed., edited by L. D. Braverman and R. D. Utiger, 1052–55 (Philadelphia: Lippincott, 1991).

4. C. Longcope, "The Male and Female Reproductive Systems in Thyrotoxicosis," in *Werner and Ingbar's The Thyroid,* 6th ed., edited by L. D. Braverman and R. D. Utiger, 828–35.

5. W. F. Bergfeld, "Androgenetic Alopecia: An Overview," Seventh Symposium on Alopecia, in *Dermatology: Capsule and Comment,* edited by H. P. Badin, 1–10 (New York: HP Publishing, 1988).

6. J. Lever and P. Schwartz, "When Sex Hurts: Finding the Causes of Your Pain during Intercourse," *Sexual Health* 1 (1997): 64–66.

7. A. J. Wright, "Lichen Sclerosus and Thyroid Disease," letter to the *Journal of Reproductive Medicine* 43 (1998): 240.

8. C. Penner and J. Penner, *The Gift of Sex: A Guide to Sexual Fulfillment* (Waco, Tex.: Word Publishing, 1981).

9. B. B. Sherwin, "Affective Changes with Estrogen and Androgen Replacement Therapy in Surgically Menopausal Women," *Journal of Affective Disorders* 14 (1988): 177–87.

CHAPTER 9:
"YOU'VE CHANGED": WHEN THE THYROID AND RELATIONSHIPS COLLIDE

1. J. Gray, *Men Are from Mars, Women Are from Venus* (New York: HarperCollins, 1992).

2. P. H. Rockey and R. J. Griep, "Behavioral Dysfunction in Hyperthyroidism," *Archives of Internal Medicine* 140 (1980): 1194–97.

CHAPTER 10:
OVERLAPPING SYMPTOMS AND SYNDROMES:
FATIGUE, CHRONIC FATIGUE, HYPOGLYCEMIA, AND FIBROMYALGIA

1. G. Lewis and S. Wessely, "The Epidemiology of Fatigue: More Questions Than Answers," *Journal of Epidemiology and Community Health* 46 (1992): 92–97.

2. K. Kroenke, D. R. Wood, A. D. Mangelsdorff, et al., "Chronic Fatigue in Primary Care: Prevalence, Patient Characteristics, and Outcome," *Journal of the American Medical Association* 260 (1988): 929–34.

3. R. C. Cuneo, F. Salomon, G. A. McGauley, et al., "The Growth Hormone Deficiency Syndrome in Adults," *Clinical Endocrinology* 37 (1992): 387–97.

4. R. M. Bennett, S. R. Clark, S. M. Campbell, et al., "Low Levels of Somatomedin C in Patients with the Fibromyalgia Syndrome: A Possible Link between Sleep and Muscle Pain," *Arthritis and Rheumatism* 35 (1992): 1113–16.

5. L. B. Krupp and D. Pollina, "Neuroimmune and Neuropsychiatric Aspects of Chronic Fatigue Syndrome," *Advances in Neuroimmunology* 6 (1996): 155–67.

6. M. B. Gonzalez, J. C. Cousins, and P. M. Doraiswamy, "Neurobiology of Chronic Fatigue Syndrome," *Progress in Neuro-Psychopharmacology and Biological Psychiatry* 20 (1996): 749–59.

7. W. K. Cho and G. H. Stollerman, "Chronic Fatigue Syndrome," *Hospital Practice* 27 (1992): 221–45.

8. S. R. Pillemer, "Identifying and Treating Fibromyalgia," *Contemporary Internal Medicine* 5, no. 12 (1993): 24–30.

9. D. Skuse, A. Albanese, R. Stanhope, et al., "A New Stress-Related Syndrome of Growth Failure and Hyperphagia in Children, Associated with Reversibility of Growth-Hormone Insufficiency," *Lancet* 348 (1996): 353–58.

10. F. Wolfe, H. A. Smythe, M. B. Yunus, et al., "The American College of Rheumatology 1990 Criteria for the Classification of Fibromyalgia: Report of the Multicenter Criteria Committee," *Arthritis and Rheumatism* 33 (1990): 160–72.

11. J. B. Shiroky, M. Cohen, M. L. Ballachey, et al., "Thyroid Dysfunction in Rheumatoid Arthritis: A Controlled Prospective Survey," *Annals of the Rheumatic Diseases* 52 (1993): 454–56.

12. J. C. Lowe, R. L. Garrison, A. Reichman, et al., "Triiodothyronine (T3) Treatment of Euthyroid Fibromyalgia: A Small-N Replication of a Double-Blind Placebo-Controlled Crossover Study," *Clinical Bulletin of Myofascial Therapy* 2, no. 4 (1997): 71–88.

13. R. M. Bennett, S. C. Clark, and J. Walczyk, "A Randomized, Double-Blind, Placebo-Controlled Study of Growth Hormone in the Treatment of Fibromyalgia," *American Journal of Medicine* 104 (1998): 227–31.

14. A. Schluderberg, S. E. Strauss, P. Peterson, et al., "NIH Conference on Chronic Fatigue Syndrome Research: Definition and Medical Outcome Assessment," *Annals of Internal Medicine* 117 (1992): 325–31.

15. D. S. Bell, "Chronic Fatigue Syndrome Update: Findings Now Point to CNS Involvement," *Postgraduate Medicine* 96, no. 6 (1994): 73–81.

16. D. W. Bates, W. Schmitt, D. Buchwald, et al., "Prevalence of Fatigue and Chronic Fatigue Syndrome in a Primary Care Practice," *Archives of Internal Medicine* 153 (1993): 2759–65.

17. S. E. Langer and J. F. Scheer, *Solved: The Riddle of Illness* (New Canaan, Conn.: Keats Publishing, 1984).

18. B. L. Farris, "Prevalence of Post–Glucose-Load Glycosuria and Hypoglycemia in a Group of Healthy Young Men," *Diabetes* 23 (1974): 189.

19. J. Yager and R. T. Young, "Nonhypoglycemia Is an Epidemic Condition," *New England Journal of Medicine* 291 (1974): 907.

20. S. E. Langer and J. F. Scheer, *Solved: The Riddle of Illness*.

CHAPTER 11:
PREMENSTRUAL SYNDROME AND MENOPAUSE: TUNING THE CYCLES

1. R. Arem and D. Escalante, "Subclinical Hypothyroidism: Epidemiology, Diagnosis, and Significance," *Advances in Internal Medicine* 41 (1996): 213–50.

2. D. I. W. Phillips, J. H. Lazarus, and B. R. Butlano, "The Influence of Pregnancy and

Reproductive Span on the Occurrence of Autoimmune Thyroiditis," *Clinical Endocrinology* 32 (1990): 301–6.

3. American Psychiatric Association, *Diagnostic and Statistical Manual of Mental Disorders,* 4th ed. (Washington, D.C.: American Psychiatric Association, 1994).

4. Columbia University College of Physicians and Surgeons, *Complete Home Guide to Mental Health* , eds. F. I. Kass et al. (New York: Henry Holt, 1995).

5. P. J. Schmidt, G. N. Grover, P. P. Roy-Byrne, et al., "Thyroid Function in Women with Premenstrual Syndrome," *Journal of Clinical Endocrinology and Metabolism* 76 (1993): 671–74.

6. N. D. Brayshaw and D. D. Brayshaw, "Thyroid Hypofunction in Premenstrual Syndrome," *The New England Journal of Medicine* 315 (1986): 1486-87.

7. P. J. Schmidt, D. Rosenfeld, K. L. Muller, et al., "A Case of Autoimmune Thyroiditis Presenting as Menstrual Related Mood Disorder," *Journal of Clinical Psychiatry* 51 (1990): 434–36.

8. A. Kadri, "Attitudes to HRT," *Practitioner* 234 (1990): 880–84.

9. C. Northrup, *Women's Bodies, Women's Wisdom* (New York: Bantam Books, 1994).

10. N. E. Avis, P. A. Kaufert, M. Lock, et al., "The Evolution of Menopausal Symptoms," *Balliere's Clinical Endocrinology and Metabolism* 7 (1993): 17–32.

11. D. J. Cooke and J. G. Green, "Types of Life Events in Relation to Symptoms at the Climacterium," *Journal of Psychosomatic Research* 25 (1981): 5–11.

12. A. Holte and A. Mikkelson, "Psychosocial Determinants of Menopausal Complaints," *Maturitas* 13 (1991): 193–203.

13. M. S. Hunter, "The SE England Longitudinal Study of the Climacteric and Postmenopause," *Maturitas* 14, no. 2 (1992): 117–26.

14. P. A. Kaufert, P. Gilbert, and R. Tate, "The Manitoba Project: A Reexamination of the Link between Menopause and Depression," *Maturitas* 14, no. 2 (1992): 143–56.

CHAPTER 12:
INFERTILITY AND MISCARRIAGE: IS YOUR THYROID A FACTOR?

1. L. P. Salzer, *Surviving Infertility* (New York: Harper Perennial, 1991).

2. E. Erickson, *Childhood and Society* (New York: Norton, 1950).

3. I. Gerhard, T. Becker, W. Eggert-Kruse, et al., "Thyroid and Ovarian Function in Infertile Women," *Human Reproduction* 6 (1991): 338–45.

4. I. Gerhard, W. Eggert-Kruse, K. Merzoug, et al., "Thyrotropin-Releasing Hormone (TRH) and Metoclopramide Testing in Infertile Women," *Gynecological Endocrinology* 5, no. 1 (1991): 15–32.

5. T. Maruo, K. Katayama, H. Matuso, et al., "Maintaining Early Pregnancy in Threatened Abortion," *Acta Endocrinologica* 127 (1992): 118–22.

6. A. Singh, Z. N. Dantas, S. C. Stone, et al., "Presence of Thyroid Antibodies in Early Reproductive Failure: Biochemical versus Clinical Pregnancies," *Fertility and Sterility* 63, no. 2 (1995): 277–81.

7. D. Glinoer, "The Regulation of Thyroid Function in Pregnancy: Pathways of Endocrine Adaptation from Physiology to Pathology," *Endocrine Reviews* 18, no. 3 (1997): 404–33.

8. A. S. Leung, L. K. Millar, P. P. Koonings, et al., "Perinatal Outcome in Hypothyroid Pregnancies," *Obstetrics and Gynecology* 81, no. 3 (1993): 349–53.

CHAPTER 13:
POSTPARTUM DEPRESSION: THE HORMONAL LINK

1. Columbia University College of Physicians and Surgeons, *Complete Home Guide to Mental Health*, ed. F. I. Kass et al. (New York: Henry Holt, 1995).

2. J. E. D. Esquirol, *Des maladies mentales considerées sous les rapports médical, hygiénique et médico-légal,* vol. 1 (Paris: J. B. Bailliere, 1838).

3. I. F. Brockington and R. Kumar, eds., *Motherhood and Mental Illness* (London: Academic Press, 1982).

4. B. Harris, S. Othman, J. A. Davies, et al., "Association between Postpartum Thyroid Dysfunction and Thyroid Antibodies and Depression," *British Medical Journal* 305, no. 6846 (1992): 152–56.

5. V. J. M. Pop, H. A. M. deRooy, H. L. Vader, et al., "Microsomal Antibodies during Gestation in Relation to Postpartum Thyroid Dysfunction and Depression," *Acta Endocrinologica* 129 (1993): 26–30.

6. M. T. Vargas, R. Broines-Urbina, D. Gladman, et al., "Antithryoid Microsomal Autoantibodies and HLA-DR5 Are Associated with Postpartum Thyroid Dysfunction: Evidence Supporting an Autoimmune Pathogenesis," *Journal of Clinical Endocrinology and Metabolism* 67 (1988): 327–33.

7. J. A. Hamilton and P. N. Harberger, eds., *Postpartum Psychiatric Illness: A Picture Puzzle* (Philadelphia: University of Pennsylvania Press, 1992).

8. W. M. Ord, "Report of a Committee of the Clinical Society of London, Nominated December 14, 1883, to Investigate the Subject of Myxoedema," *Transactions of the Clinical Society of London* (suppl.) 21, no. 18 (1888).

9. H. C. Gerstein, "How Common Is Postpartum Thyroiditis? A Methodologic Overview of the Literature," *Archives of Internal Medicine* 150 (1990): 1397–1400.

10. T. F. Nikolai, S. L. Turney, and R. C. Roberts, "Postpartum Lymphocytic Thyroiditis: Prevalence, Clinical Course, and Long-Term Follow-up," *Archives of Internal Medicine* 147 (1987): 221–24.

11. S. Othman, D. I. W. Phillips, A. B. Parkes, et al., "A Long-Term Follow-up of Postpartum Thyroiditis," *Clinical Endocrinology* 32 (1990): 559–64.

12. C. C. Hayslip, H. G. Fein, V. M. O'Donnell, et al., "The Value of Serum Antimicrosomal Antibody Testing in Screening for Symptomatic Postpartum Thyroid Dysfunction," *American Journal of Obstetrics and Gynecology* 159 (1988): 203–9.

13. D. E. Stewart, A. M. Addison, G. E. Robinson, et al., "Thyroid Function in Psychosis following Childbirth," *American Journal of Psychiatry* 145, no. 12 (1988): 1579–81.

CHAPTER 14:
WHAT YOU NEED TO KNOW ABOUT THYROID TESTS

1. D. S. Ross, G. H. Daniels, and D. Gouveia, "The Use and Limitations of a Chemiluminescent Thyrotropin Assay as a Single Thyroid Function Test in an Outpatient Endocrine Clinic," *Journal of Clinical Endocrinology and Metabolism* 71, no. 3 (1990): 764–69.

2. K. W. Geul, I. L. L. van Sluisveld, D. E. Grobbee, et al., "The Importance of Thyroid Microsomal Antibodies in the Development of Elevated Serum TSH in Middle-Aged Women: Associations with Serum Lipids," *Clinical Endocrinology* 39 (1993): 275–80.

3. G. Michalopoulou, M. Alevizaki, G. Piperingos, et al., "High Serum Cholesterol Levels in Persons with 'High-Normal' TSH Levels: Should One Extend the

Definition of Subclinical Hypothyroidism?" *European Journal of Endocrinology* 138, no. 2 (1998): 141–45.

4. R. Arem and D. Escalante, "Subclinical Hypothyroidism: Epidemiology, Diagnosis, and Significance," *Advances in Internal Medicine* 41 (1996): 213–50.

5. J. G. Eales, "Iodine Metabolism and Thyroid-Related Functions in Organisms Lacking Thyroid Follicles: Are Thyroid Hormones Also Vitamins?" *Proceedings Society for Experimental Biology and Medicine* 214 (1997): 302–17.

6. G. R. B. Skinner, R. Thomas, M. Taylor, et al., "Thyroxine Should Be Tried in Clinically Hypothyroid but Biochemically Euthyroid Patients," *British Medical Journal* 314 (1997): 1764.

7. L. Wartofsky, "The Scope and Impact of Thyroid Disease," *Clinical Chemistry* 42 (1996): 121–24.

8. M-F. Poirier, H. Lôo, A. Galinowski, et al., "Sensitive Assay of Thyroid-Stimulating Hormone in Depressed Patients," *Psychiatry Research* 57 (1995): 41–48.

9. R. A. Dickey and H. W. Rodbard, "American Association of Clinical Endocrinologists 'Neck Check' Promoted during Thyroid Awareness Month," *First Messenger* 5, no. 1 (1997): 1.

10. S. Morita, T. Arima, and M. Matsuda, "Prevalence of Nonthyroid Specific Autoantibodies in Autoimmune Thyroid Diseases," *Journal of Clinical Endocrinology and Metabolism* 80, no. 4 (1995): 1203–6.

11. B. Lindberg, U-B. Ericsson, R. Ljung, et al., "High Prevalence of Thyroid Autoantibodies at Diagnosis of Insulin-Dependent Diabetes Mellitus in Swedish Children," *Journal of Laboratory and Clinical Medicine* 130 (1997): 585–89.

12. J. Heward and S. C. L. Gough, "Genetic Susceptibility to the Development of Autoimmune Disease," *Clinical Science* 93 (1997): 479–91.

13. M. S. Rosenthal, *The Thyroid Source Book: Everything You Need to Know*, 2d ed. (Los Angeles: Lowell House, 1996), 57.

14. P. F. Peerboom, E. A. M. Hassink, R. Melkert, et al., "Thyroid Function 10–18 Years after Mantle Field Irradiation for Hodgkin's Disease," *European Journal of Cancer* 28A, no. 10 (1992): 1716–18.

15. A. Leznoff and G. L. Sussman, "Syndrome of Idiopathic Chronic Urticaria and Angioedema with Thyroid Autoimmunity: A Study of 90 Patients," *Journal of Allergy and Clinical Immunology* 84, no. 1 (1989): 66–71.

16. L. C. Hofbauer, C. Spitzweg, S. Schmauss, et al., "Graves' Disease Associated with Autoimmune Thrombocytopenic Purpura," *Archives of Internal Medicine* 157 (1997): 1033–36.

17. A. Pinchera, E. Martino, and G. Faglia, "Central Hypothyroidism," in *Werner and Ingbar's The Thyroid*, 6th ed., edited by Lewis E. Braverman and R. D. Utiger, 968–84 (Philadelphia: Lippincott, 1991).

18. M. Mori, Y. Shoda, M. Yamada, et al., "Case Report: Central Hypothyroidism Due to Isolated TRH Deficiency in a Depressive Man," *Journal of Internal Medicine* 229 (1991): 285–88.

CHAPTER 15: TREATING THE IMBALANCE

1. U. M. Kabadi, "Optimal Daily Levothyroxine Dose in Primary Hypothyroidism: Its Relation to Pretreatment Thyroid Hormone Indexes," *Archives of Internal Medicine* 149 (1989): 2209–12.

2. M. I. Surks, "Treatment of Hypothyroidism," in *Werner and Ingbar's The Thyroid*,

6th ed., edited by Lewis E. Braverman and R. D. Utiger, 1099–1103 (Philadelphia: Lippincott, 1991).

3. E. Roti, R. Minelli, and E. Gardini, "The Use and Misuse of Thyroid Hormone," *Endocrine Reviews* 14, no. 4 (1993): 401–23.

4. P. C. Whybrow, "Behavioral and Psychiatric Aspects of Hypothyroidism," in *Werner and Ingbar's The Thyroid,* 1078–83.

5. D. S. Ross, G. H. Daniels, and D. Gouvela, "The Use and Limitations of a Chemiluminescent Thyrotropin Assay as a Single Thyroid Function Test in an Outpatient Endocrine Clinic," *Journal of Clinical Endocrinology and Metabolism* 71, no. 3 (1990): 764–69.

6. B. Biondi, S. Fazio, A. Cuocolo, et al., "Impaired Cardiac Reserve and Exercise Capacity in Patients Receiving Long-Term Thyrotropin Suppressive Therapy with Levothyroxine," *Journal of Clinical Endocrinology and Metabolism* 81 (1996): 4224–28.

7. B. Uzzan, J. Campos, M. Cucherat, et al., "Effects on Bone Mass of Long-Term Treatment with Thyroid Hormones: A Meta-Analysis," *Journal of Clinical Endocrinology and Metabolism* 81 (1996): 4278–89.

8. B. Scholte, B. Nowotny, L. Schaaf, et al., "Subclinical Hyperthyroidism: Physical and Mental State of Patients," *European Archives of Psychiatry and Clinical Neuroscience* 241 (1992): 357–64.

9. G. B. Anker, P. E. Lønning, A. Aakvaag, et al., "Thyroid Function in Postmenopausal Breast Cancer Patients Treated with Tamoxifen," *Scandinavian Journal of Clinical Laboratory Investigation* 58 (1998): 103–7.

10. E. Lesho and R. E. Jones, "Hypothyroid Graves' Disease," *Southern Medical Journal* 90, no. 12 (1997): 1201–3.

11. N. Takasu, T. Yamada, A. Sato, et al., "Graves' Disease following Hypothyroidism Due to Hashimoto's Disease: Studies of Eight Cases," *Clinical Endocrinology* 33 (1990): 687–89.

12. R. Comtois, L. Faucher, and L. Lafleche, "Outcome of Hypothyroidism Caused by Hashimoto's Thyroiditis," *Archives of Internal Medicine* 155 (1995): 1404–8.

13. A. H. Saliby, C. Larosa, R. Rachid, et al., "Changes in Levothyroxine Dose Requirements in the Follow-up of Patients with Primary Hypothyroidism" (abstract presented at the Sixty-ninth Annual Meeting of the American Thyroid Association, November 13, 1996).

14. R. Arem, "When to Choose Radioactive Iodine, Drugs, or Surgery," *Consultant* 28, no. 9 (January 1989): 21–35.

15. J. A. Franklyn, "The Management of Hyperthyroidism," *New England Journal of Medicine* 330, no. 24 (1994): 1731–38.

16. N. L. Gittoes and J. A. Franklyn, "Hyperthyroidism: Current Treatment Guidelines," *Drugs* 55, no. 4 (1998): 543–53.

17. J. M. H. Deklerk, J. W. Van Isselt, A. Van Dijk, et al., "Iodine-131 Therapy in Sporadic Nontoxic Goiter," *Journal of Nuclear Medicine* 38, no. 3 (1997): 372–76.

18. R. E. Imseis, L. Vanmiddlesworth, J. D. Massie, et al., "Pretreatment with Propylthiouracil but Not Methimazole Reduces the Therapeutic Efficacy of Iodine-131 in Hyperthyroidism," *Journal of Clinical Endocrinology and Metabolism* 83, no. 2 (1998): 685–87.

19. R. A. Hegele and R. Volpe, "Relapse of Graves' Disease 23 Years after Treatment

with Radioactive Iodine (131I)," *Journal of Clinical and Laboratory Immunology* 18 (1985): 103–5.

20. J. A. Franklyn, P. Maisonneuve, M. C. Sheppard, et al., "Mortality after the Treatment of Hyperthyroidism with Radioactive Iodine," *New England Journal of Medicine* 338, no. 11 (1998): 712–18.

21. L. E. Holm, P. Hall, K. Wiklund, et al., "Cancer Risk after Iodine-131 Therapy for Hyperthyroidism," *Journal of the National Cancer Institute* 83 (1991): 1072–77.

22. S. T. Tietgens and M. C. Leinung, "Thyroid Storm," *Medical Clinics of North America* 79, no. 1 (1995): 169–84.

23. M. T. Gladwin and P. B. Duell, "Inappropriate Thyroid Gland Ablation in Patients with Generalized Resistance to Thyroid Hormone," *Archives of Internal Medicine* 156, no. 8 (1996): 106–9.

24. M. A. Emanuele, M. H. Brooks, D. L. Gordon, et al., "Agoraphobia and Hyperthyroidism," *American Journal of Medicine* 86 (1989): 484–86.

25. S. Benvenga, "Benzodiazepine and Remission of Graves' Disease," *Thyroid* 6, no. 6 (1996): 659–60.

26. J. H. Lazarus, "Antithyroid Drug Treatment," *Clinical Endocrinology* 45 (1996): 517–18.

27. A. Toft, "Transient Hypothyroidism," *Clinical Endocrinology* 46 (1997): 7–8.

28. D. Glinoer, "The Regulation of Thyroid Function in Pregnancy: Pathways of Endocrine Adaptation from Physiology to Pathology," *Endocrine Reviews* 18, no. 3 (1997): 404–33.

29. T. Maruo, K. Katayama, H. Matuso, et al., "Maintaining Early Pregnancy in Threatened Abortion," *Acta Endocrinologica* 127 (1992): 118–22.

30. E. Roti, S. Minelli, and M. Salvi, "Management of Hyperthyroidism and Hypothyroidism in the Pregnant Woman," *Journal of Clinical Endocrinology and Metabolism* 81, no. 5 (1996): 1679–82.

CHAPTER 16:
CURING THE LINGERING EFFECTS OF THYROID IMBALANCE

1. H. Leigh, "Cerebral Effects of Endocrine Disease," in *Principles and Practice of Endocrinology and Metabolism,* 2d ed., edited by K. L. Becker et al. (Philadelphia: Lippincott, 1995), 1695.

2. P. C. Whybrow, "Behavioral and Psychiatric Aspects of Hypothyroidism," in *Werner and Ingbar's The Thyroid,* 6th ed., edited by Lewis E. Braverman and R. D. Utiger, 1078–83 (Philadelphia: Lippincott, 1991).

3. R. A. Stern, B. Robinson, A. R. Thorner, et al., "A Survey Study of Neuropsychiatric Complaints in Patients with Graves' Disease," *Journal of Neuropsychiatry and Clinical Neurosciences* 8 (1996): 181–85.

4. M. Bommer, T. Eversmann, R. Pickardt, et al., "Psychopathological and Neuropsychological Symptoms in Patients with Subclinical and Remitted Hyperthyroidism," *Klinische Wochenschrift* 68 (1990): 552–58.

5. P. Thygesen, K. Hermann, and R. Willanger, "Concentration Camp in Denmark: Persecution, Disease, Disability, Compensation. A 23-Year Follow-Up. A Survey of the Long-Term Effect of Severe Environmental Stress," *Danish Medical Bulletin* 17 (1970): 65–108.

6. S. A. Green, "Office Psychotherapy for Depression in the Primary Care Setting," *The American Journal of Medicine* 101, no. 6A, suppl. (1996): 37–44.

7. I. Elkin, M. Shea, J. Warkins, et al., "National Institute of Mental Health Treatment

of Depression: Collaborative Research Program: General Effectiveness of Treatments," *Archives of General Psychiatry* 46 (1989): 971–83.

8. M. Mennemeier, R. D. Garner, and K. M. Heilman, "Memory, Mood, and Measurement in Hypothyroidism," *Journal of Clinical and Experimental Neuropsychology* 15, no. 5 (1993): 822–31.

9. H. Perrild, J. M. Hansen, K. Arnung, et al., "Intellectual Impairment after Hyperthyroidism," *Acta Endocrinologica* 112 (1986): 185–91.

10. L. S. Chia, J. E. Thompson, and M. A. Moscarello, "Changes in Lipid Phase Behaviour in Human Myelin during Maturation and Aging," letter to *Federation of European Biochemical Societies* 157 (1983): 155–58.

11. J. M. Pasquini and A. M. Adamo, "Thyroid Hormones and the Central Nervous System," *Developmental Neuroscience* 16 (1994): 1–8.

12. L. A. Videla, T. Sir, and C. Wolff, "Increased Lipid Peroxidation in Hyperthyroid Patients: Suppression by Propylthiouracil Treatment," *Free Radical Research Communications* 5 (1988): 1–8.

13. J. Bernal and J. Nunez, "Thyroid Hormones and Brain Development," *European Journal of Endocrinology* 133 (1995): 390–98.

14. I. Skoog, L. Nilsson, B. Palmertz, et al., "A Population-Based Study of Dementia in 85-Year-Olds," *New England Journal of Medicine* 328 (1993): 153–58.

15. J. S. Meyer, B. W. Judd, T. Tawakina, et al., "Improved Cognition after Control of Risk Factors for Multi-Infarct Dementia," *Journal of the American Medical Association* 256 (1986): 2203–9.

16. N. Pancharuniti, C. A. Lewish, H. E. Sauberlich, et al., "Plasma Homocysteine, Folate, and Vitamin B_{12} Concentrations and Risk for Early Onset Coronary Artery Disease," *American Journal of Clinical Nutrition* 59 (1994): 940–48.

17. P. A. Bastenie, L. Van Haelst, M. Bonnyns, et al., "Preclinical Hypothyroidism: A Risk Factor for Coronary Heart Disease," *Lancet* 1 (1971): 203–4.

18. M. Singh, E. M. Meyer, W. J. Millard, et al., "Ovarian Steroid Deprivation Results in a Reversible Learning Impairment and Compromised Cholinergic Function in Female Sprague-Dawley Rats," *Brain Research* 644 (1994): 305–12.

19. L. S. Schneider, M. R. Farlow, V. W. Henderson, et al., "Effects of Estrogen Replacement Therapy on Response to Tacrine in Patients with Alzheimer's Disease," *Neurology* 46 (1996): 1580–84.

20. B. B. Sherwin, "Estrogen and/or Androgen Replacement Therapy and Cognitive Functioning in Surgically Menopausal Women," *Psychoneuroendocrinology* 13 (1988): 345–57.

21. S. R. Lindheim, R. S. Legro, L. Bernstein, et al., "Behavioral Stress Responses in Premenopausal and Postmenopausal Women and the Effects of Estrogen," *American Journal of Obstetrics and Gynecology* 167 (1992): 1831–36.

22. B. B. Sherwin, "Affective Changes with Estrogen and Androgen Replacement Therapy in Surgically Menopausal Women," *Journal of Affective Disorders* 14 (1988): 177–87.

23. M. M. Rice, A. B. Graves, and E. B. Larson, "Estrogen Replacement Therapy and Cognition: Role of Phytoestrogens," abstract, *Gerontologist* 35, special issue 1 (1995): 169.

24. M. Holzbauer and M. B. Youdim, "The Oestrous Cycle and Monoamine Oxidase Activity," *British Journal of Pharmacology* 48 (1973): 600–8.

CHAPTER 17:

THE NEW T4/T3 PROTOCOL: "IT MADE ME FEEL BETTER ALL OVER"

1. M. I. Surks, "Treatment of Hypothyroidism," in *Werner and Ingbar's The Thyroid,* 6th ed., edited by Lewis E. Braverman and R. D. Utiger, 1099–1103 (Philadelphia: Lippincott, 1991).

2. R. W. Rees-Jones and P. R. Larsen, "Triiodothyronine and Thyroxine Content of Desiccated Thyroid Tablets," *Metabolism* 26 (1977): 1213–18.

3. S. C. Kaufman, G. P. Gross, and G. L. Kennedy, "Thyroid Hormone Use: Trends in the United States from 1960 through 1988," *Thyroid* 1 (1991): 285–91.

4. J. C. Lowe, R. L. Garrison, A. Reichman, et al., "Triiodothyronine (T3) Treatment of Euthyroid Fibromyalgia: A Small-*N* Replication of a Double-Blind Placebo-Controlled Crossover Study," *Clinical Bulletin of Myofascial Therapy* 2, no. 4 (1997): 71–88.

5. J. C. Lowe, "Results of an Open Trial of T3 Therapy with 77 Euthyroid Female Fibromyalgia Patients," *Clinical Bulletin of Myofascial Therapy* 2, no. 1 (1997): 35–37.

CHAPTER 18:

LIVING A THYROID-FRIENDLY LIFE: HEALTHFUL CHOICES DAY BY DAY

1. W. J. W. Morrow, J. Homsy, and J. A. Levy, "The Influence of Nutrition on Experimental Autoimmune Disease," in *Nutrient Modulation of the Immune Response,* edited by S. Cunningham-Rundles, 153–67 (New York: Dekker, 1993).

2. H. L. Steward, M. C. Bethea, S. S. Andrews, et al., *Sugar Busters!: Cut Sugar to Trim Fat* (New York: Ballantine Books, 1998).

3. R. Lozano, S. A. Chalew, A. A. Kowarski, "Cornstarch Ingestion after Oral Glucose Loading: Effect on Glucose Concentrations, Hormone Response, and Symptoms in Patients with Postprandial Hypoglycemic Syndrome," *American Journal of Clinical Nutrition* 52 (1990): 667–70.

4. V. E. Kelley, A. Ferretti, S. Izui, et al., "A Fish Oil Diet Rich in Eicosapentaenoic Acid Reduces Cyclooxygenase Metabolites and Suppresses Lupus in MRL/1pr Mice," *Journal of Immunology* 134 (1985): 1914–19.

5. S. Iossa, M. P. Mollica, L. Lionetti, et al., "Effect of a High-Fat Diet on Energy Balance and Thermic Effect of Food in Hypothyroid Rats," *European Journal of Endocrinology* 136 (1997): 309–15.

6. M. J. Müller, "Thyroid Hormones and Energy and Fat Balance," *European Journal of Endocrinology* 136 (1997): 267–68.

7. V. Kamat, W. L. Hecht, and R. T. Rubin, "Influence of Meal Composition on the Postprandial Response of the Pituitary-Thyroid Axis," *European Journal of Endocrinology* 133 (1995): 75–79.

8. B. D'Avanzo, E. Ron, C. La Vecchia, et al., "Selected Micronutrient Intake and Thyroid Carcinoma Risk," *Cancer* 79 (1997): 2186–92.

9. B. Contempre, J. E. Dumont, J. F. Denef, et al., "Effects of Selenium Deficiency on Thyroid Necrosis, Fibrosis, and Proliferation: A Possible Role in Myxoedematous Cretinism," *European Journal of Endocrinology* 133 (1995): 99–109.

10. G. M. Reid and H. Tervit, "Sudden Infant Death Syndrome and Placental Disorders: The Thyroid-Selenium Link," *Medical Hypotheses* 48 (1997): 317–24.

11. R. B. Gillie, "Endemic Goitre," *Scientific American* 22 (1978): 213–19.

12. F. Licastro, E. Mocchenegiani, M. Zannotti, et al., "Zinc Affects the Metabolism of Thyroid Hormones in Children with Down's Syndrome: Normalisation of Thyroid-Stimulating Hormone and of Reverse Triiodothyronine Plasmic Levels by Dietary Zinc Supplementation," *International Journal of Neuroscience* 65 (1992): 259–68.

13. R. P. Gupta, P. C. Verma, and S. L. Garg, "Effect of Experimental Zinc Deficiency on Thyroid Gland in Guinea Pigs," *Annals of Nutrition and Metabolism* 41 (1997): 376–81.

14. G. Di Martino, M. G. Matera, B. De Martino, et al., "Relationship between Zinc and Obesity," *Journal of Medicine* 24 (1993): 177–83.

15. O. Olivieri, D. Girelli, M. Azzini, et al., "Low Selenium Status in the Elderly Influences Thyroid Hormones," *Clinical Science* 89 (1995): 637–42.

16. J. F. Bach, "The Multi-Faceted Zinc Dependency of the Immune System," *Immunology Today* 2 (1981): 225–27.

17. M. J. Berry and P. R. Larsen, "The Role of Selenium in Thyroid Hormone Action," *Endocrine Reviews* 13 (1992): 207–19.

18. K. Asayama and K. Kato, "Oxidative Muscular Injury and Its Relevance to Hyperthyroidism," *Free Radical Biology and Medicine* 8 (1990): 293–303.

19. M. D. Edden and M. S. Torre, "Physician's Guide to Herbs," *Practical Diabetology* 16, no. 1 (1997): 10–20.

20. M. Auf'mkolk, J. C. Ingbar, K. Kubota, et al., "Extracts and Auto-Oxidized Constituents of Certain Plants Inhibit the Receptor-Binding and the Biological Activity of Graves' Immunoglobulins," *Endocrinology* 116, no. 5 (1985): 1687–93.

21. J. G. Eales, "Iodine Metabolism and Thyroid-Related Functions in Organisms Lacking Thyroid Follicles: Are Thyroid Hormones Also Vitamins?" *Proceedings Society for Experimental Biology and Medicine* 214 (1997): 302–17.

22. N. R. Rose, A. M. Saboori, L. Rasooly, et al., "The Role of Iodine in Autoimmune Thyroiditis," *Clinical Reviews in Immunology* 17 (1997): 511–17.

23. H. R. Harach and E. D. Williams, "Thyroid Cancer and Thyroiditis in the Goitrous Region of Salta, Argentina, before and after Iodine Prophylaxis," *Clinical Endocrinology* 43 (1995): 701–6.

24. J. Kabat-Zinn, *Full Catastrophe Living: Using the Wisdom of Your Body and Mind to Face Stress, Pain, and Illness* (New York: Dell, 1990).

25. D. R. Brown, Y. Wang, A. Ward, et al., "Chronic Psychological Effects of Exercise and Exercise Plus Cognitive Strategies," *Medicine and Science in Sports and Exercise* 27, no. 5 (1995): 765–75.

26. C. C. Chow and C. S. Cockram, "Thyroid Disorders Induced by Lithium and Amiodarone: An Overview," *Adverse Drug Reactions and Acute Poisoning Reviews* 9, no. 4 (1990): 207–22.

27. K. C. McCowen, J. R. Garber, and R. Spark, "Elevated Serum Thyrotropin in Thyroxine-Treated Patients with Hypothyroidism Given Sertraline," letter to *New England Journal of Medicine* 337, no. 14 (1997): 1010-11.

28. R. D. Utiger, "Effects of Smoking on Thyroid Function," *European Journal of Endocrinology* 138 (1998): 368–69.

29. G. D. Braunstein, R. Koblin, M. Sugawara, et al., "Unintentional Thyrotoxicosis Factitia Due to a Diet Pill," *Western Journal of Medicine* 145 (1986): 388–91.

30. F. Ohno and K. Miyoshi, "Clinical Observations on Thyreoidismus Medicamentosus Due to Weight-Reducing Pills in Japan," *Endocrinologica Japonica* 18 (1971): 321–23.

CHAPTER 19:
LIVING WITH THYROID EYE DISEASE

1. C. A. Gorman, R. S. Bahn, and J. A. Garrity, "Ophthalmopathy," in *Werner and Ingbar's The Thyroid,* 6th ed., edited by L. E. Braverman and R. D. Utiger, 657–76 (Philadelphia: Lippincott, 1991).

2. B. J. Major, B. E. Busuttil, and A. G. Frauman, "Graves' Ophthalmopathy: Pathogenesis

and Clinical Implications," *Australian and New Zealand Journal of Medicine* 28 (1998): 39–45.

3. D. L. Kendler, J. Lippa, and J. Rootman, "The Initial Clinical Characteristics of Graves' Orbitopathy Vary with Age and Sex," *Archives of Ophthalmology* 111 (1993): 197–201.

4. L. Tallstedt, G. Lundell, O. Tørring, et al., "Occurrence of Ophthalmopathy after Treatment of Graves' Hyperthyroidism," *New England Journal of Medicine* 326 (1992): 1733–38.

5. B. Bush, *Barbara Bush: A Memoir* (New York: St. Martin's Paperbacks, 1994).

6. P. Perros, A. L. Cromble, P. Kendall-Taylor, "Natural History of Thyroid-Associated Ophthalmopathy," *Clinical Endocrinology* 42 (1995): 45–50.

7. R. S. Bahn, "Assessment and Management of the Patient with Graves' Ophthalmopathy," *Endocrine Practice* 1, no. 3 (1995): 172–78.

8. I. B. Hales and F. F. Rundle, "Ocular Changes in Graves' Disease: A Long-Term Follow-up Study," *Quarterly Journal of Medicine* 29 (1960): 113–26.

9. G. B. Bartley, V. Fatourechi, E. F. Kadrmas, et al., "The Treatment of Graves' Ophthalmopathy in an Incidence Cohort," *American Journal of Ophthalmology* 121 (1996): 200–6.

10. I. A. Petersen, J. P. Kriss, I. R. McDougall, et al., "Prognostic Factors in the Radiotherapy of Graves' Ophthalmopathy," *International Journal of Radiation Oncology/Biology/Physics* 19 (1990): 259–64.

11. M. F. Prummel, W. M. Wiersinga, M. Mourits, et al., "Effect of Abnormal Thyroid Function on the Severity of Graves' Ophthalmopathy," *Archives of Internal Medicine* 150 (1990): 1098–1101.

12. L. Bartalena, C. Marocci, F. Bogazzi, et al., "Use of Corticosteroids to Prevent Progression of Graves' Ophthalmopathy after Radioiodine Therapy for Hyperthyroidism," *New England Journal of Medicine* 321 (1989): 1349–52.

13. N. Sonino, M. E. Girelli, M. Boscaro, et al., "Life Events in the Pathogenesis of Graves' Disease," *Acta Endocrinologica* 128 (1993): 293–96.

14. B. Shine, P. Fells, O. M. Edwards, et al., "Association between Graves' Ophthalmopathy and Smoking," *Lancet* 335 (1990): 1261–63.

CHAPTER 20:
THYROID CANCER: CURABLE BUT ANGUISHING

1. T. Zheng, T. R. Holford, Y. Chen, et al., "Time Trend and Age-Period-Cohort Effect on Incidence of Thyroid Cancer in Connecticut, 1935–1992," *International Journal of Cancer* 67 (1996): 504–9.

2. B. L. Solomon, L. Wartofsky, and K. D. Burman, "Current Trends in the Management of Well-Differentiated Papillary Thyroid Carcinoma," *Journal of Clinical Endocrinology and Metabolism* 81 (1996): 333–39.

3. R. L. Rossi, B. Cady, and M. L. Silverman, "Surgically Incurable Well-Differentiated Thyroid Carcinoma: Prognostic Factors and Results of Therapy," *Archives of Surgery* 123 (1988): 569–74.

4. D. Zimmerman, I. D. Hay, and I. R. Gough, "Papillary Thyroid Carcinoma in Children and Adults: Long-Term Follow-up of 1,039 Patients Conservatively Treated at One Institution during Three Decades," *Surgery* 104 (1988): 1157–66.

5. A. Schindler, G. Van Melle, B. Evequoz, et al., "Prognostic Factors in Papillary Carcinoma of the Thyroid," *Cancer* 68 (1991): 324–30.

6. D. P. Aiello and A. Manni, "Thyroglobulin Measurements vs. Iodine 131 Total-Body

Scan for Follow-up of Well-Differentiated Thyroid Cancer," *Archives of Internal Medicine* 150 (1990): 437–39.

7. A. Brander, P. Viikinkoski, J. Nickels, et al., "Thyroid Gland: U.S. Screening in a Random Adult Population," *Radiology* 181 (1991): 683–87.

8. F. S. Greenspan, "The Role of Fine-Needle Aspiration Biopsy in the Management of Palpable Thyroid Nodules," *Pathology Patterns* 108, no. 4, suppl. (1997): S26–S30.

9. M. Boignon and D. Moyer, "Solitary Thyroid Nodules: Separating Benign from Malignant Conditions," *Postgraduate Medicine* 98, no. 2 (1995): 73–80.

10. R. M. Tuttle, H. Lemar, and H. B. Burch, "Clinical Features Associated with an Increased Risk of Thyroid Malignancy in Patients with Follicular Neoplasia by Fine-Needle Aspiration," *Thyroid* 8, no. 5 (1998): 377–83.

11. E. Papini, L. Petrucci, R. Guglielmi, et al., "Long-Term Changes in Nodular Goiter: A 5-Year Prospective Randomized Trial of Levothyroxine Suppressive Therapy for Benign Cold Thyroid Nodules," *Journal of Clinical Endocrinology and Metabolism* 83 (1998): 780–83.

12. A. E. Schwartz, O. H. Clark, P. Ituarte, et al., "Therapeutic Controversy: Thyroid Surgery—The Choice," *Journal of Clinical Endocrinology and Metabolism* 83, no. 4 (1998): 1097–1105.

13. L. A. Burmeister, R. P. du Cret, and C. N. Mariash, "Local Reactions to Radioiodine in the Treatment of Thyroid Cancer," *American Journal of Medicine* 90 (1991): 217–22.

14. P. W. Ladenson, L. E. Braverman, E. L. Mazzaferri, et al., "Comparison of Administration of Recombinant Human Thyrotropin with Withdrawal of Thyroid Hormone for Radioactive Iodine Scanning in Patients with Thyroid Carcinoma," *New England Journal of Medicine* 337, no. 13 (1997): 888–96.

15. J. D. Pineda, T. Lee, K. Ain, et al., "Iodine-131 Therapy for Thyroid Cancer Patients with Elevated Thyroglobulin and Negative Diagnostic Scan," *Journal of Clinical Endocrinology and Metabolism* 80 (1995): 1488–92.

16. P. Hall, L. E. Holm, G. Lundell, et al., "Cancer Risks in Thyroid Cancer Patients," *British Journal of Cancer* 64 (1991): 159–63.

CHAPTER 21:
EIGHT STEPS FOR THE FUTURE:
HOW TO PROMOTE A BETTER UNDERSTANDING OF THYROID, MIND, AND MOOD

1. S. I. Sherman, P. Nadkarni, and R. Arem, "Outcomes of a Community TSH Screening Program" (abstract presented at the Seventy-ninth Annual Meeting of the Endocrine Society, Minneapolis, June 11, 1997).

2. M. D. Danese, N. R. Powe, C. T. Sawin, et al., "Screening for Mild Thyroid Failure at the Periodic Health Examination: A Decision and Cost-Effectiveness Analysis," *Journal of the American Medical Association* 276 (1996): 285–92.

3. L. H. Fish, "The Role of the Endocrinologist in Patient Care: Indications for Specialty Consultations and Management," *Endocrine News* 20, no. 2 (1995): 3.

4. L. Wartofsky, "The Scope and Impact of Thyroid Disease," *Clinical Chemistry* 42 (1996): 121–24.

RESOURCES

SUGGESTED BOOKS ON THYROID DISORDERS

Baskin, H. Jack, M.D. *How Your Thyroid Works.* 3d ed. Chicago: Adams Press, 1991.

Bayliss, R. I. S., and W. M. G. Tunbridge. *Thyroid Disease: The Facts.* New York: Oxford University Press, 1991.

Hamburger, Joel I., M.D., F.A.C.P. *The Thyroid Gland: A Book for Thyroid Patients.* 7th ed. Self-published by Joel I. Hamburger, M.D., Southfield, Michigan, 1991.

Rosenthal, M. S. *The Thyroid Source Book: Everything You Need to Know.* 2d ed. Los Angeles: Lowell House, 1996.

Rubenfeld, Sheldon, M.D. *Could It Be My Thyroid?* Self-published by Sheldon Rubenfeld, M.D., Houston, 1996.

Surks, Martin I. *The Thyroid Book: What Goes Wrong and How to Treat It.* Yonkers, N.Y.: Consumer Reports Books, 1994.

Wood, Lawrence C., M.D., F.A.C.P., and Chester Ridgway, M.D., F.A.C.P. *Your Thyroid: A Home Reference.* New York: Ballantine, 1995.

NATIONAL THYROID ORGANIZATIONS

American Foundation of Thyroid Patients
P.O. Box 820195
Houston, TX 77282-0195
Phones: (888) 996-4460 and (281) 496-4460
Fax: (281) 496-0369
Web site: www.thyroidfoundation.org

Gland Central
Web site: www.glandcentral.com

The Magic (Major Aspects of Growth in Children)
1327 North Harlem Ave.
Oak Park, IL 60302
Phone: (800) 3MAGIC3
Fax: (708) 383-0899
E-mail: Mary@magicfoundation.org
Web site: www.magicfoundation.org

National Graves' Disease Foundation
2 Tsitsi Ct.
Brevard, NC 28712
Phone: (828) 877-5251
Fax: (828) 877-5251
E-mail: ngdf@citcom.net
Web site: www.ngdf.org
Send SASE with your information request.

Thyroid Foundation of America
Ruth Sleeper Hall, RSL 350
40 Parkman St.
Boston, MA 02114-2698
Phones: (800) 832-8321 and
(617) 726-8500
Fax: (617) 726-4136
E-mail: tfa@clark.net
Web site: www.tfaweb.org/pub/tfa

Thyroid Society for Education and Research
7515 S. Main St., Suite 545
Houston, TX 77030
Phones: (800) THYROID and
(713) 799-9909
Fax: (713) 779-9919

INTERNATIONAL THYROID ORGANIZATIONS

Associazione Italiana Basedowiani e Tiroidei
c/o Centro Minerva
7 Via Mazzini
43100 Parma
Italy
Phone: 39-521-207771
Fax: 39-521-207771

Australian Thyroid Foundation
P.O. Box 186
Westmead
NSW 2145
Australia
Phone: 61-2-890-6962

British Thyroid Foundation
P.O. Box HP22
Leeds LS6 3RT
England

Nederlandse Vereniging van Graves Patenten
Heemskerk Klein Elsbroek 3
2182 TE Hillegom
Holland

Schilddrusen Liga
Peter-Samder Strasse 15
D55252 Mainz-Kastel
Germany

Schilddrusen Liga Deutschland e.V.
Postfach 800 740
65907 Frankfurt
Germany
Phone: 49-69-31-40-53-76
Fax: 49-69-31-40-53-16
Web site: www.thyrolink.com/sd-liga

Thyreoidea Landsforeningen
c/o Lis Larsen
Abakkevej 55, st. tv.
2720 Vanlose
Denmark
E-mail: Lis Larsen@net.dialog.dk

T.E.D. (Thyroid Eye Disease)
Lea House
21 Troarn Way
Chudleigh
Devon TQ13 OPP
England
Phone: 06-26-852980

Thyroid Eye Disease Association
34 Fore St.
Chudleigh
Devon TQ13 0HX
England
Phone: 44-1626-852980
Fax: 44-1626-852980

Thyroid Federation International
96 Mack St.
Kingston
Ontario K7L 1N9
Canada
Phone: (613) 544-8364
Fax: (613) 544-9731
E-mail: thyroid@limestone.kosone.com
Web site: www.thyroid-fed.org

Thyroid Foundation of Canada/La Fondation Canadienne de la Thyroide
96 Mack St.
Kingston
Ontario K7L 1N9
Canada
Phone: (613) 544-8364
Fax: (613) 544-9731
E-mail: thyroid@limestone.kosone.com
Web site: home.ican.net/~thyroid/
    Canada.html

Vastsvenska Patientforeningen for Skoldkortelsjoka
Mejerivalen 8
439 36 Onsala
Sweden
Phone: 46-30-06-39-12
Fax: 46-30-06-30-12

DIRECTORIES FOR THYROID SPECIALISTS

American Association of Clinical Endocrinologists
2589 Park St.
Jacksonville, FL 32204-4554
Phone: (904) 384-9490
Fax: (904) 384-8124

American Thyroid Association, Inc.
Mentefiore Medical Center
111 E. 210th St.
Bronx, NY 10467
Phone: (718) 882-6047
Phone (physician referral): (800) 542-6687
Fax: (718) 882-6085

The Endocrine Society
4350 East West Highway, Suite 500
Bethesda, MD 20814-4410
Phone: (301) 941-0200
Fax: (301) 941-0259

FIBROMYALGIA ORGANIZATIONS

The American Fibromyalgia Syndrome Association, Inc.
6380 E. Tanque Verde, Suite D
Tucson, AZ 85715
Phone: (520) 733-1570
Web site: www.afsafund.org

Fibromyalgia Network
P.O. Box 31750
Tuscon, AZ 85751
Phone: (800) 853-2929
Web site: www.fmnetnews.com

National Fibromyalgia Research
Association
P.O. Box 500
Salem, OR 97302
Web site: www.teleport.com/~nfra

CHRONIC FATIGUE SYNDROME ORGANIZATIONS

**American Association for Chronic
Fatigue Syndrome**
P.O. Box 895
Olney, MD 20830

CFIDS Activation Network (CAN)
P.O. Box 726
Onadell, NY 07649
Phone: (201) 599-0770

**Chronic Fatigue and Immune
Dysfunction Syndrome Association of
America**
P.O. Box 220398
Charlotte, NC 28222-0398
Phone: (800) 442-3437

**National Chronic Fatigue Syndrome and
Fibromyalgia Association**
P.O. Box 18426
Kansas City, MO 64133
Phone: (816) 931-4777

AUTOIMMUNE DISORDER ORGANIZATIONS

**American Autoimmune-Related Diseases
Association, Inc.**
21200 Gratiot Ave.
Detroit, MI 48201-2227
Phones: (800) 598-4668 and
(810) 776-3900
Fax: (810) 776-3903
E-mail: aarda@aol.com
Web site: www.aarda.org

American Diabetes Association
1660 Duke St.
Alexandria, VA 22314
Phone: (800) 232-3472

Arthritis Foundation
1314 Spring St. NW
Atlanta, GA 30309
Phone: (800) 283-7800

Lupus Foundation of America
4 Research Pl., Suite 180
Rockville, MD 20850
Phones: (800) 558-0121 and
(301) 670-9292

National Adrenal Diseases Foundation
505 Northern Blvd.
Great Neck, NY 11021
Phone: (516) 487-4992
E-mail: nadf@aol.com

**National Organization for Rare
Disorders (NORD)**
P.O. Box 8923
New Fairfield, CT 06812-1783
Phone: (800) 999-NORD
Web site: www.rarediseases.org

**National Sjögren's Syndrome
Foundation, Inc.**
3333 N. Broadway
Jericho, NY 11753
Phones: (800) 4 SJOGRENS and
(516) 933-6365
Web site: www.sjogrens.com

MOOD DISORDER ORGANIZATIONS

Bipolar Disorder Online Support Group
Web site: www.moodswing.org

**Depression and Related Affective
Disorders Association (DRADA)**
Meyer 3-18
600 North Wolfe St.
Baltimore, MD 21287-7381
Phones: (410) 955-4647 (Baltimore) and
(202) 955-5800 (Washington, DC)
Fax: (410) 614-3241
E-mail: drada@welchlink.welch.jhu.edu
Web site: www.med.jhu.edu/drada/

**National Depressive and Manic-
Depressive Association**
730 North Franklin St., Suite 501
Chicago, IL 60610
Phones: (800) 826-3632 and
(312) 642-0049
E-mail: myrtis@aol.com

**National Foundation for Depressive
Illness, Inc.**
P.O. Box 2257
New York, NY 10116
Phones: (800) 248-4344 and
(212) 268-4260
Fax: (212) 268-4434
E-mail: NAFDI@pipeline.com

National Institute of Mental Health
Depression Awareness, Recognition, and
Treatment (DART)
5600 Fishers La., Room 10-85
Rockville, MD 20857
Phones: (800) 421-4211 and
(301) 443-4140

National Mental Health Association
1021 Prince St.
Alexandria, VA 22314-2971
Phones: (800) 969-6642 and
(703) 684-5968

**National Organization for Seasonal
Affective Disorder**
P.O. Box 40133
Washington, DC 20016

Society for Manic Depression
P.O. Box 22
Bonsall, CA 22003
Web site: www.theport.com

The Synergy Group of Canada
Web site: www.lethbridgelife.com

What's New in Depression
Web site: www.mediconsult.com/
depression/

ANXIETY DISORDER ORGANIZATIONS

Anxiety Disorders of America
600 Executive Blvd., Suite 513
Rockville, MD 20852
Phone: (301) 231-9350

Mental Health Clinical Research Center
New York State Psychiatric Institute
722 W. 168th St.
New York, NY 10032
Phone: (212) 960-2442

INFERTILITY ORGANIZATIONS

**National Infertility Network Exchange
(NINE)**
P.O. Box 204
East Meadow, NY 11554

Resolve of Michigan
P.O. Box 2185
Southfield, MI 48037
Phone: (248) 680-0093
E-mail: kae@mediat.com
Web site: www.mediat.com/resolve

IODINE DEFICIENCY DISORDER ORGANIZATION

**International Council for Control of
Iodine Deficiency Disorders (ICCIDD)**
J. T. Dunn, M.D.
P.O. Box 511
University of Virginia Medical Center
Charlottesvile, VA 22908

NUCLEAR MEDICINE ORGANIZATION

Society of Nuclear Medicine
1850 Samuel Morse Dr.
Reston, VA 20190-5316
Phone: (703) 708-9000
Fax: (703) 708-9015
Web site: www.snm.org

SUPPORT FOR SPOUSES ORGANIZATIONS

**The American Association of Sex
Educators, Counselors, and Therapists**
P.O. Box 238
Mt. Vernon, IA 52314-0238
Phone: (319) 895-8407
Fax: (319) 895-6203
E-mail: info@aasect.org

Well Spouse Foundation
P.O. Box 801
New York, NY 10023
Phones: (212) 664-1241 and
(800) 838-0879
Fax: (212) 644-1338

BIBLIOGRAPHY

BOOKS

American Psychiatric Association: Diagnostic and Statistical Manual of Mental Disorders. 4th ed. Washington, D.C.: American Psychiatric Association, 1994.

Chopra, D. *Ageless Body, Timeless Mind: The Quantum Alternative to Growing Old.* New York: Harmony Books, Random House, 1993.

Columbia University College of Physicians and Surgeons: Complete Home Guide to Mental Health. New York: Henry Holt, 1992.

Domar, A. D., and H. Dreher. *Healing Mind, Healthy Woman: Using the Mind-Body Connection to Manage Stress and Take Control of Your Life.* New York: Henry Holt, 1996.

Ediger, B. *Coping with Fibromyalgia.* Toronto: LRH Publications, 1991.

Fieve, R. R. *Moodswing.* New York: Bantam Books, Morrow, 1989.

Ford, G. *Listening to Your Hormones.* Rocklin, Calif.: Prima Publishing, 1997.

Gold, M. S. *The Good News about Depression: Breakthrough Medical Treatments That Can Work for You.* New York: Bantam Books, 1995.

Gorman, J. M. *The New Psychiatry: The Essential Guide to State-of-the-Art Therapy, Medication, Emotional Health.* New York: St. Martin's Press, 1996.

Greist J. H., and J. W. Jefferson. *Depression and Its Treatment.* New York: Warner Books, 1992.

Hamilton, J. A., and P. N. Harberger, eds. *Postpartum Psychiatric Illness: A Picture Puzzle.* Philadelphia: University of Pennsylvania Press, 1992.

Hart, C. *Secrets of Serotonin: The Natural Hormone That Curbs Food and Alcohol Cravings, Elevates Your Mood, Reduces Pain, and Boosts Energy.* New York: St. Martin's Paperbacks, 1996.

Hoffman, R. L. *Tired All the Time: How to Regain Your Lost Energy.* New York: Pocket Books, 1993.

Kabat-Zinn, J. *Full Catastrophe Living: Using the Wisdom of Your Body and Mind to Face Stress, Pain, and Illness.* New York: Dell, 1990.

Kernodle, William O. *Panic Disorder.* 2d ed. Richmond, Va.: William Byrd Press, 1993.

Langer, S. E., and J. F. Scheer. *Solved: The Riddle of Illness.* New Canaan, Conn.: Keats Publishing, 1995.

Lickey, M. E., and B. Gordon. *Medicine and Mental Illness: The Use of Drugs in Psychiatry.* New York: Freeman, 1991.

Mason, L. J. *Guide to Stress Reduction.* Berkeley, Calif.: Celestial Arts, 1985.

Morrison, J. *DSM-IV Made Easy: The Clinician's Guide to Diagnosis.* New York: Guilford Press, 1995.

Ratey, J. J., and C. Johnson. *Shadow Syndromes: Recognizing and Coping with the Hidden Psychological Disorders That Can Influence Your Behavior and Silently Determine the Course of Your Life.* New York: Pantheon Books, Random House, 1997.

Salzer, L. P. *Surviving Infertility: A Compassionate Guide through the Emotional Crisis of Infertility.* New York: HarperCollins, 1991.

Scherbaum, W. A., U. Bogner, B. Weinheimer, and G. F. Bottazzo, eds. *Autoimmune Thyroiditis: Approaches towards Its Etiological Differentiation.* Heidelberg, Germany: Springer-Verlag Berlin, 1991.

Sears, B., with B. Lawren. *Enter the Zone: A Dietary Road Map to Lose Weight Permanently, Reset Your Genetic Code, Prevent Disease, Achieve Maximum Physical Performance, Enhance Mental Productivity.* New York: Regan Books, HarperCollins, 1995.

Shils, M. E., J. A. Olson, and M. Shike. *Modern Nutrition in Health and Disease.* 8th ed. Philadelphia: Lea and Febieger, 1994.

Somer, E. *Food and Mood: The Complete Guide to Eating Well and Feeling Your Best.* New York: Henry Holt, 1995.

Steward, H. L., M. C. Bethea, S. S. Andrews, and L. A. Balart. *Sugar Busters! Cut Sugar to Trim Fat.* New York: Ballantine, 1998.

Teitelbaum, J. *From Fatigued to Fantastic! A Guide to Overcoming Severe Chronic Fatigue, Poor Sleep, Achiness, "Brain Fog," Increased Thirst, Bowel Disorders, Recurrent Infections, and Exhaustion.* Garden City Park, N.Y.: Avery Publishing Group, 1996.

ARTICLES

Ahrén, B. "Thyroid Neuroendocrinology: Neural Regulation of Thyroid Hormone Secretion." *Endocrine Reviews* 7, no. 2 (1986): 149–55.

Arem, R. "When to Choose Radioactive Iodine, Drugs, or Surgery." *Consultant* 28, no. 9 (1989): 21–35.

Arem, R., and D. Escalante. "Subclinical Hypothyroidism: Epidemiology, Diagnosis, and Significance." *Advances in Internal Medicine* 41 (1996): 213–50.

Beall, G. N. "Immunologic Aspects of Endocrine Diseases." *Journal of the American Medical Association* 258, no. 20 (1987): 2952–56.

Beck, P. "Acute Therapy of Depression." *Journal of Clinical Psychiatry* 54, no. 8, suppl. (1993): 18–27.

Bergeron, E., A. Mitchell, F. Heyen, et al. "Acute Colonic Surgery and Unrecognized Hypothyroidism: A Warning." *Disease of Colon and Rectum* 40 (1997): 859–61.

Bhatia, S. K., N. R. Rose, B. Schofield, et al. "Influence of Diet on the Induction of Experimental Autoimmune Thyroid Disease." *Proceedings Society for Experimental Biology and Medicine* 213 (1996): 294–300.

Burch, E. A., and T. W. Messervy. "Psychiatric Symptoms in Medical Illness: Hyperthyroidism Revisited." *Psychosomatics* 19, no. 2 (1978): 71–75.

Calabrese, J. R., M. A. Kling, and P. W. Gold. "Alterations in Immunocompetence during Stress, Bereavement, and Depression: Focus on Neuroendocrine Regulation." *American Journal of Psychiatry* 144 (1987): 1123–34.

Campbell, A. J. "Thyroid Disorders in the Elderly: Difficulties in Diagnosis and Treatment." *Drugs* 31 (1986): 455–61.

Dayan, C. M., and G. H. Daniels. "Chronic Autoimmune Thyroiditis." *New England Journal of Medicine* 335, no. 2 (1996): 99–107.

Dratman, M. B., and J. T. Gordon. "Thyroid Hormones as Neurotransmitters." *Thyroid* 6, no. 6 (1996): 639–47.

Esposito, S., A. J. Prange Jr., and R. N. Golden. "The Thyroid Axis and Mood Disorders: Overview and Future Prospects." *Psychopharmacology Bulletin* 33, no. 2 (1997): 205–17.

Ettigi, P. G., and G. M. Brown. "Brain Disorders Associated with Endocrine Dysfunction." *Psychiatric Clinics of North America* 1 (1978): 117–36.

Forchetti, C. M., G. Katsamakis, and D. C. Garron. "Autoimmune Thyroiditis and a Rapidly Progressive Dementia: Global Hypoperfusion on SPECT Scanning Suggests a Possible Mechanism." *Neurology* 49 (1997): 623–26.

Geringer, E. S., and C. Wool. "Recognizing and Treating Depression." *Contemporary Internal Medicine* 6, no. 12 (1994): 19–28.

Giddings, A. E. B. "Thyroidectomy and Parathyroidectomy: A Guide for Patients." *Journal of the Royal Society of Medicine* 91, suppl. 33 (1998): 33–35.

Gittoes, N. J. L., and J. A. Franklyn. "Hyperthyroidism: Current Treatment Guidelines." *Drugs* 55, no. 4 (1998): 543–53.

Gomberg-Maitland, M., and W. H. Frishman. "Thyroid Hormone and Cardiovascular Disease." *American Heart Journal* 135 (1998): 187–96.

Greer, M. A. "Treating Graves' Disease." *Endocrinologist* 4, no. 1 (1994): 69–76.

Haggerty, J. J., D. L. Evans, and A. J. Prange Jr.. "Organic Brain Syndrome Associated with Marginal Hypothyroidism." *American Journal of Psychiatry* 143 (1986): 785–86.

Haggerty, J. J., J. C. Garbutt, D. L. Evans, et al. "Subclinical Hypothyroidism: A Review of Neuropsychiatric Aspects." *International Journal of Psychiatry in Medicine* 20, no. 2 (1990): 193–208.

Haggerty, J. J., and A. J. Prange Jr. "Borderline Hypothyroidism and Depression." *Annual Review of Medicine* 46 (1995): 37–46.

Hall, R. C. W. "Psychiatric Effects of Thyroid Hormone Disturbance." *Psychosomatics* 24, no. 1 (1983): 7–18.

Hennessey, J. V., and I. M. D. Jackson. "The Interface between Thyroid Hormones and Psychiatry." *Endocrinologist* 6 (1996): 214–23.

Herbert, T. B., and S. Cohen. "Depression and Immunity. A Meta-Analytic Review." *Psychological Bulletin* 133, no. 3 (1993): 472–86.

Jackson, I. "Does Thyroid Hormone Have a Role as Adjunctive Therapy in Depression?" *Thyroid* 6, no. 1 (1996): 63–66.

Jodar, S., M. Munoz-Torres, F. Escobar-Jiménez, et al. "Antiresorptive Therapy in Hyperthyroid Patients: Longitudinal Changes in Bone and Mineral Metabolism." *Journal of Clinical Endocrinology and Metabolism* 82, no. 6 (1997): 1989–94.

Joffe, R. T., and A. J. Levitt. "Major Depression and Subclinical (Grade 2) Hypothyroidism." *Psychoneuroendocrinology* 17, nos. 2–3 (1992): 215–21.

Klein, I., D. V. Becker, and G. S. Levey. "Treatment of Hyperthyroid Disease." *Annals of Internal Medicine* 121 (1994): 281–88.

Lidz, T. "Emotional Factors in the Etiology of Hyperthyroidism Occurring in Relation to Pregnancy." *Psychosomatic Medicine* 17 (1955): 420–27.

MacCrimmon, D. J., J. E. Wallace, W. M. Goldberg, et al. "Emotional Disturbance and Cognitive Deficits in Hyperthyroidism." *Psychosomatic Medicine* 41, no. 4 (1979): 331–41.

Mazzaferri, E. L. "Evaluation and Management of Common Thyroid Disorders in Women." *American Journal of Obstetrics and Gynecology* 176 (1997): 507–14.

Miller, F. W., G. F. Moore, B. D. Weintraub, et al. "Prevalence of Thyroid Disease and Abnormal Thyroid Function Test Results in Patients with Systemic Lupus Erythematosus." *Arthritis and Rheumatism* 30, no. 10 (1987): 1124–31.

Muller, M. J. "Thyroid Hormones and Energy and Fat Balance." *European Journal of Endocrinology* 136 (1997): 267–68.

Musselman, D. L., and C. B. Nemeroff. "Depression and Endocrine Disorders: Focus on the Thyroid and Adrenal System." *British Journal of Psychiatry* 168, suppl. 30 (1996): 123–28.

Nemeroff, C. B. "Augmentation Regimens for Depression." *Journal of Clinical Psychiatry* 52, suppl. 5 (1991): 21–27.

Noth, R. H., and E. L. Mazzaferri. "Age and the Endocrine System." *Clinics in Geriatric Medicine* 1, no. 1 (1985): 223–50.

Olivieri, O., D. Girelli, A. M. Stanzial, et al. "Selenium, Zinc, and Thyroid Hormones in Healthy Subjects. Low T3/T4 Ration in the Elderly is Related to Impaired Selenium Status." *Biological Trace Element Research* 51 (1996): 31–41.

Pillemer, S. R. "Identifying and Treating Fibromyalgia." *Contemporary Internal Medicine* 5, no. 12 (1993): 24–30.

Prummel, M. F., and W. M. Wiersinga. "Smoking and Risk of Graves' Disease." *Journal of the American Medical Association* 269 (1993): 479–82.

Reus, V. I. "Behavioral Aspects of Thyroid Disease in Women." *Psychiatric Clinics of North America* 12, no. 1 (1989): 153–65.

Ridgway, E. C. "Modern Concepts of Primary Thyroid Gland Failure." *Clinical Chemistry* 42, no. 1 (1996): 179–82.

Schlumberger, M. J. "Papillary and Follicular Thyroid Carcinoma." *New England Journal of Medicine* 338, no. 5 (1998): 297–305.

Seven, A., O. Seymen, S. Hatemi, et al. "Antioxidant Status in Experimental Hyperthyroidism: Effect of Vitamin E Supplementation." *Clinica Chimica Acta* 256 (1996): 65–74.

Sussman, N., and S. Stahl. "Update in the Pharmacotherapy of Depression." *American Journal of Medicine* 101, suppl. 6A (1996): 26S–36S.

Szabadi, E. "Thyroid Dysfunction and Affective Illness." *British Medical Journal* 302 (1991): 923–24.

Wang, C., and L. M. Crapo. "The Epidemiology of Thyroid Disease and Implications for Screening." *Endocrinology and Metabolism Clinics of North America* 26, no. 1 (1997): 189–218.

Westphal, S. A. "Unusual Presentations of Hypothyroidism." *American Journal of the Medical Sciences* 314, no. 5 (1997): 333–37.

Woeber, K. A. "Subclinical Thyroid Dysfunction." *Archives of Internal Medicine* 157 (1997): 1065–68.

INDEX

abuse
  child, 170
  verbal, 159
acetylcholine, 277
Achilles reflex time, 222
activities, lack of interest in, 49, 85, 156–57
acupuncture, 172
Addison's disease, 32, 167, 234, 235
adrenal glands, 167, 235
adrenaline, 299
aggression, 67, 159–60
aging, 56–58, 80–82, 272–74, 302
agoraphobia, 48, 73, 257
agranulocytosis, 252
alcohol, 107, 313–14
allergies, 320
alopecia areata, 238, 239
alprazolam, 258
Alzheimer's disease, 57–58, 238, 274, 275, 277
American Foundation of Thyroid Patients,
  266
amiodarone, 45, 226, 306, 312–13
amitriptyline, 172, 270
amygdala, 107
anemia, 235
anger, 70–71, 153–55, 158–59
anorexia nervosa, 37–38, 118
antibodies
  antithyroid, 35, 209, 210, 211, 232–34
  markers for autoimmune diseases, 31,
    233–34
antidepressants, 95, 216, 313
  atypical, 269, 270
  and hyperthyroidism, 33
  potentiation of, 111–12
  selecting, 268–71
  SSRIs, 96, 106, 109, 110, 268–71
  and T4/T3 therapy, 292–94
  thyroid hormones as, 4, 105–20
  tricyclic, 111, 172, 268–69, 270
antioxidants, 274, 300–302, 308
anxiety, 25, 49–51, 66, 67, 71–74
  and infertility, 201–3
  persistent, 264
  and thyroid dose, 245–46
  work-related, 157–58
anxiety disorders, 19, 88, 96–99, 188
aplasia cutis, 261

appearance
  concerns about, 19, 318, 320
  of thyroid patients, 15, 44
appetite
  changes in, 54, 85, 92, 166
  regulation of, 125–26, 131–32
  suppressants, 129, 133
  and thyroid hormone, 126–28
arthritis, 32, 171, 234, 235
Asher, R., 45
aspirin, 248
asthma, 312
atherosclerosis, 57, 275
Ativan, 271
attention, need for, 156
attention deficit hyperactivity disorder
  (ADHD), 83, 107–8
autoimmune disorders, 31, 32, 40, 233–36, 296

bacteria, 301
Barnes, Broda O., 117–18
behavior, irrational, 159–60
benzodiazepines, 271
beta-blockers, 80, 257, 312
beta-endorphin, 126
biofeedback, 172, 266, 310
biopsy, 256, 332, 333–34
biopsychiatry, 87
bipolar disorders, 101, 113, 115.
  See also depression, manic; mood swing
    disorders
blinking, 318
block-replace regimen, 259, 326–27
blood pressure, 46, 54, 275
blood sugar. *See* insulin
body mass index (BMI), 133
bone, loss of, 65, 76, 246, 284
brain
  chemistry of, 2, 87–89, 109–11, 181
  hypothyroidism, 109, 119, 289
  and mood swings, 100
  response to stress, 30
  serotonin levels, 93–94, 109–10, 127
  and sexual desire, 140
  and T3, 107, 109, 114
  and thyroid function, 15–16, 37–38
  and thyroid imbalance, 15, 29, 273–74
  See also cognitive abilities

About the Author

Ridha Arem, M.D., is an associate Professor of Medicine in the Division of Endocrinology and Metabolism at Baylor College of Medicine in Houston, Texas. He is also Chief of Endocrinology and Metabolism at Ben Taub General Hospital, a major teaching hospital affiliated with Baylor College of Medicine, and Medical Director of the Endocrine Laboratory at Methodist Hospital, another major teaching hospital affiliated with Baylor.

Dr. Arem has greatly contributed to thyroid-related research and is author of many articles published in prestigious medical journals. Since 1988 he has been editor and author of an educational periodical on thyroid disorders, *Clinical Thyroidology,* which is read by approximately 25,000 physicians nationwide.

In addition to teaching medical students and physicians-in-training at Texas Medical Center, Dr. Arem is often asked to speak at continuous medical educational programs for primary-care physicians and specialists at other institutions and annual meetings. Dr. Arem has also served as the Medical Director of the American Foundation of Thyroid Patients, a national support organization for thyroid patients. He often gives lectures to the public on thyroid disorders and contributes to the writing of articles and educational topics for the public.

Dr. Arem lives in Houston with his wife and their two sons.